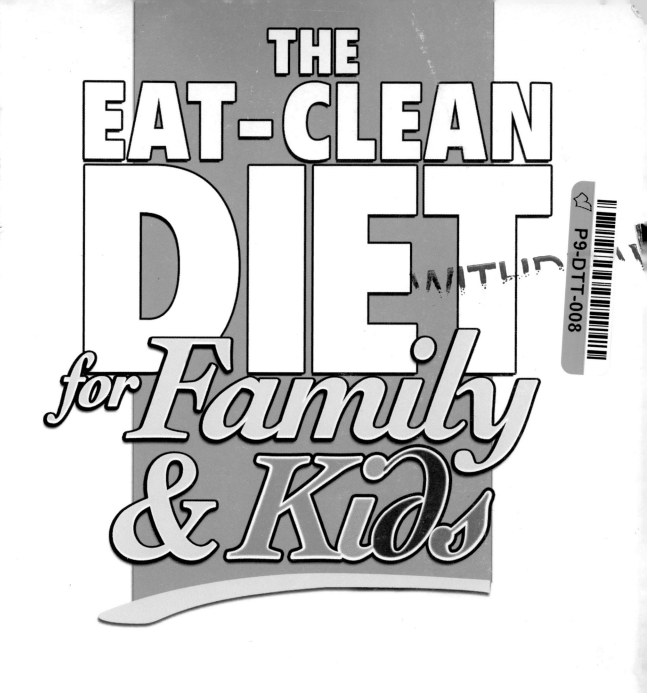

THE EAT-CLEAN DIET for Family & Kids

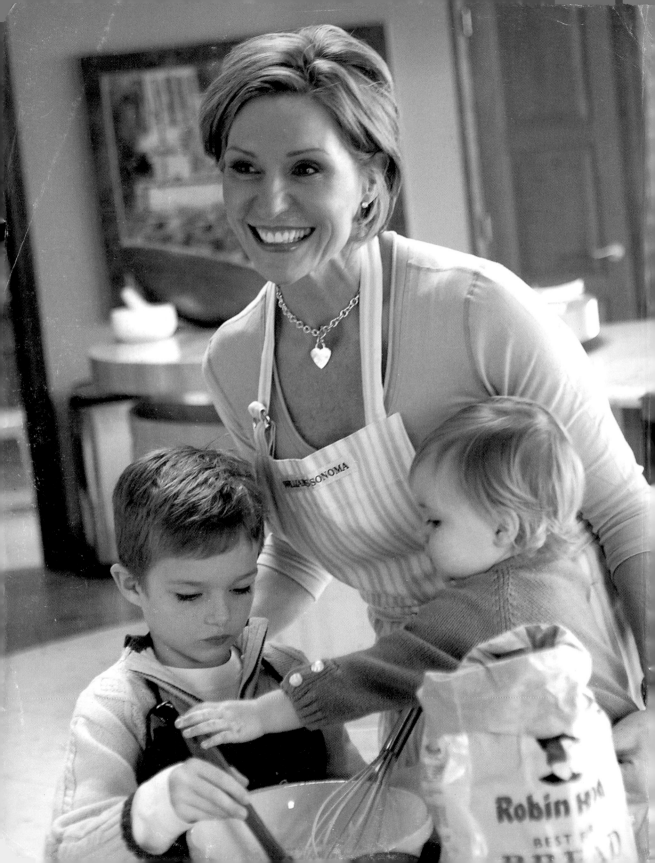

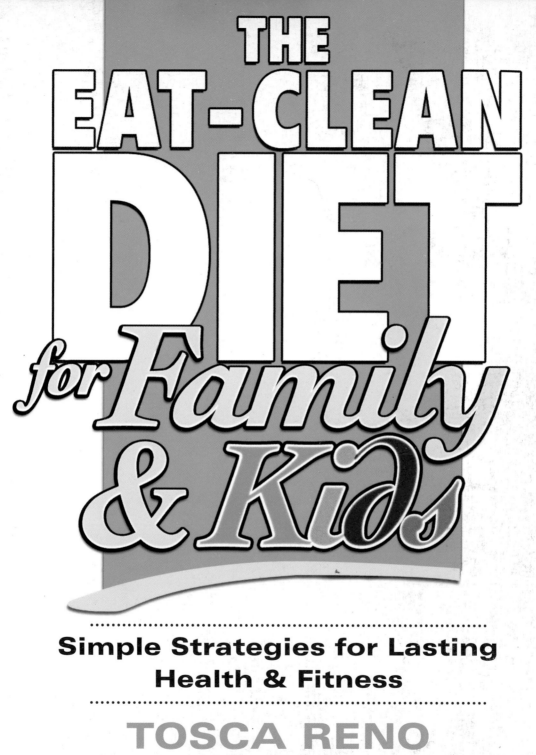

THE EAT-CLEAN DIET for Family & Kids

Simple Strategies for Lasting Health & Fitness

TOSCA RENO

FOREWORD BY Bobbi Brown

RKP ROBERT KENNEDY PUBLISHING

Published by Robert Kennedy Publishing
5775 McLaughlin Road
Mississauga, ON
L5R 3P7 Canada
Visit us at **www.eatcleandiet.com**
or **www.toscareno.com**

Design by Gabriella Caruso Marques
Edited by Wendy Morley and Rachel Corradetti

Library and Archives Canada Cataloguing in Publication

Reno, Tosca, 1959-
    The Eat-Clean Diet for Family and Kids : *Simple Strategies for Lasting
Health & Fitness* / Tosca Reno ; foreword by Bobbi Brown.

Includes index.
ISBN 978-1-55210-050-9

    1. Family--Health and hygiene. 2. Children--Health and hygiene.
3. Physical fitness. 4. Health. I. Title.

RA777.7.R46 2008   613.2   C2008-903856-8

10 9 8 7 6 5 4 3 2 1

Distributed in Canada by
NBN (National Book Network)
67 Mowat Avenue, Suite 241
Toronto, ON
M6K 3E3

Distributed in USA by
NBN (National Book Network)
15200 NBN Way
Blue Ridge Summit, PA
17214

Printed in Canada

IMPORTANT

The information in this book reflects the author's experiences and opinions and is not intended to replace medical advice.

Before beginning this or any nutritional or exercise regimen, consult your physician to be sure it is appropriate for you. Ask for a physical stress test.

I dedicate this book to the health and wellness of our children. They are our legacy and our future.

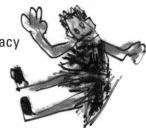

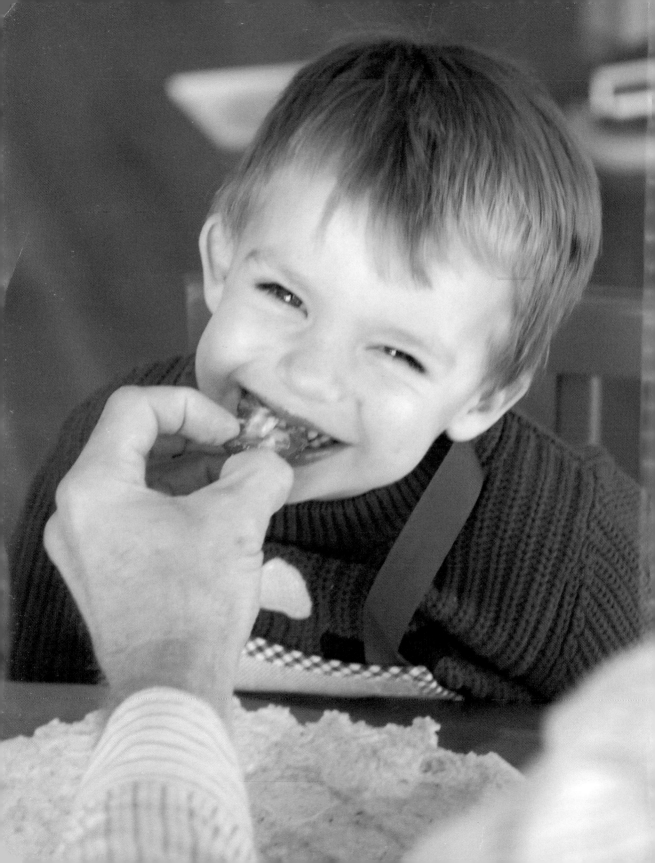

Contents

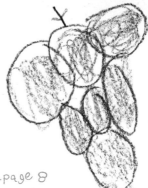

Foreword

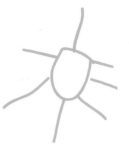

BY BOBBI BROWN, CEO BOBBI BROWN COSMETICS, BESTSELLING AUTHOR & MOTHER OF THREE

When I stumbled on Tosca Reno's first book, *The Eat-Clean Diet*, I was instantly hooked. Her advice was simple, sensible and focused on what you could eat, rather than on what you couldn't eat. I've always believed in the connection between healthy living and well-being – and Reno has helped me take my nutrition and fitness to a whole new level. Thanks to her I've discovered what it means to eat really clean; I've learned the amazing benefits of flax seed and bee pollen.

Reno's newest book, *The Eat-Clean Diet for Family and Kids*, could not come at a better time. Juggling the demands of work, home and school, many families now rely on fast food and processed food as their main sources of nutrition. As a result, a lot of kids are growing up unhealthy, overweight or obese. Healthy eating needs to start at home and it is our obligation as parents to set the right example for our kids. Involve your family with food shopping and food preparation. Nourish your family with meals loaded with natural, good-for-you ingredients. Assume responsibility for what goes in your grocery cart and ultimately in the stomachs of your loved ones.

There are no quick fixes in Reno's book. She does not sell gimmicks. She believes – as I do – that true health requires an attitude and lifestyle shift. While this may sound like an overwhelming undertaking, it's not. Change your eating habits one meal at a time. Before you know it, you and your family will be Eating Clean all the time. Here's to looking and feeling your best, for life.

Bobbi Brown

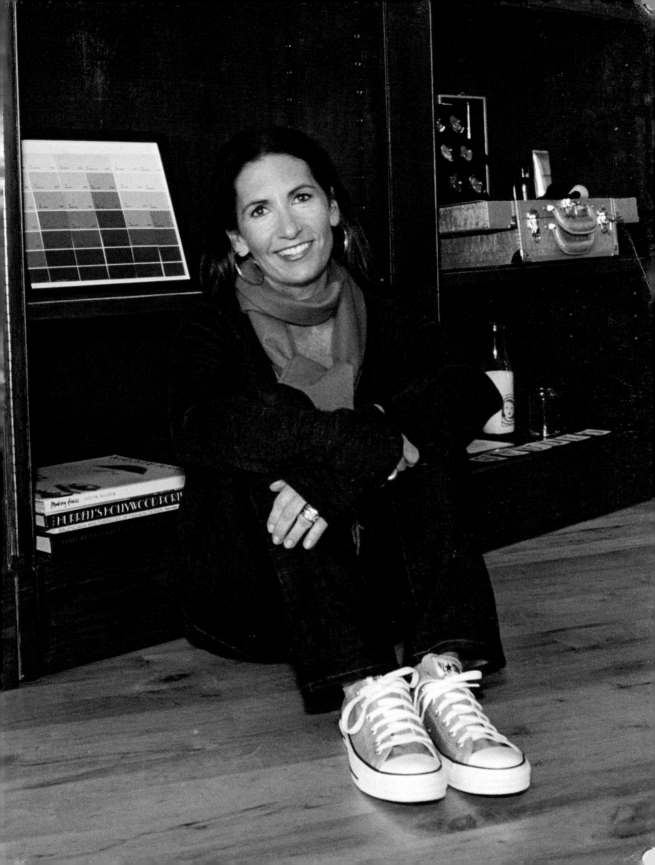

Introduction

Necessity is the mother of all invention it's true, but fear can be a wonderful motivator as well. Fear is the reason I wrote this book. I am afraid of many things, but nothing frightens me more than what is happening across the face of this planet at this very moment. Not only is our environment falling into ruin, thanks to broad sweeping disregard for preserving our Earth, the same is true for the health of our citizens, particularly our children.

How did I become so frightened? Not long ago I spent several weeks visiting a family member who was recovering from surgery in an intensive care unit at a prominent hospital. The ordeal was itself significant and worrying, but my concern grew as I came to know other patients also temporarily residing here. As I wandered the halls of the hospital I noticed something. From day one I saw that more than 50 percent of the folks either visiting or staying at the hospital were overweight, and I am being generous with that term. Many were actually obese. In this population I include not only patients, young and old, but also visitors and, unfortunately, staff. I always considered the hospital to be a bastion of health for the uniformed angels who minister to the sick. In-

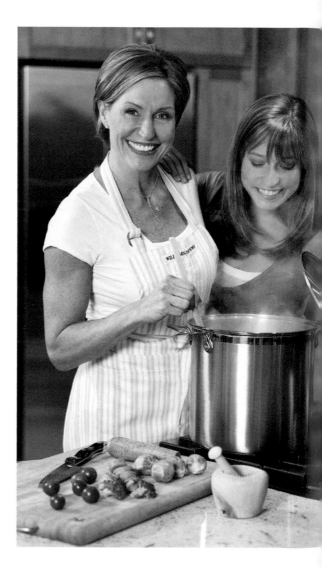

creasingly those who run the hospital are as apt to be obese as those to whom they minister. And what of the children? It seemed to me it was more often the case to see an overweight child than not. If our children are indeed the future of our country then we are certainly heading for disaster. Overweight and obesity are robbing us of our future. It is foolish to think carrying a few extra pounds of weight is a light matter. The costs, both economical and health wise, are staggering.

How did this happen? It's similar to collecting clutter in a house you have lived in for many years. Little by little stuff accumulates. Putting each item away every time you use it is a simple act of keeping things

"If our children are indeed the future of our country then we are certainly heading for disaster."

tidy, but you get a little lazy. You don't notice the bits piling up at the beginning, but once you have a great heap it's hard to ignore and even harder to clean up. A house full of junk is overwhelming. Believe it or not, living with so much stuff can be detrimental to your health — think along the lines of mold, fungus, mildew and even infestations of various kinds of vermin in the worst cases. And that brings me to my point about overweight. One or two pounds may not seem to matter much at the outset. But as the pounds pile up, destructive eating habits become further entrenched (like the habit of not putting things away in your house) and virtually impossible to break. Robust health, once taken for granted, erodes. Hormones go askew, and the body becomes misshapen. If the decline in health is serious enough, you may end up in the very hospital where I saw enough to make me want to write this book.

At the root lies my worry that we have been misled about how to nourish ourselves and our families. In the agrarian days of our country there was no question that what was served on our tables had come from the earth and was indeed nourishing. The same is not always true today. We have lost contact with our food's origins, because it now comes from the shelves of grocery stores in colorful packages. It no longer seems to come from our good earth — and unfortunately the food we end up with is often far removed from how it started out.

This book is my answer for you. If even one or two families will take up my call to return to more informed food decisions in the form of Clean Eating, then my efforts will have been worthwhile. Let these pages serve as your guide to rethink the simplest of all human needs, to eat and to eat well.

My best wishes for you and your loved ones.
I am always listening,

Tosca Reno

CHAPTER ONE

What is Clean Eating?

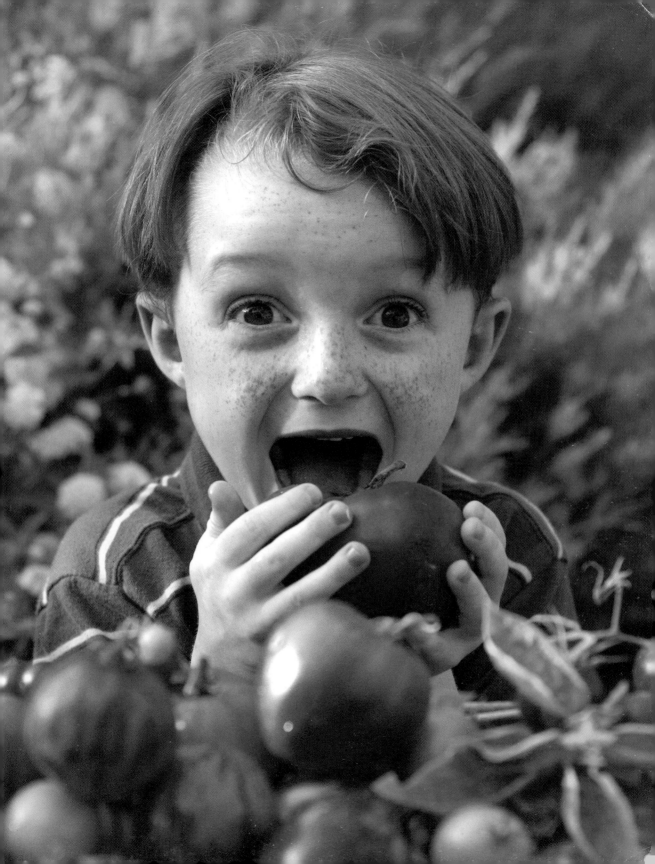

HOW IT STARTED

Not long ago I wrote the first in a series of books. *The Eat-Clean Diet* is a title charged with meaning for me, since I used the principles of Clean Eating to change my entire life. At 40 I went from frumpy, unhappy, out-of-shape and overweight to having the time of my life writing and modeling for health and fitness publications. This first little book told my story. It explained in friendly, simple terms how I ate my way to a lean and healthy physique. It became such a grand idea that others noticed, and now hundreds of thousands of you are also Eating Clean. I knew I was onto something when I realized the life-altering experience Clean Eating was offering me, but to have a nation behind me is quite another feeling altogether. I am honored.

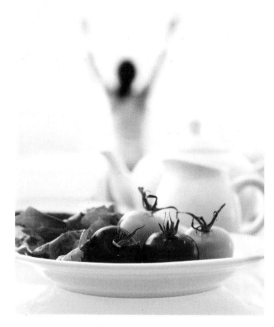

YOU ARE FEELING BETTER

As you embraced the Clean-Eating lifestyle I began to hear the stories of how this simplest of acts, eating, could alter your life in such a powerful way. Your nourishment became a thing of beauty as you ditched sugars, unhealthy fats, chemically charged foods and other garbage. Soon your letters shared with me how much weight you had lost, or that the headaches you had always experienced were now gone. Some of you told me that the afternoon naps you once took had been replaced with an afternoon walk or run. People who had suffered from irritable bowel syndrome no longer had it. Others could reduce cholesterol or heart medication. More of you could reduce or go off of insulin altogether. The stories kept coming. It was a revolution of sorts. Apparently North Americans wanted to be told what to eat, when to eat it and why. Clean Eating gave them the answer.

CAN I DO IT?

One question kept popping up. Virtually everyone wanted to know if Clean Eating was intended for families and kids too. The answer is a resounding yes! Everyone can and should Eat Clean. Why? Quite simply because this way of eating is safe, healthy and smart — in fact, it's the way we should all be eating in the first place. I had already practiced Clean Eating with my family and I knew how powerful the results were for my children. As growing young teenagers and adults who ate the Clean healthy food I

ROY'S STORY
A reader's testimonial

Hey Tosca,

I just thought I would pop you an email and let you know of my progress. I really enjoyed my success with the Clean-Eating change. I used to take a nap almost every day when I would get home from work and it really is quite a rarity at this point! My energy has gone through the roof since I started [Eating Clean] the week of Christmas. It's not that I don't take a nap on certain occasions but now I look at it as a treat for certain days when I really feel like I need it. Not all treats have to be food related!

To date I have lost 35 pounds and I'm having a great time watching my body change. I never did get that photo of me at my heaviest because I did a lot of reflection on it. I never wanted to be there again and I really have no need to see myself that way ever again either. I like to focus my energies to the future and know that I'm going in the right direction. I started in size 52 pants and have finally gotten into my 44's this week. WooHoo! I knew it would happen at some point so I never threw those old pants away. My goal is to eventually get back into my 36's and dare I say, try for 34's. With this new Live-It change, I feel that even this will be a possibility some time in the next year!

I have been on just about every program and diet in my life and many of them have gotten the weight off and I have looked incredible but I always knew that something was missing. Some small part just didn't fit into the puzzle and it wasn't until I heard you, and yes, I say heard you because I feel like you wrote the book for me, that everything started to click! This is not something I will only do until the weight comes off, this is the way I will eat for the rest of my life, which I feel will be much longer thanks to Clean Eating!

All my blessings,
Roy Everhart

prepared for them I saw that they did not suffer what so many other young people did. Instead of having blemished skin and misshapen bodies, my children have glowing, clear skin, healthy thick hair and none of the diseases that seem to be creeping up on our youth at alarming rates – especially diabetes Types 1 and 2. Where other young folks were overweight and plagued with ill health, my children had lean, athletic bodies and rarely suffered from any illnesses at all. A zest for life radiated from them. Clean Eating was paying off. Even the dentist noticed. When the girls went in for checkups they never had cavities and their gums were healthy. I took it as a sign of good health and good eating.

A LIVE-IT, NOT A DIE-IT!

One of the strongest reasons Clean Eating works is that it is not a diet. In fact many people refer to it as a Live-It and not a Die-It. One of my readers sent me that line and I have happily borrowed it when trying to explain what Clean Eating means (see below). It helps a lot, because some people get a funny look on their face when they read the title. I can tell they are thinking, "What is Clean Eating? And if I am not Eating Clean then am I Eating Dirty?" I get a laugh out of that one.

Clean Eating is a set of good eating habits which, when combined with exercise, makes for a lifestyle of health and happiness because you are the owner of a lean, vital and robust physique. There are no

ANGIE'S STORY
A reader's testimonial

Hey there Tosca!

Just wanted to write and tell you that you put the wrong title on your book. You should not have called it a diet. Clean Eating is more of a lifestyle. Why not call it a Live-It rather than a Die-It? I feel so wonderful eating this way, I just know my children, husband and myself are going to stick to this for life. We all feel more energy and it is easy to do. Your recipes and lifestyle coaching tips are working in this house.

Thanks for writing this book!
Angie, Bob, Tracy and Jeff – the Underwood family.

 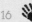

cute gimmicks, you don't have to bring a change of clothes to work in case of embarrassing and smelly leaks (as with the fat-blocker pills), you don't have to eat only protein, and you can actually eat both healthy fats and carbohydrates. You never go hungry and you feel elated as your body responds to the vibrant foods you put into it. I know you are probably expecting something fancy or gimmicky because the word "diet" is in the title, but you won't find a fad diet here. Clean Eating is all about making smarter food choices, eating more often and stimulating the most effective fat-burning mechanism you already possess, your metabolism.

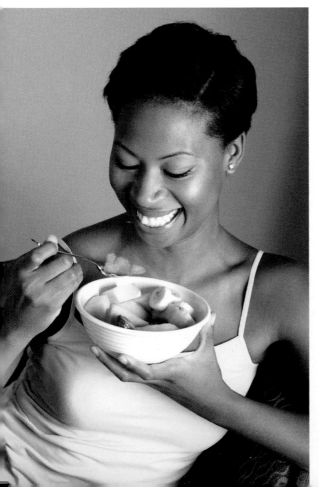

CLEAN-EATING
PRINCIPLES

1 Eat 6 small meals each day.

2 Eat every 2 to 3 hours.

3 Eat a combination of lean protein plus complex carbohydrates at each meal.

4 Drink 2 to 3 liters of water each day.

5 Depend on fresh fruits and vegetables for complex carbs, enzymes and fiber.

6 Eat whole grains, not refined, over-processed, chemically charged foods.

7 Choose lean protein from poultry, fish, wild game, soy products and legumes.

8 Eat healthy fats every day from fish, healthy oils, nuts, seeds and grains.

9 Never miss a meal, especially breakfast.

10 Stick to reasonable portion sizes.

AVOID THESE

- Over-processed, refined foods.
- Chemicals and perservatives.
- White flour.
- White sugar.
- Artificial sugars.
- Saturated and trans fats.
- Alcohol – avoid or minimize intake.
- Calorie-dense foods with little or no nutritional food value.

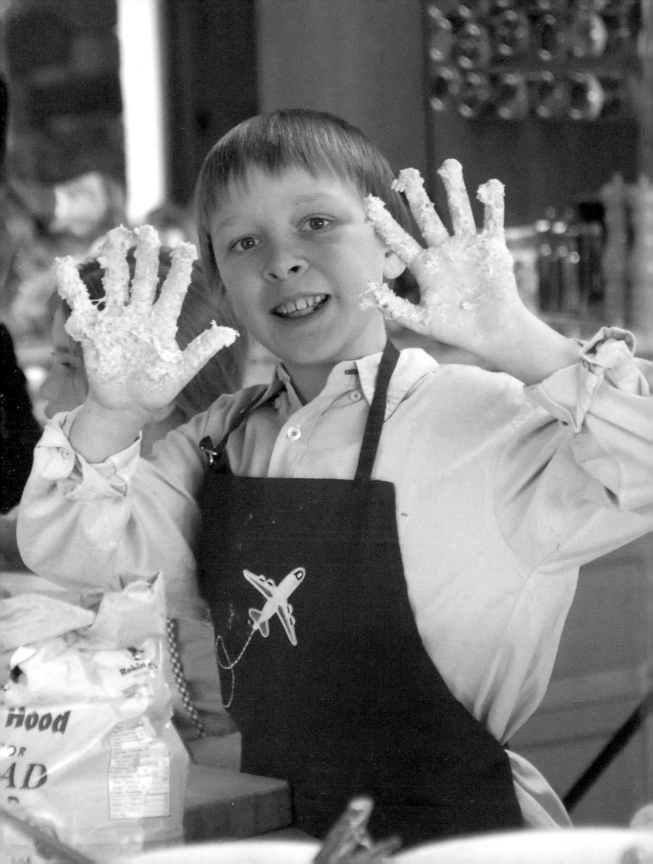

HOW DOES CLEAN EATING WORK?

You will have noticed as you read the Clean-Eating principles that the list does not include foolish behaviors such as restricting food intake. At first glance you may think there is a lot of eating involved, and there is, but no more than you are probably already doing if you think about it. The difference lies in what you are eating and how often, and this is a crucial element of Clean Eating. It may surprise you that you can actually eat more often and still lose weight. You are probably wondering how that works. I did not believe it until I tried it myself, and now of course I am hooked. My family and I have eaten this way for several years and counting, with no intention of stopping. It is the only way to eat as far as I can tell.

Many of us eat only two or three meals per day and wonder why, with so little apparent eating, we are still overweight. But think about it. When you put off eating for longer than four or five hours, you begin to feel pretty lousy. Physical and chemical changes take place in response to this lack of food. Now, the body is pretty smart. If you repeatedly skip meals and restrict food intake, your body learns to be perpetually prepared for a crisis that it reads as a food shortage or starvation. It has been set up that way via the process of evolution to protect us from periods of food shortages. The metabolism slows and any food energy is tightly preserved in the body as a source of fuel for these desperate times. You don't

get fat from skipping one meal one time, but you do get heavy and sluggish from repeating this pattern of not eating on a regular basis. On the other hand, if you eat too much too often you become overweight and in extreme cases obese, which appears to be the current trend in North America.

EATING MORE FREQUENTLY

Depositing regular helpings of good-quality food into your system keeps your body chemistry at an even keel. You won't have wild hormonal swings, shakiness, cravings, or uncontrollable hunger. When we eat inconsistently our body has no reliable source of fuel, so the inherent fat-burning mechanism in us goes to sleep. As you begin to eat quality food every three hours or so, your body begins to expect this and rebalances its inner workings. That dependability helps you to reestablish optimal health. From there, anything is possible.

HIGH-GRADE FUEL

It is also important to consider the quality of fuel you are putting into your engine, which in this case is your body. One of the key principles of Clean Eating is to make sure you eat two very important food macronutrients together at each meal. You must combine lean protein and complex carbohydrates to help drive the metabolism, which in turn burns fuel in the form of fat or glucose. Before I learned how to Eat Clean I often felt dizzy, sweaty and fatigued. I suffered from hypoglycemia, a condition in which my blood sugar dropped so low that on occasion I would actually pass out. The solution before Clean Eating was always to eat or drink something very sugary, which made me feel better for a short while and then completely exhausted afterwards. It is not pleasant. Once I learned how to Eat Clean I never experienced a hypoglycemic attack again. Hooray! The solution to my situation and so many other hormonally based problems lay in regularly and consistently eating the correct combination of nutrients: lean protein and complex carbohydrates. The body cannot digest these macronutrients quickly and that helps to keep blood chemistry in check.

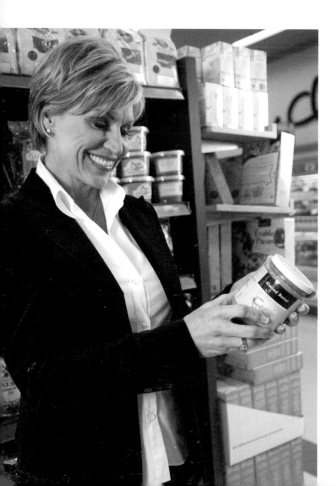

DRINK IT DOWN

Virtually all of us are under-hydrated. This is so even if you currently carry a bottle of water with you. It is difficult to picture how much water 2 or 3 liters is unless you fill a few liter bottle containers and see it for yourself. That's how I manage my water intake for the day. I fill my containers ahead of time and know that is my allotment. Water is absolutely essential because it assists in removing toxins and waste while it keeps the body, which is approximately 75 percent water already, in a well-hydrated and efficiently functioning state. If you constantly feel funny, headachy, tired, or generally unwell, your problem may be as simple as not drinking enough water. Try my little plan. Fill three 1-liter bottles with water at the start of your day and make sure by the end of the day these bottles are empty. See if you don't feel better.

NATURAL FOODS

My general rule of thumb is that food needs to be as natural as possible. I can't imagine what a processed cheese slice is made of, and what do they put in a Twinkie that prevents it from breaking down in a garbage dump (according to urban legends)? Who knows, but I won't be eating it anyway. The more processing a food has been through, the less chance it will be good for you.

When I am doing my groceries I aim for efficient shopping but I do read labels. If a food has a label with a long ingredient list that I can't read or pronounce then I am not going to buy it or eat it. I give myself that challenge every time I shop. Guess what? Produce and other natural unprocessed foods have either no ingredient list or a very short one indeed. Sticking to natural foods makes Clean Eating a breeze. Many of us think popcorn is the perfect snacking choice. But take a look below at a few different popcorn choices. The first example is popcorn you pop yourself in a pot or hot air popper. One ingredient. Now look at the ingredients in a few different flavors of microwave popcorn. In fact, any microwave popcorn will at the very least contain oils you probably do not want. Guess which one is the healthiest snack option for you?

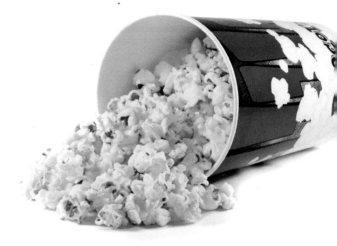

Orville Redenbacher brand
Popping Corn for Hot Air Poppers
INGREDIENTS: Popping corn.

Orville Redenbacher brand
Extra Buttery
INGREDIENTS: Popping corn, hydrogenated soybean oil, salt, natural and artificial butter flavor, color, butter. Contains Milk.

Orville Redenbacher brand
Corn on the Cob Flavor
POPCORN INGREDIENTS: Popping corn, palm oil, salt
PACKET: Whey powder, dextrose, natural flavors, onion powder, sour cream, hydrogenated soybean oil, sugar, salt, corn syrup solids, garlic powder, spice, disodium inosinate, disodium guanylate, artificial flavors

Orville Redenbacher brand
BBQ Flavor
POPCORN INGREDIENTS: Popping corn, palm oil, salt
PACKET: sugar, dextrose, onion powder, tomato powder, maltodextrin, salt, malted barley flour, spices, garlic powder, honey, fermented whey solids, caramel, yeast, spice extractive, disodium isonate, disodium guanylate.

LEAN PROTEIN

Very few of us eat enough of the right kinds of protein each day. North Americans do have a love affair with beef, however. We eat staggering amounts. Beef is a good source of protein, but because we raise our beef differently today than years ago – think concentrated feed lots, antibiotics, hormones … and sometimes even animal products that have no place in the diet of a herbivore – beef simply does not have the same nutritional value it once did. Unhealthy processed meats are also extremely popular. It is wise to vary your sources of protein. I incorporate legumes, nuts, seeds, soy products, quinoa, fish, lean turkey, chicken, bison, elk, pork tenderloin, whole grains, dairy and egg whites into my diet. Be sure to vary your proteins, as well.

EAT FAT! GET LEAN!

Fat is a concentrated source of energy. We need some fat for optimal health but we have become scared of fat today. We have to keep in mind that there are two kinds of fats – good and bad! Obviously you need to maximize your healthy fat intake and limit the other. You may be surprised to learn that in order to build a lean body full of healthy muscle you need healthy fat.

So who is the Bad Guy and who is the Good Guy? Trans and saturated fats are both bad guys. Many processed and fast foods contain these because they contribute to a longer shelf life and a better

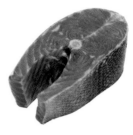

You may be surprised to learn that in order to build a lean body full of healthy muscle you need healthy fat.

"mouthfeel," which is important to food manufacturers (but not good for us). Unfortunately, both of these translate into weight gain and high cholesterol when consumed in excess. Sadly we are seeing more and more of these problems in younger and younger children since we have launched our love affair with convenience foods. Diseases that normally appear in adults, including high cholesterol and heart disease, are now showing up in our youth, especially in very overweight children. It is a no-brainer, then, to stay away from unhealthy fats.

Healthy fats, including Essential Fatty Acids, or EFA's, are very important in the diet. So EFA's are definitely the good guys. Adequate essential fatty acids help to super charge the burning of fat inside you and me. When cells are bathed in a rich environment of these necessary fats they burn more oxygen – think how brightly a fire burns in the presence of oxygen. This is ideal because it enhances the body's own way of dealing with fuel or, as you and I know it, food. Healthy fat acts as a catalyst for burning fat and fuel.

FISH AND TOMATO SEEDS

You and I have to make a point of eating EFA's every day, because the body cannot make them on its own. We have to help and do our part by eating foods containing plenty of these efficient little fat burners. Look for such oils as flax seed, pumpkin seed, avocado, olive, tomato seed, rice bran, sesame, grape seed and fish. Of course you could also include the source of these oils in your diet, namely sesame, pumpkin, flax, tomato seeds, avocado, whole-grain rice, and olives. And you should make a point of eating cold-water fish such as salmon at least once or twice a week, since there are plenty of healthy fats in fish, too. Just be careful about which fish you purchase, as there is some concern lately that fish contains concentrated chemical toxins and environmental pollutants in its flesh when it is at or near the top of its food chain.

WHY SHOULD YOU CARE?

Isn't it funny how little we think of health until we lose it? I realize this is human nature. I never used to think of my health. I know what it's like to feel unwell and when I contrast that against how I feel today I always experience a jolt – a physical reaction in my gut and my bones that reminds me I need to continue taking good care of myself. I got a second chance. I passed that on to my children and now I am passing it on to you.

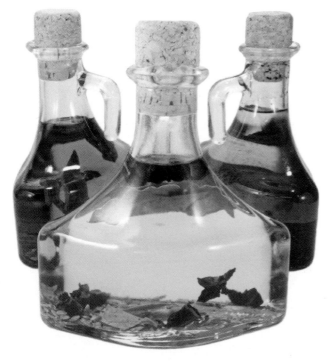

EAT-CLEAN COOKING SPRAY

Cooking sprays such as Pam and others are very handy, but I have become concerned about the presence of isobutane as an ingredient. My solution is to put healthy oils such as extra-virgin olive oil inside a spritz bottle, and simply spritz my pans and baking sheets when ready to use. Voilà! Healthy Eat-Clean cooking spray with no questionable ingredients.

There is a sense of urgency these days regarding how and what to eat. We have not been doing a good job of it and this is beginning to show. Never before has our very future faced a threat as dire as this. Indeed, a vibrant future is not possible if we continue at this rate. North Americans are among the fattest people on earth. Oddly, we are both over- and under-nourished at the same time. Food just isn't food anymore.

OUR RELATIONSHIP WITH FOOD

We have to remind ourselves that what we feed our children today influences not only their health during childhood but also during adulthood. It also affects how they will feed their own children. One hundred years ago most people on this great continent grew their own food. Ninety percent of the population lived on farms and ate every meal at the family dinner table. Today the picture is very different. We have moved away from the farm and cluster around fast-food dinner tables with strangers. We zoom through drive-thrus and eat our food at breakneck speed as we race through our busy lives. Rather than picking our food from the rich earth in the garden, we pick colorful boxes off grocery-store shelves. And more dis-

tressing is that few of us eat the recommended daily servings of fresh fruit and vegetables anymore – we are supposed to eat at least 2 ½ cups of vegetables

TIP Bring it to your children's school! If the school has a lunch plan and cafeteria, talk to the principal of the school about getting healthier options. Speak to the health and physical education teachers to create lesson plans on healthy eating and activities. If Clean-Eating is implemented in your child's education it will encourage them to make healthier choices as they grow.

each day and 2 cups of an array of fresh fruits. We get so lazy about eating properly we call ketchup and French fries vegetables and we call juice a fruit!

References:

www.mypyramid.gov

www.hc-sc.gc.ca

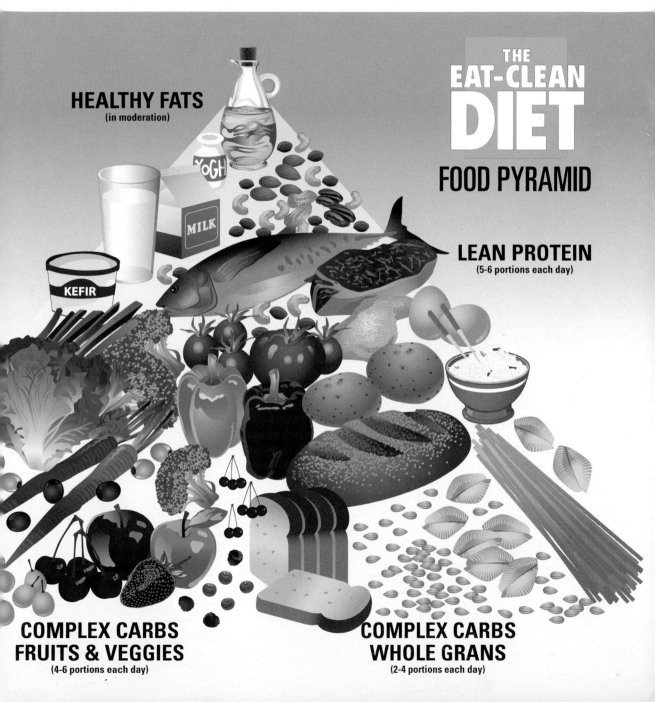

HEALTHY FATS
(in moderation)

THE EAT-CLEAN DIET
FOOD PYRAMID

LEAN PROTEIN
(5-6 portions each day)

MILK

YOGH

KEFIR

COMPLEX CARBS FRUITS & VEGGIES
(4-6 portions each day)

COMPLEX CARBS WHOLE GRANS
(2-4 portions each day)

CHAPTER TWO

Our kids' Failing Health

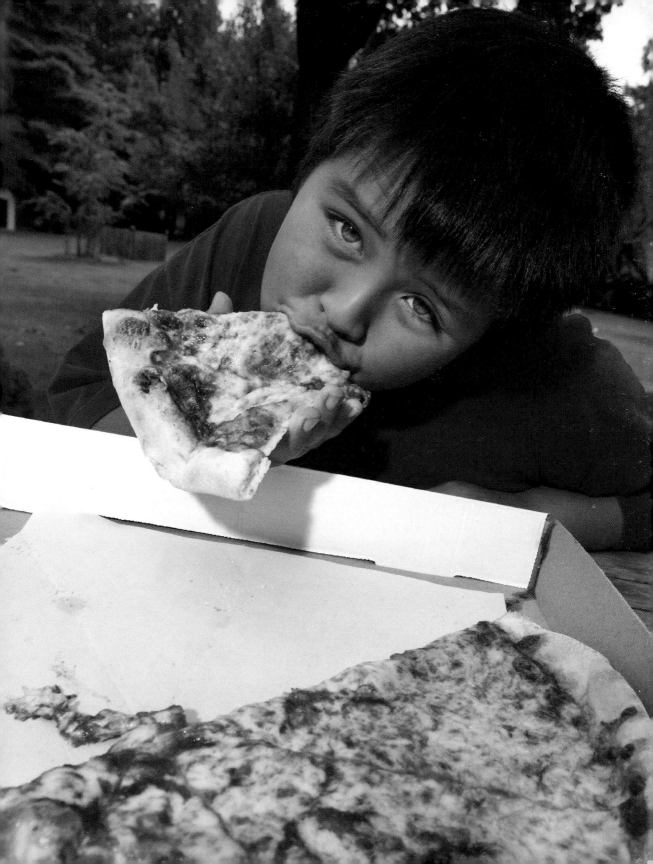

OUR CHILDREN ARE PAYING THE PRICE

The poor food choices we have made in the last few decades are beginning to show up today; not just because our children are heavier, but also because they are sicker. It used to be the odd child that had diabetes. The frightening trend today is that one third of young children have some form of this disease – Type 1, Type 2, pre-diabetes or metabolic syndrome X. Overweight kids also have greater chances of suffering from a variety of other health conditions including heart disease, high cholesterol, high blood pressure, fatty liver disease and even cancer. A weight gain of as little as five pounds can set off a series of "overweight" changes in the body. You may see only the tighter waistband or the chubby tummy, but much more is happening on the inside. This is where the danger is. The common denominator? Excess fat!

When I talk about Clean Eating I don't necessarily place emphasis on the outward appearance of my body, or especially my children's. I know that if we eat well, which to me means Eating Clean, we are taking care of ourselves from the hair on the top of our heads down to the tiniest cell in the deepest part of our body. The fact that most people lose weight on this program is just an added benefit.

MAKING A MENTAL CONNECTION

I try to make a mental connection between the food I am eating and my insides because it helps me to visualize complex carbohydrates and protein flowing through my intestinal tract and from there into my cells. I picture nutrients being exchanged from the blood into my cells and imagine how happy those little cells are to receive these nutrients. Perhaps they do a little cell dance when they are charged with energy and goodness from the well-chosen Clean food I just ate! I don't know, but I do know that good food makes for happy people.

Kids eat too much sugar and it is a nasty business!

SUGAR MAKES US SICK

I see what Clean Eating does for my kids and I can see what excess sugar does, too. Occasionally we will celebrate a birthday or other happy event and of course there will be cake and sweets. Often this cake will have frosting dripping with cups of confectioner's sugar. This evil white poison then seeps into my child's body and transforms what had been moments before a calm, pleasant person into a vibrating, erratic, sugar-charged creature. I am sure that teachers reading this can relate, as I have seen it in the classroom myself. Kids eat too much sugar and it is a nasty business!

Picture those cells way down inside us again. Here comes a flood of sugar, which now must be mopped up by insulin, which is secreted by the pancreas. Insulin plays an important role because its job is to break down sugar and make it usable by the body. This is hard work. Insulin must be manufactured and then delivered to each of the trillions of cells in the body. Sometimes the pancreas loses its ability to manufacture enough insulin. This is called Type 1 diabetes. At other times there is too much fatty tissue in the body for the insulin to travel through. Excess fat prevents insulin from doing its job correctly. Very heavy children place an excessive demand on their body to produce insulin. The pancreas just can't keep up the pace and gets fatigued or loses its ability to generate enough insulin. The child then has a condition known as Type 2 diabetes.

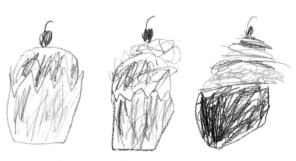

Eating too many cupcakes makes me feel sick.

Many obese children who have Type 2 diabetes also have a family history of the condition. This kind of diabetes is most commonly found in children who have already gone through puberty (excess fat actually encourages the body to go through puberty earlier). In children who have not yet reached puberty the condition is known as pre-diabetes. This is the stage just before diabetes occurs. Metabolic syndrome X is another precursor to diabetes, but it also is a precursor to heart disease, and guess what? Fifty percent of obese children have this syndrome. These are disease states and are a source of concern for parents and children. Once you have diabetes there is little you can do to change things. The most you can do is prevent it from getting worse by at least eating better or preferably by Eating Clean. However, even if you are at the pre-diabetic stage you can still prevent diabetes by Eating Clean right now!

"UNHEALTHIEST" FOODS

It is hard to deny that some foods out there must be avoided. We are all a little guilty of noshing on no-no's – or gorging on one-pound bags of potato chips or a tub of ice cream, for that matter. Most of these foods are no longer foods – they are so chemically charged and heavily processed you can hardly figure out the ingredients from which they were made. In general, if you can't pronounce the ingredient list you should steer clear away. To the right is a list of "foods" you might want to avoid. Be sure to read the ingredient list of every product you buy.

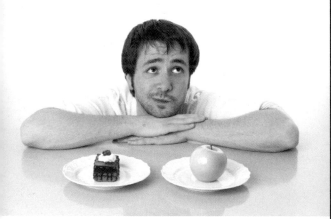

⭐ Keep in mind this list is of foods available commercially, which are usually refined and processed. If you prepare some or all of these foods from scratch with Clean-Eating ingredients you will significantly increase their nutritional content and decrease the danger caused by eating them.

AVOID
THESE★

- **White sugar – and any foods containing this**
- **White flour – and any foods containing this**
- **White fat – and any foods containing this**
- **Soft drinks**
- **Many breads and bread products**
- **Most crackers**
- **Pastries**
- **Pastry fillings**
- **Cakes and cake icings**
- **Margarine and other bread "spreads"**
- **Jams and jellies**
- **Commercial peanut butter**
- **Candy**
- **Candy bars**
- **Junk food**
- **Frozen and TV dinners**
- **Hamburgers and buns**
- **Hot dogs and buns**
- **Snack foods**
- **Fast foods**
- **Pizza**
- **Pies**
- **Doughnuts**
- **Muffins (unless made from scratch with healthy ingredients)**
- **Most cookies**

WHAT SYMPTOMS SHOULD YOU LOOK FOR?

As a parent you should keep a close eye on your child and watch for certain symptoms. You can also do what I have always done with my children: I schedule a yearly physical to track my child's health. I like to do this just before the school year starts. Having a yearly physical provides many benefits, including the following:

• Tracks your child's growth and development

• Provides a record of your child's progress or any changes

• Provides a record of your child's medical history

• Provides a safe atmosphere for both your child and you to learn about taking care of the body

• A urine test is normally taken to screen for certain conditions, including diabetes

• Blood pressure is measured

• An exchange of information will occur if the doctor discovers something

• Further tests can be ordered

• A verbal assessment of your child's mental status is usually undertaken

In general, visiting your doctor on an annual basis is a healthy habit to get into for both you and your kids. If the subject arises that your child may be overweight, a doctor is often the ideal person to deliver the news. Parents don't have to look like the bad guys.

SYMPTOMS OF DIABETES

+ **Blurred vision**

+ **Increased urination**

+ **Rapid weight loss or gain**

+ **Increased fatigue**

+ **Increased irritability**

+ **Increased infections**

+ **Prolonged wound-healing time**

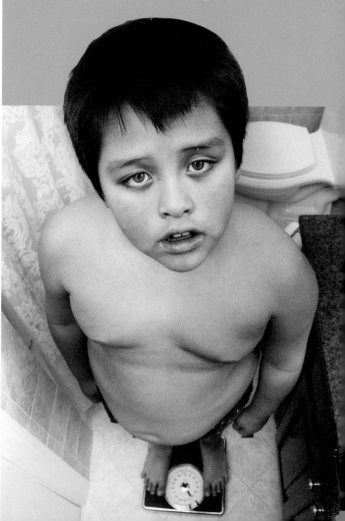

OVERWEIGHT AND ITS DANCING PARTNERS

Diabetes is not the only disease to worry about if your child or someone in your family is overweight. With excess fatty tissue comes an increase in blood pressure. If your child has high blood pressure it means his or her heart is working like crazy to push blood through the vessels in the body. A poor diet contributes to this dangerous condition, as does a lack of physical exercise. While a child will not likely die from high blood pressure, over time the damage done to the organs in the body takes its toll and the child's adult life will be one filled with ill health, disease, and in all probability an early death. The fatty liver disease mentioned earlier eventually turns to cirrhosis of the liver. We think this disease occurs only with older alcoholics, but it is now occurring in young children – because of eating junk food.

Overweight and obesity can cause other problems too. Think how hard it is to carry groceries from your car, especially when the bags are full of canned goods, weighty produce and other items. Now imagine carrying the equivalent of a few bags of groceries around with you all day long. It is exhausting. The body complains aloud with physical aches and pains, strains and other problems. As I mentioned earlier, a gain of even five pounds causes physical and chemical changes in the body. These would be magnified many times over, depending on how much excess weight you are carrying. Some overweight children also suffer from breathing problems, including asthma and sleep apnea.

Unfortunately, overweight also brings many psychological issues to the table too. Seriously heavy children will be made fun of. Those who suffer this cruelty are often ostracized and isolated. Growing up with self-confidence is hard enough under any circumstances, but when you complicate things with overweight it gets far worse.

DON'T WAIT!

In short, it is a mistake to think that a weight gain of a few pounds is not a problem. To avoid the burden of disease now and later in life parents need to assume responsibility for a healthy nutritional strategy today. Don't wait. Clean Eating can happen at this very moment in your house. Clean out your cupboards, refrigerator and freezer and fill garbage bags with nutritionally empty, chemically charged, calorie-loaded foods. Toss them right out the door! Chuck anything that comes in a box with words you can't pronounce. Give your child an apple and a few unsalted almonds instead of a Fruit Roll Up. Dump out sodas and drink loads of water. Put a water cooler in your house as I did and see how easily your family can quench their thirst with water. The minute you start making even the simplest changes, your body will "notice" and respond. You may not see it right away but believe me, your microscopic cells will be dancing for joy!

No more junk food!

THE EDWARDS FAMILY'S STORY

A reader's testimonial

"

Hello Tosca.

Thanks for writing your Eat-Clean Diet book. My children were soda-holics. We could down two liters of soda-pop at the dinner table in one sitting. They even started their day with soda. I happened upon your book when my sister told me how she used it to get her family off of sugar. My thoughts raced to my own kids, who can do serious damage in the sugar department. I went straight home that day and ditched every pop bottle we had. Then I bought a water cooler and got hardnosed with my kids – two teenaged boys and a 12-year-old daughter. No more sugar for them, at least not in my house. Already I can see and feel a difference. They aren't nearly so "teenagerish" to me. I actually like my kids again.

Thanks Tosca for bringing my family back to me.

"

Sincerely,
Tina Edwards

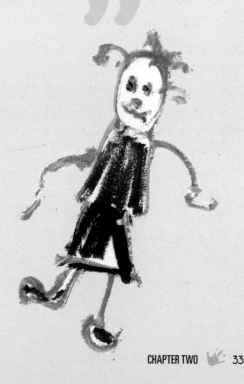

CHAPTER THREE

Get Your Family on Board

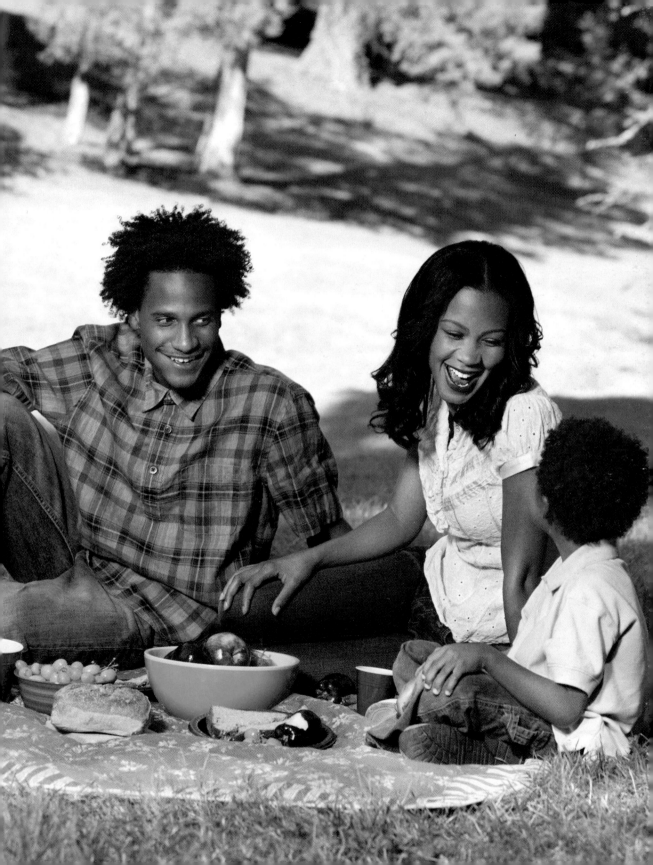

IN THE BEGINNING

It isn't easy bringing the news of change to your little world. Change means things have to be done differently and that is uncomfortable for most of us. I recall the days when I first brought Clean Eating home to my family. I had already experienced my first success with this lifestyle by dropping excess fat and not experiencing those terrible hypoglycemic attacks again. I felt so good I knew I would have to share it with my family. At that time I was newly divorced, and the new life for my three daughters and me was full of changes already. All three of them rebelled at the idea of Clean Eating. They did it because they were scared they were going to lose the mom they knew so well and I understood that. Still, their rebellion did not prevent me from continuing to incorporate Clean Eating into my home on Evans Terrace those years ago. Breakfast, lunch and supper were Clean-Eating meals and so were the mini-meals in between. My Clean-Eating lifestyle soon became that of my family too, and no one is complaining now!

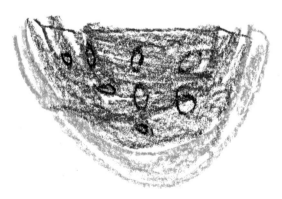

SMALL CHANGES, BIG SUCCESSES

Making changes, no matter how good these changes may be, is a daunting task. But as the old saying goes: "Question: How do you eat an elephant? Answer: One bite at a time." If we can change little bites one at a time we will be more successful. I found that to be true for me, and for my family as well. I did not hit my girls over the head with lectures about how to eat and when and so on. I quietly went about my business making little changes in the kitchen. A new dish made with Clean-Eating foods was never announced like this: "Boy are you girls going to love this new protein-rich ancient grain I have just discovered!" I just put the quinoa on the table as part of the meal and let the girls try what I made. (And by the way, most kids love quinoa.) I made a mental note of whether they liked the food or not, made variations, and kept going until we had a happy agreement on the age-old question, "MOM!! What's for supper!!??"

START WITH A CHANGE YOU KNOW YOU AND YOUR FAMILY CAN MAKE

Since change is a difficult thing to usher into your world it is always smart to start with a change you know for sure you can make. A good example would be to start by cleaning out your cupboards. When you do that you can go whole hog and toss it all, which I recommend and did in my own house, or you can

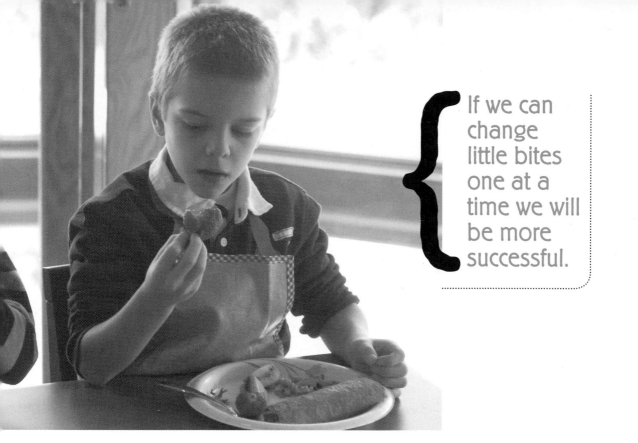

> { If we can change little bites one at a time we will be more successful.

make gradual changes if you have a cohort of resistant family members. By choosing the strategies your gang is most likely to stick to, you are more likely to be successful, which is, after all, what you want.

If your family currently quenches its collective thirst with soda and other carbonated, sugary beverages, this would be the place to begin. I installed a water cooler in my kitchen when I cleaned out the kitchen cupboards in preparation for Clean Eating. Instead of drinking gallons of sugar-loaded drinks, my family began satisfying their thirst with ice-cold water. Part of the success, of course, was having a neat gadget from which my children could dispense their own

water. Whatever the reason, it worked and I spent a lot less money on soda pop. In fact, it did not take long to make up for the cost of the water cooler and then some. I am not suggesting you have to buy a water cooler, but this is an example of how you can make a small change that yields a big difference for your family.

MAKING THE CHANGES

1 Eat several small meals instead of three or fewer large meals.

This is easy enough to do since it simply requires that you make meals a regular habit in the first place. Set regular times for meals in your house.

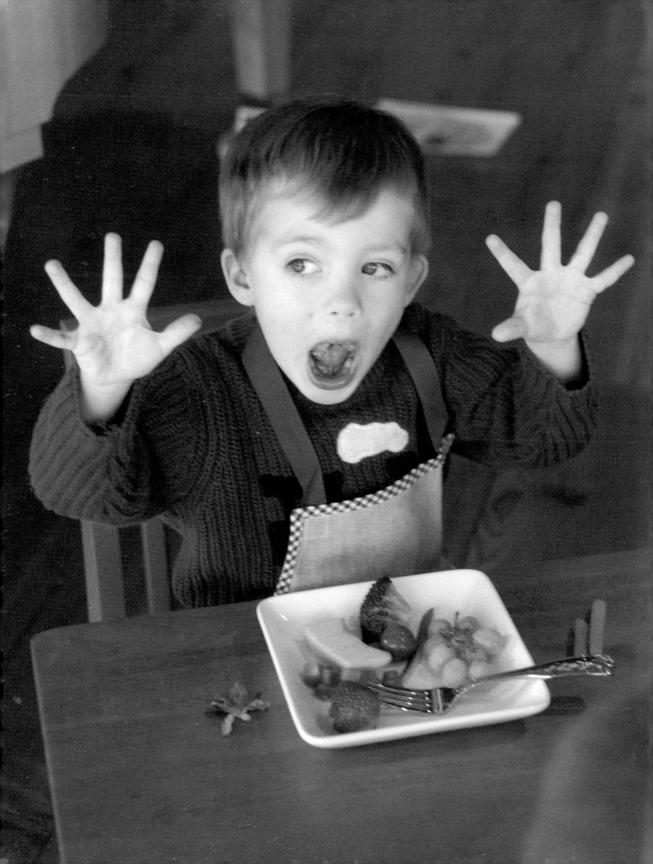

Have breakfast with as many family members as possible. Find a time that works for dinner and set that too. The remaining meals are probably those that need to be transported to and from school and/ or work. Pack small snack-like meals for your family members. Even better? Have them help you or do it themselves.

2 Eat every 2 to 3 hours.

This will be slightly harder to control, since most family members walk out the door every day to their various roles in life, whether that includes school or a job, and you don't see each other for the next few hours. Part of the success of Clean Eating is to listen to your tummy and decide if you are hungry or full. If you really get on board with Clean Eating you will soon notice that pangs of hunger will arrive knocking on your stomach walls approximately every two-and-a-half to three hours like clockwork. The more you Eat Clean the more pronounced these feelings will be, and the easier it becomes to recognize when that three-hour timeframe is up and you must eat again. I was amazed to discover this. I had been raised to eat only three times per day and yet I was truly and undeniably hungry more often than that. Eating this way keeps you consistently nourished and feeling well as a result.

Of course many of you have e-mailed me and complained that frequent eating is not provided for in traditional work or school settings and I know this is a problem. I have told my own children to keep small amounts of clean foods in their pockets or backpacks so that when they are switching classes at school they can nibble on pieces of fruit or un-salted nuts (where allowed). Or I will give them one Clean protein or granola bar, which they can eat in pieces between classes. The same would work for someone in a work environment. Most workplaces allow for a short break in the mid-morning and mid-afternoon. This is the perfect time to give up that calorie-loaded Starbucks Frappucino and have a proper Clean-Eating snack instead. I have nothing against Starbucks but I do worry about those 500-plus-calorie drinks people are guzzling instead of getting the nutrition that comes from Clean food. Protein shakes (smoothies) can be a great alternative at these times.

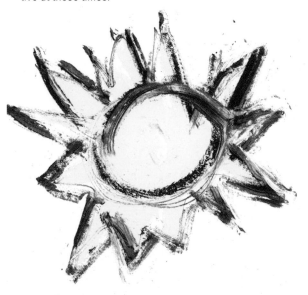

For most jobs, even if you are on the road a lot, you can ensure Clean-Eating success by packing a cooler, another principle I advocate strongly.

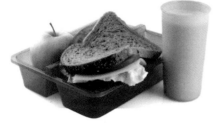

3 Eat lean protein and complex carbohydrates at each meal.

This is a change that you must practice a little before you get the hang of it. It helps if you choose the appropriate products right at the grocery store. If you bring home Clean-Eating groceries, this food will also end up as a Clean-Eating meal. The point is to be sure to partner these two macronutrients: lean protein and complex carbs.

THINGS TO PACK IN A COOLER

+ **A variety of raw fresh fruits and vegetables**

+ **Raw leafy greens and sprouts to toss into a salad**

+ **Raw unsalted nuts and seeds**

+ **Natural nut butters**

+ **Hummus and other legume-based spreads**

+ **Whole-grain wraps, bagels, breads and crackers**

+ **Water stored in a stainless steel container**

+ **Plain yogurt**

+ **Dried fruit**

+ **Hardboiled eggs**

+ **Leftovers from dinner the night before**

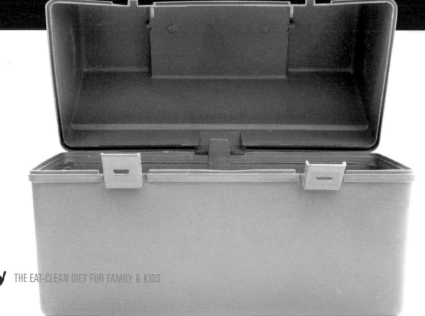

MOM AND DAD ARE DRIVING THE BUS

I remember mealtimes spent with cranky children not wanting to eat broccoli or squash. An exhausted parent can be no match for a stubborn whining child. It's easy to give in and let them eat at McDonald's. But reconsider. Very young children won't need a lengthy explanation from you about why you are now serving Clean-Eating food. Just serve and eat.

If your kids are older, involve them in aspects of food preparation. I'm no chef, but I loved to cook even as a young person because I got to spend time with Mom and Dad. You are the parents. You make the food choices. Introduce Clean Eating slowly if you have to, so your kids don't mutiny. Prepare Clean, healthy alternatives to kid-friendly foods: switch greasy deep-fried French fries for oven-baked fries; make healthier homemade pizza options featuring less processed meat and sauce and more veggies and lean grilled chicken or turkey. The recipes found in Chapter 15 will help you accomplish this. Make Clean Eating a family priority. Don't serve unhealthy options alongside Clean options. That's sending mixed messages.

TELEZA'S STORY
A reader's testimonial

Hi Tosca,

We purchased The Eat-Clean Diet *book and believe it or not I am finished reading it! As a wife and mother of three, it is my responsibility to make sure my family eats healthy. We typically eat pretty healthy but the children were getting bored with the same recipes. Thanks to you and* The Eat-Clean Diet *book I can incorporate every-thing I just learned into our Eat-Clean lifestyle. What others need to know is that eat-ing clean is not only for adults, but also for the entire family.*

Thank you Tosca,
Marvin and Teleza Thomas

CHILDREN EAT ACCORDING TO HABIT

For thousands of years prior to this century (and still today in most of the world), children ate what their parents ate. If they didn't, they went hungry. These days in the wealthy western world, parents can indulge a child's food preferences and often do. Worse, parents have less control over the quality of what their kids eat thanks to the "ingenuity" of modern food manufacturing. The child of today appears to be in the driver's seat, directing food choices at every turn. Families spend less time preparing food and less time eating together.

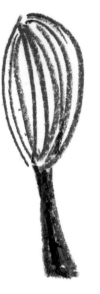

It's so much fun to whisk eggs!

Children, creatures of habit like their parents, develop food preferences based on familiarity. The more processed, suspect, chemically charged, nutrient-deficient foods they are exposed to, the more they recognize these as their diet. The more they eat such foods, the more they become hardwired to adopt them as a dietary pattern. Don't be surprised that your kids love salt, sugar, and fat. Most adults do, too. We are programmed to like calorie-dense and water-retaining foods because throughout history we were often short on food and water. However, these days we are anything but short on food, and eating these foods regularly reinforces the habit. Since these ingredients are put in practically every processed food, it is easy to consume them unwittingly, and often.

TIP Get your kids in the kitchen to help prepare Clean-Eating meals. Not only will you have memorable together time, you can teach your children at an early age the benefits of healthy eating.

Parents, you have in your hands at this moment a powerful tool to help guide you and your family in the right direction of more healthful eating. Clean Eating advocates eating plenty of fresh fruits and vegetables, whole grains and lean protein. Food intake is not restricted and calories are not counted. Meals are eaten at regular, frequent intervals, which correlate to a growing child's hunger patterns (as well as a busy adult's). Remember, if you are Eating Clean you are setting the positive example for your children to Eat Clean too.

GET THEM INVOLVED

There are many ways to get your kids and family members excited about Clean Eating. Generally, the more involved your family is in the process of selecting food and preparing it, the more energized they'll be about participating in this new healthy lifestyle. Try the following strategies with your own Clean-Eating team to keep them committed. The more your family members get to play with the foods, and the pots and pans, the more likely they will be to stick to healthy eating.

MY KIDS WON'T EAT IT! EVEN *MY* KID WON'T EAT IT!

Just because I am known as the Clean-Eating Lady does not mean I had an easy time getting my family to Eat Clean. I have managed to change countless ingredients in recipes to healthier options but there are few things I can't fiddle with and I still have resisters in the ranks. Siggghhh!! I am certain many of you will relate to the difficulties of convincing your loved ones to participate in this new way of eating.

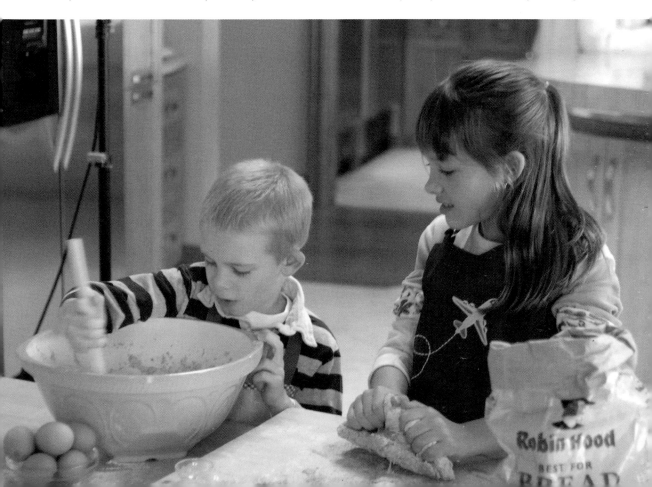

Sometimes going about it in a quiet but dedicated way is best. You know who is shopping and preparing the meals!

I encourage my family to at least try new fruits and vegetables and other Clean foods. I became so desperate with my daughter Kelsey-Lynn's resistance to eating fruit

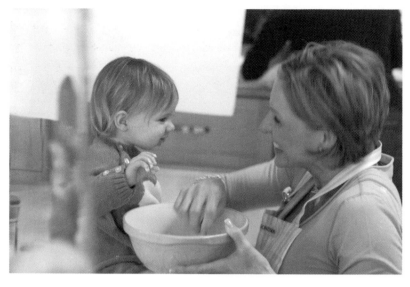

that I even went to our family physician for help. Kelsey avoids all fruit. No exceptions! I had hoped the good doctor could scare some sense into Kelsey. We have a good, longstanding relationship with our family doctor. The doctor reminded Kelsey of the need for fiber, enzymes and anti-cancer agents that fruit could provide. For a while things went well. We began with apples. The doctor suggested them because Kelsey loved sweet carrots and apples were, in her opinion, quite similar as far as texture and taste. The doctor suggested we visit the grocery store and let Kelsey choose any apples she liked and then go home and try them. We brought home apples of every color, shape and size. Before long Kelsey was eating half an apple a day and I felt a surge of happiness, thinking I had won this battle. That lasted until Kelsey was selected to attend a ballet school away from home. At the young age of 11 my little

girl left home to learn how to become a classically trained ballerina. Fruit is back on her "disgusting" list and I have very little control over how she eats when she's not home, since she must rely on her billet "mother" for her food.

At this point I have come to the conclusion Kelsey may never love fruit. Regardless, her taste for it will develop at her own pace when she is good and ready. I can't fight it. My only option is to capitalize on the fact that she loves vegetables and will eat a wide variety of them. This I have done with a vengeance. I still can't believe how much my kid loves vegetables but I count my blessings that she does.

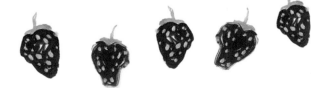

CHANGE AND HOW TO MAKE IT

Getting your loved ones to eat healthy foods is, in some cases, more work than you would like to shoulder. You must try to put the task into perspective. Moms, dads, caregivers, you are responsible for what ultimately lands in the stomachs of those you care for and love, and how they eat has everything to do with their health, growth and physical condition. It may be difficult to introduce change into your home, but you will get immense satisfaction from knowing how much good you are doing for them. And remember, even the small step of encouraging your child to eat half an apple each day is a victory. The best approach to making changes for those who are resistant is to make small, subtle changes. As with any changes in life baby steps and small victories add up to big successes.

MANAGING THE TRANSITION

Experts will tell you transition is the most difficult aspect of making changes. Teachers know this too. When I was a teacher I found that the best way to manage change, particularly for little people, was to let them know what was on the agenda. When kids (and adults) know what is going to happen they seem better able to cope. You can have a short family meeting to discuss in a non-confrontational way how this family is going to eat from now on. Make it an open forum where everyone gets to have a say, and have some examples of the foods you plan on introducing so kids can see what you mean. Be sure to put a positive spin on the discussion and don't threaten your family with frightening "must do's" and "if you don'ts." You want everyone on your side and you need to have a smooth transition if you are going to be successful at this.

When I sat down with my family and introduced Clean Eating to them I assured them I would go easy and help them make the transition. I did not harp on the antioxidant power and fiber – kids don't care so much about that. I did talk about how good these foods taste and I garnered participation by having them each choose a night when they could make the meal choice. They could choose their veggies and main-course ideas, and I "cleaned" them up from my end. Now my kids are familiar with vegetables such as aspiration, brocolirabe, brocoflower, golden beets and rutabagas. Who knew? More importantly they love these foods and eat them happily. I am sure it is because I instilled a positive, cooperative attitude into our family. You as the parent are the guide, there to shepherd your gang on this nutritional path. Provide loads of variety in healthy foods to promote the feeling of choice rather than restriction.

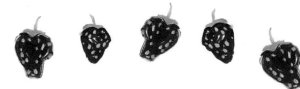

SIMPLE CHANGES YOU CAN
MAKE IMMEDIATELY

Don't hesitate to make these changes. You can do them today without so much as stepping out of your home.

- Switch Froot Loops and any other sugary cereals to oatmeal.

- Top oatmeal with unsweetened applesauce, berries, sliced banana or chopped apples and cinnamon rather than tablespoons of sugar.

- Switch regular heavily sweetened peanut butter to natural nut butters – they are delicious!

- Switch string cheese to yogurt.

- Switch white bread to whole-grain breads, wraps, Ezekiel bread and crackers.

- No more processed crackers! Switch to Salba crackers or flatbread.

- Got a can of chickpeas? Garlic? Lemon juice? Sesame seeds? Then whizz it up in the food processor and make hummus as your favorite new bread spread.

- No more fruit juice! Whatever juice you plan to serve your family, make it with one part juice and two parts water.

- Toss soda and other heavily sweetened beverages. Do it now! Drink more water instead.

- Candy, junk food and other processed, nutritionally lacking foods should be tossed immediately.

- Be aware of unhealthy fats in your family's diet and cut them out right away. Trans and saturated fats are killers.

- Eat more EFAs, especially those from seeds, nuts, nut butters and healthy oils such as pumpkin, olive and safflower.

- Eat meals together. You can do this today. Make your next meal a family event.

- Switch off TVs, video games, computers, iPods and any other distractions so you are fully engaged in each other and the food. Make mealtime pleasant. This is not a time to lecture your kids on homework; it's a time to get to know one another better.

- Do not use food as reward or punishment. Food serves the purpose of nourishment.

- Include your children in the shopping process. Be sure to take them not just on trips to grocery stores, but farmer's markets and stalls as well.

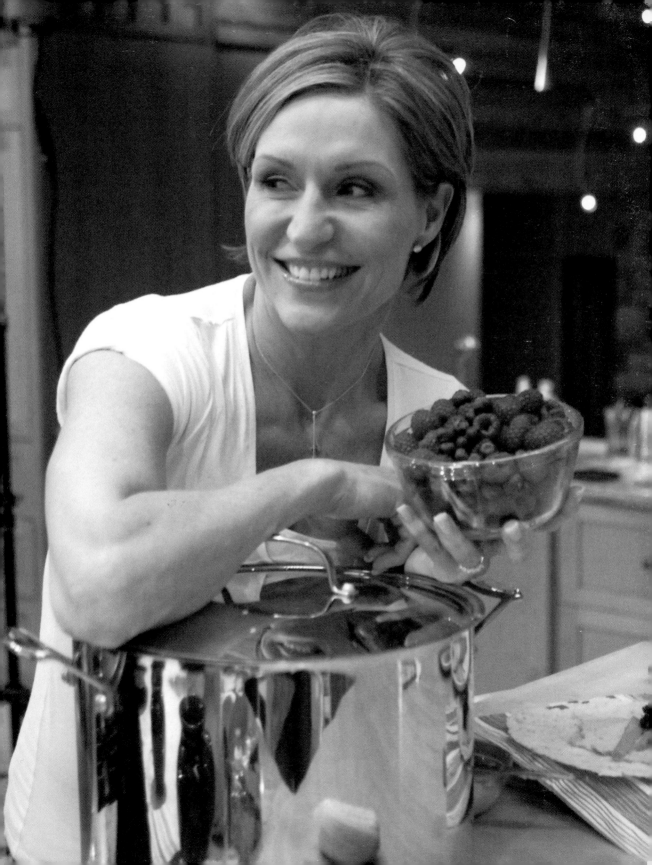

CHAPTER FOUR

Making it Work at Home

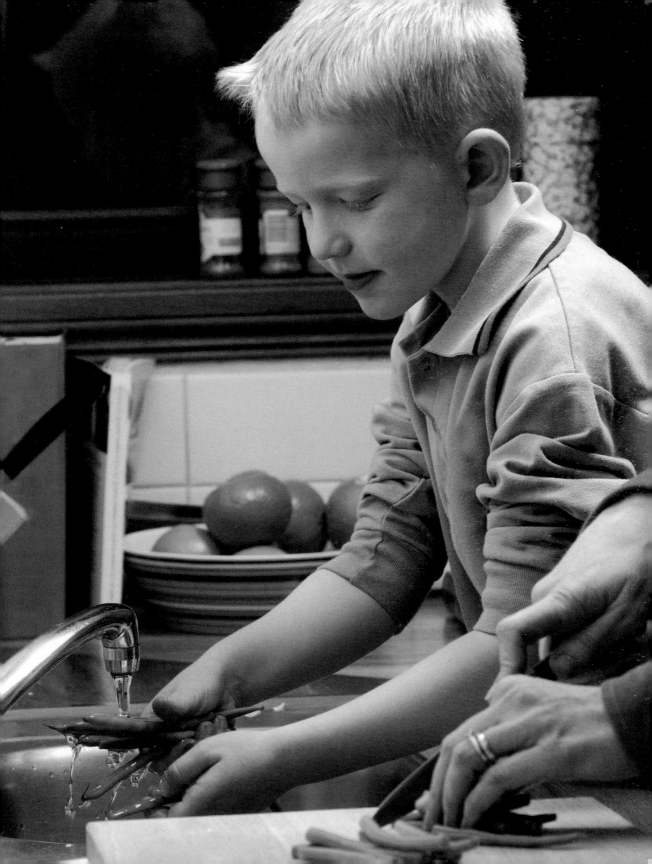

MAKING IT WORK AT YOUR HOUSE

1 BE A GOOD ROLE MODEL.

Set the Clean-Eating example yourself. Children learn by imitation and they're probably modeling you right now whether you are eating an apple or a sticky doughnut. Study after study shows that when Mom and Dad eat fruits and vegetables, exercise and take good care of their health, so do the kids. Conversely, when parents smoke, drink alcohol, take drugs or eat garbage foods, the children are more likely to follow.

My children and their friends call me the Clean-Eating Lady. They know I will prepare nourishing food for them no matter what. We recently celebrated New Year's Eve at our home with 35 guests, most of them our children and their friends. We prepared a beautiful dining-room setting with enough seating for all and enjoyed a Clean-Eating celebratory meal they are still talking about today. They raved about pumpkin soup, roasted fingerling potatoes, roasted tenderloin and an assortment of delicious sides from my *Eat-Clean Diet Cookbook*, and then cheered when the glorious Chocolate Tofu Mousse was served with intensely colored fresh berries.

2 TAKE KIDS SHOPPING WITH YOU.

Let them be part of the process of selecting both everyday and new foods. I'm nearly 50 and I still get a thrill out of seeing the rainbow of foods in the produce section. I try to pass that on to my kids. Just recently I discovered the joys of golden beets and rutabagas. I have known about them for a long time but didn't serve them very often until I mastered roasting them. The more food experiences you share with your family members the more interested they will be in a variety of foods.

As crazy as this may sound to you, when our family travels out of the country we make a point of visiting a grocery store or local market in that new culture.

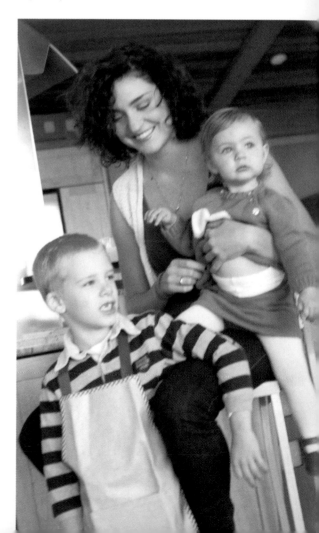

We like to immerse ourselves in foods that are foreign to us. I remember planning to go shopping for food when we were visiting the town of Sapri (not Capri) in Italy. We set off just before lunchtime on a hot August day and were completely shocked to find the local market closed. To our surprise we learned all businesses closed their doors during the hottest hours of the day. We had to settle for some plums from a local farmer who was making his way home for his siesta!

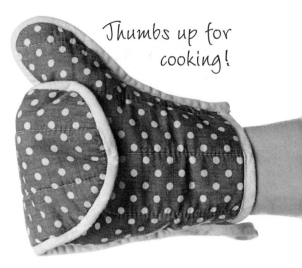

Thumbs up for cooking!

 ### 3 GET FAMILY MEMBERS IN THE KITCHEN.

I learned to cook at my mother's elbow. Her patient teaching helped me enjoy the process of creating meals then and now. Children love to eat what they have created. Let them make a mess and experiment right along with you. They can measure, mix, pour, assemble, and stir with little trouble and will enjoy the results more. They will take pleasure in the experience and carry that with them into their adulthood. My own three girls love to be in the kitchen, something I have fostered from their early years.

I always encouraged my girls to join me in the kitchen and some of our happiest hours were spent together there. We all have to eat – why not make the best of it? When we gather around the stove it gives us an opportunity to reconnect while creating a meal. I still get a good laugh when I recall some of the kitchen disasters they conjured up. Once

Rachel baked a cake with one cup of salt instead of sugar. The cake was inedible of course but we laughed ourselves silly when the first person took a bite and made a horrible face. Then there was the time Chelsea used Shake 'n Bake instead of flour to make oatmeal cookies and wondered why the cookies tasted so weird. There were plenty of times when the end result of the children's efforts in the kitchen was memorable, and they are preserved forever in photographs and countless reminiscences.

4 WHAT MESSAGES ARE YOU SENDING?

"Finish your food! Eat it all! You can't go and play until you have finished every morsel on your plate!"

These commands are familiar to many families. Such instructions may mean well, but they don't translate well. Kids read them as threats and inevitably take confusion about eating into their adult years. They get mixed messages about what to eat, when to eat and how much. They no longer know what hunger and satiety feel like. Let them become familiar with these physical feelings. These are the most reliable pieces of information for any of us to depend on when feeding ourselves. Clean Eating helps us get back in touch with these important signs. If you think about it, your body is constantly talking to you. All you have to do is listen.

Don't use food as a reward. Many of us, from parents to teachers to caregivers, rely on food as a reward for positive behavior. Since when does food have anything to do with how we behave (unless you are talking about a sugar high, of course)? Food is food, and not a reward. Use the six small meals advocated in Clean Eating as opportunities to nourish your loved ones with substantial, wholesome foods as well as small snacks. If you must give a reward, stick to simple, enjoyable things like a day at the park or a new book. Besides, most kids just want recognition for their accomplishments; they don't need a reward.

5 PROVIDE NUTRITIOUS CLEAN-EATING FOODS – LEAVE TEMPTATION IN THE GROCERY STORE.

Clean Eating suggests eating healthy foods from the Food Pyramid or the Food Guide. These include complex carbohydrates from whole grains as well as from fresh fruits and vegetables. Does that sound familiar to you? It should, since by now you know these are the kinds of foods I recommend for Clean Eating. Stock up on these first as you make your way through the supermarket. I like to call this Perimeter Shopping because most of the produce, dairy and meat you need are found on the perimeter or outside aisles. That's because they need to be kept refrigerated and the walls are where the outlets are. Don't be tempted by the bakery, junk food or cookie aisles. These aisles hold all kinds of temptation, and I steer clear. The best treats are those you make together anyway. And make snack choices wisely – which means read the ingredients.

6 MAKE ONE MEAL. THAT'S IT.

Don't make a special meal for Johnny and another for Susie. This sends a confusing message that one child is special or different than the other, and that special foods are entitled. Preparing the same food for everyone unites the family in the Clean-Eating cause. Everyone shares the same nutritious food and benefits together. Obviously if a family member has food allergies or intolerances you must avoid those foods for that person. But I find if I start preparing something different for everyone it gets crazy in the kitchen and at the dinner table. In my house, it's one meal and that is it.

7 DON'T YIELD!

Stay firm with whining kids when they demand the "old" foods loaded with unhealthy fats, sugars and other chemical calories. Initially

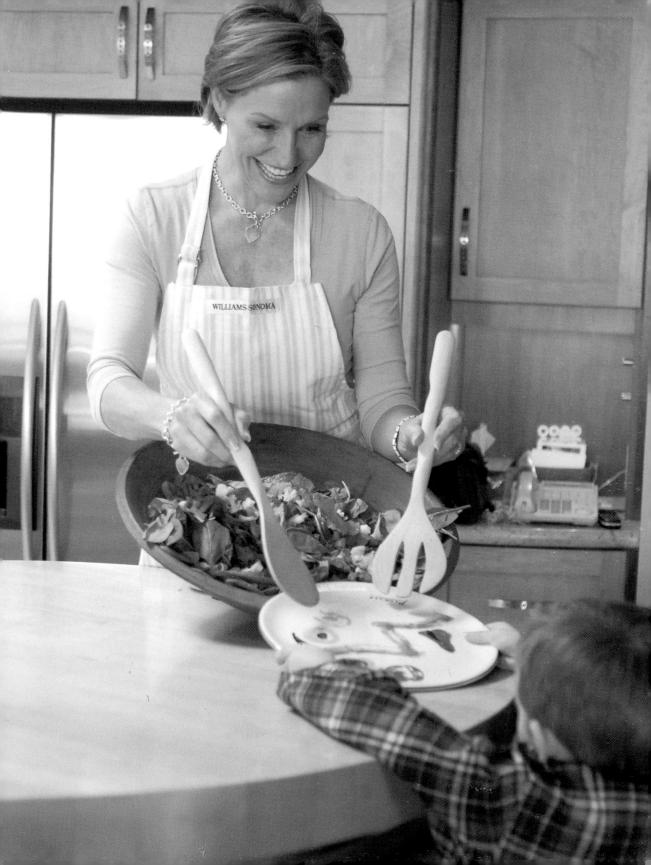

they may challenge you and dig their heels in but you will prevail as you set the positive example of tough love and Clean Eating.

My daughters fought me initially because they thought what they had been eating was food. When I explained that it wasn't they thought I was losing my mind. I stayed the course and kept introducing more Clean foods into every meal. They grew to love vegetables, grains and other nutritious foods that appeared on their plates more and more frequently. Soon they were noticing how much better they felt. They had more energy, less blemished skin, and their hair looked great all the time. Before long, Clean Eating was how we ate, no questions asked.

8 TAKE YOUR FOCUS OFF THE TV SET.

There are 150 channels and nothing good on. Choose a particular show that you will allow the kids to watch or that you watch as a family. Don't make TV the permanent electronic babysitter in your house. North Americans watch far too much TV, and this habit shortens the time available for sports, outdoor activity, play, conversation, games, and so many other healthy, productive pursuits.

I make a point of turning the TV off, especially at mealtimes. There is nothing I hate more than distractions at mealtimes. I want to enjoy the dining experience and reconnect with my family after a busy day. The less time we spend in front of the TV set the more we connect. Our family has become very good at communicating.

9 PLAN FAMILY OUTINGS THAT INVOLVE EXERCISE.

The more you get out of the house for organized family activities that include hiking, skiing, swimming or any other interests, the less time you will have to spend in front of the television or the fridge. You will build healthy muscles, heart and lungs in the process and enjoy time spent together, too. Exercise done this way doesn't feel like punishment; it's simply an enjoyable family activity.

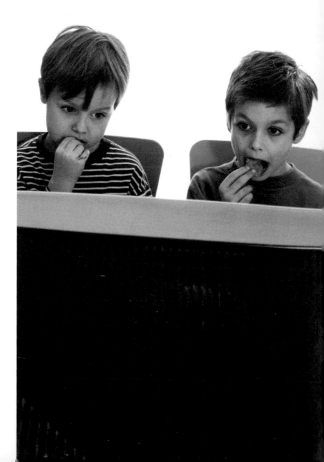

THE EAT-CLEAN DIET FOR FAMILY & KIDS

There hasn't been a holiday yet when our family has not gone for a hike or some other activity. When I think about it, holidays are enhanced by our spending physical time together.

10 WHEN PROGRESS IS MADE, RECOGNIZE IT.

Acknowledge positive changes without using food as the reward. This may be a hard habit to break: food is ingrained in the process of raising and educating our children, particularly as a reward. However, movie tickets, a book or a favorite outing are all excellent items with which to recognize your child, especially when he or she has given up a pack-a-day cookie habit. And remember, just that you noticed and remarked upon the change is a reward in itself.

11 BE PATIENT WHEN EXPOSING YOUR CHILD TO NEW FOODS.

Studies show it takes as many as 10 tries to make the leap from YUCKY to YUMMY. Experiment with different textures. Some kids like crunchy while others prefer smooth. Something as simple as a change in texture can convert a food from yuck to yum in one serving. You may also want to revisit certain foods as your family becomes accustomed to eating a wider variety. I noticed that I could serve a vegetable such as Brussels sprouts one time and the gang would turn up their nose at it and the next time they would love it. The reason? Most often it

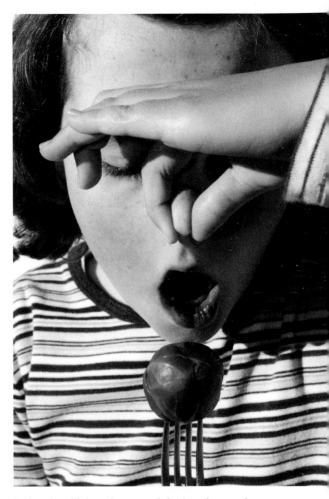

had to do with how I prepared the item in question. The Brussels sprouts were rejected when boiled, but they were a hit roasted. I also discovered that adding roasted garlic to dishes made them more readily accepted in my house. Once I learned how much the family loved the flavor, I began preparing several bulbs of roasted garlic at a time. The bonus is that I know garlic is potent disease fighter. My family simply loved the taste.

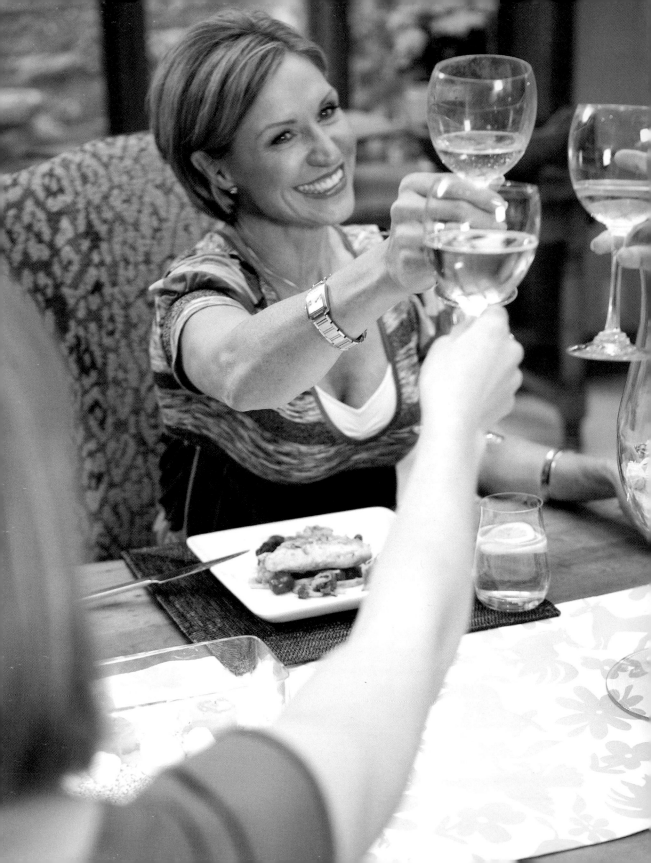

12 MAKE MEALTIMES RELAXED AND ENJOYABLE.

I love to set the table with clean linens, interesting plates, glasses and flatware and even light candles. I need the atmosphere at mealtime to promote a friendly interchange of ideas, day's events and discussion. Mealtime is social time and matters very much. Enjoy food with your family this way at least three times a week if possible. If three meals together sounds like a lot, start with one but stick to it and work towards eating together as often as possible. Try also to avoid discussing difficult or contentious subjects at the dinner table. I do my best to stay away from issues such as politics, finances and work-related concerns. I really want to hear about the day my family has had.

> **Clean Eating is the simplest, healthiest way to take care of you and yours.**

YOUR FAMILY IS WITH YOU

Clean Eating is for you and your family. Husbands, boyfriends, sons, daughters, mothers and wives can eat this way and enjoy a robust and healthy life. You should feel encouraged that you will be making positive changes for your family and that those changes will not interfere with your normal way of living. Clean Eating is the simplest, healthiest way to take care of you and yours.

THE NEED FOR SPEED – FAST FOOD IN YOUR KITCHEN

We have developed a reliance on fast food because we have become fast people. Some days I feel I'm running so hard I wish I could stop the planet for a minute and just get off. Days like that make even thinking about a meal difficult, let alone preparing one. And days like that are the reason we have developed a reliance on fast food. Of course, overwhelming evidence points to the many negatives of this dependence. We need to find a better way to get through mealtime.

In my experience, with a little planning you can easily have a nutritious meal ready in the time it takes to drive to the Golden Arches, get out of your car, order and pay for the meal, wait for it to be prepared, go back to your car and drive home with the loot. Even using the drive-thru takes about the same amount of time needed to make, say, pasta, sauce and salad at your address.

Your strongest card in the game of "Making Supper on Week Nights" is to have a well-stocked cupboard, fridge, freezer and pantry. Your second strongest card is having a game plan. That is, you need to know your schedule and that of your family members and determine which nights are going to be the most challenging. On those nights I usually serve a one-dish meal that I have prepared in advance. This could be soup, stir-fry or stew. These dishes can easily be placed in a saucepan and warmed up just before serving.

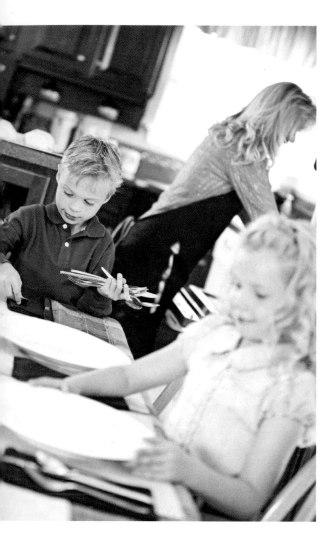

Setting the table is my favorite thing to do!

Other times I like to put ingredients into a slow cooker and find a meal ready when I get home several hours later. I also use the weekends to make extra chicken breasts, whole-grain dishes, turkey meatballs and muffins. Foods such as these will keep and can be readily used for upcoming meals.

My favorite "trick" is to make Planned Leftovers: whatever meal I am serving I consciously make twice the amount to have the remainder available for meals the next day.

Finally, you will need the cooperation of your family. Nowhere in the guidebook does it say Mom has to do all the cooking! Get help. Have your kids take some of the responsibility for food prep. Chopping veggies is easy and can be fun as long as there are no wayward knives. Children can also set the table. In my house, the cook cooks but does not do clean up afterwards. So whoever cooked the meal does not have the extra responsibility of cleaning up.

If you must visit a fast-food establishment, then make sure you pay attention to the amount of food you have been served. These restaurants tend to serve enormous portions. Decide right away not to eat all of it. Choose grilled options for your main course. Grilled foods have less fat and fewer calories than deep-fried foods. Avoid creamy, fatty salad dressings. Stay away from sugary beverages.

FAST-FOOD OPTIONS
FOR YOUR KITCHEN

➤➤ **Raw fruit.**

➤➤ **Raw vegetables** – keep prepared in the fridge to nibble on or use in stir-fries or soups when you don't have much time or energy.

➤➤ **Frozen veggies are a lifesaver.** You can add them to practically any meal when vegetable prep is just not possible. Keep a good selection on hand.

➤➤ **Yogurt, kefir, and cottage cheese.**

➤➤ **Turkey or veggie burgers** – make them in batches, freeze them with waxed paper between patties, and pull one out when you need it.

➤➤ **Rice, spelt or kamut cakes can be topped with sliced avocado and salsa.**

➤➤ **Make a hearty sandwich with Ezekiel bread, nut butters, hummus, sprouts, sliced tomato or protein from poultry, fish or soy.**

➤➤ **Brown rice** – I always make extra to have handy for a quick meal. Simply add beans to rice and you have a meal. Add cooked or frozen spinach to round out your veggie needs for the day. Try brown rice, steamed spinach, low-sodium soy sauce and toasted sesame seeds for another quick meal.

➤➤ **Couscous, orzo and quinoa are perfect whole-grain carbs for quick meal bases.** Add boiling water to grains and let steam. Mix with beans, veggies and favorite seasonings for a fast-food meal.

➤➤ **Bake a sweet or regular potato and top with homemade chili or cottage cheese with steamed broccoli.**

➤➤ **Have breakfast for dinner.** Scrambled eggs, sliced tomato, baked beans and Ezekiel bread are super fast.

➤➤ **Pasta is a great failsafe.** Keep a few jars of Clean tomato sauce on hand. Add some frozen spinach and chickpeas or other beans to the sauce, mix in with cooked whole-grain pasta. You may think this sounds crazy, but you can add a can of broken-up chunk tuna to the mix, too.

➤➤ **One of my favorite super fast meals is to make a multicolored salad with baby spinach and lettuce leaves, sprouts, nuts and seeds, sliced salad vegetables and topped with water-packed tuna.** I drizzle the whole business with ground flax seed and pumpkin oil (or any other interesting oil) and citrus juice or vinegar. Voila! Dinner is served!

CHAPTER FIVE

Clean Up Your Eating Environment

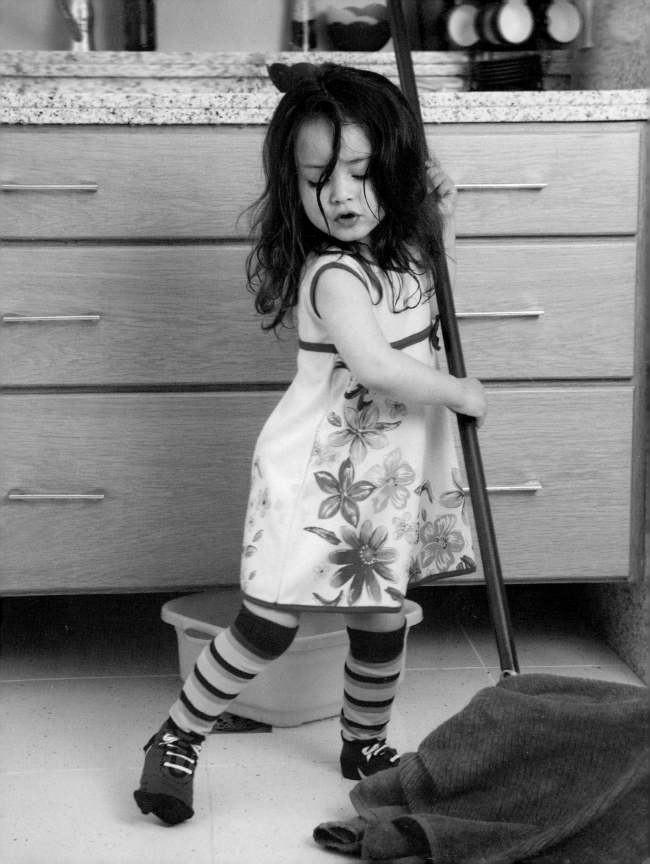

YOUR OWN EATING PHILOSOPHY

Kids soak up everything, from the good to the bad to the ugly. I have vivid memories of the way our kitchen cupboards looked when I was growing up. My mother's philosophy about fresh, healthy foods spilled over into everything she did. Her cupboards were not full of boxes neatly lined up, sporting colorful labels and ingredient lists as long as my arm. Instead she provided her own version of Clean Eating – lots of veggies, whole grains, fresh fruit and lean meats. She edited the kitchen cupboards for her family and it worked. Her strict views of limiting junk kept us lean and healthy. I thank her for it. She ran her house with an iron fist.

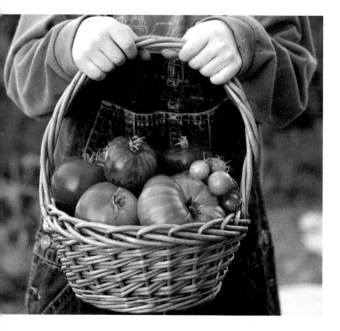

Children pick up on parental attitudes about food and body image. Whether you know it or not, your children begin absorbing verbal, emotional, and visual cues from you early on. They can sense if Mom and Dad feel good about themselves, take care of their health, get enough exercise, and don't drink too much alcohol. All things contribute to an overall "Clean Environment." So parents, you are the teachers. Do not underestimate the significance of that role.

WHAT IS THE STATE OF YOUR KITCHEN?

Consider your own environment. Does your food space support healthy clean living? Is your home filled with garbage, empty pizza boxes, empty cases of pop, half-eaten contents of doughnut boxes, and KFC barrels? What have you put in the cupboards and fridge? What have you made available for your kids to munch on when dinner isn't quite ready?

Fresh tomatoes from the market are my favorite!

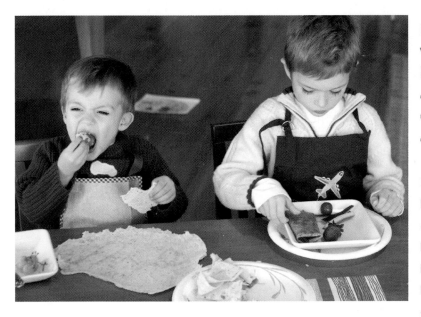

I have to relearn
what their food
likes and dislikes
are. Taste is
ever changing,
apparently.

I took my own advice and had my daughters accompany me to Whole Foods. I was surprised to learn that my 23-year-old loves zucchini, especially grilled, while my 20-year-old now despises green beans. My youngest loves all veggies, but can't do fruit. My daughters are off at university and classical dance training so they are not at home as much anymore. I have to relearn what their food likes and dislikes are. Taste is ever changing, apparently.

My childhood memories are flooded with images of a sparkling kitchen: no garbage overflowing from the bins, but a bowl of fruit shining on the table. My father would bring fresh vegetables from his garden, supplementing what Mom would bring home from the farmer's market or grocery store. A visit to the farmer's market was a family activity, done weekly when the weather was good.

FIND OUT WHAT THEY LIKE

You may not be able to provide fresh greens from your own garden, but you can visit the produce section of your grocery store and stock up on vegetables and fruits found there. Have your children join you on your shopping trip. Not only will you expose them to the possibilities existing in produce, you may discover something about your child's tastes. Recently

I realize now that I was fortunate to have a Clean-Eating environment modeled for me as I was growing up. No junk food or candy sat on the kitchen table. Meals were nutritious, but not indulgent. Vegetables formed the backbone of every meal. Protein was lean and varied and included eggs, low-fat dairy, legumes and fish, while whole grains were plentiful. I was off to a good start. Many of us today are not so lucky. It is the goal of this book to change this, one mouthful at a time.

ROBYN'S STORY

A reader's testimonial

"During my childhood healthy eating was a foreign concept. From school I knew there were foods you were supposed to eat, but I didn't necessarily know why. I never stayed at school for lunch and was too shy to stay for dinner at a friend's house. Therefore I was not exposed to the eating habits of others. I vaguely remember my mom cooking dinner, but being a normal picky kid I didn't like many foods. If I did not want what was made for dinner I was on my own, usually relying on quick meals such as eggs and toast or Kraft Dinner. With a house in which my brother and sister were gone, my dad was on shift work, and my mother had never gotten her driver's license after arriving from Britain, home-cooked dinners became scarce and take-out bags became the norm. Breakfast usually consisted of my dad's favorite sugary cereal, toast, or nothing at all. For lunch we often ate pizza that my mom had brought home from work, and dinner was from the fast-food place of the moment. Wendy's was the usual choice. We never drank water or juice with our take-out. Instead we had soda pop. Take-out meals were not eaten as a family around the dinner table. In fact, I can remember only a handful of times we ever sat at the table to eat. Once the food arrived we would grab our own bags and take off to separate corners of the house to watch TV.

As a kid I would watch my dad eat serving after serving of cookies, cake, or ice cream without any obvious ill effects. My dad is a very skinny man, and since bad eating habits were often linked to being fat, I assumed there was nothing wrong with our way of eating. My parents rarely went grocery shopping because we always ate out, but this meant there was never any fresh produce in the house. When we did manage to buy groceries there still never seemed to be anything to eat because it was all junk food. Snacks never contained vegetables, but cookies, chips, and candy were in abundance. I have vivid memories of coming home after some sporting event and sitting down to watch TV with a fruit roll-up wrapped around my finger.

I believe my parents developed our fast-food lifestyle out of convenience and perhaps a bit of nutritional ignorance. They could have bought groceries, but then someone would have to cook and I probably wouldn't like it anyway. For my family, fast food provided a quick and reliable fix to hunger.

As I got older and my shyness dissipated, I began spending some mealtimes at friends' houses and I started seeing how other families ate. I realized that other families served vegetables at most dinners. Not everyone had dessert after each meal. I began requesting that grocery shopping be done more frequently. As a result my snacks got better, but I had no idea how to cook a healthy meal, so once again take-out became the food of choice.

It was not until university that I started to make a conscious effort to eat healthfully. I picked up cooking ideas from friends and roommates, who also introduced me to new vegetables that I actually enjoyed. I began grocery shopping regularly to ensure fresh fruits and vegetables were available. Even with my new knowledge of nutrition and cooking methods, and the ability to shop for food at will, I experienced many bumps along my journey to healthy eating. Studying got in the way of grocery shopping, and I often did not feel like using my free time for cooking. Fast food reentered my life.

In my opinion the key to healthy eating is to start young. Providing your child with a good role model and the ability to make healthy food choices is a great gift. By introducing them to good foods, you establish a foundation of healthy eating that hopefully will remain with them throughout adulthood and into the next generation. Unhealthy food was my reality as a child and, as you have read, remains a hard habit to break.

”

 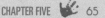

MAKING CLEAN-EATING CHANGES AT THE GROCERY STORE

Remember you, the parents, are "driving the bus" when it comes to making food decisions for your family. With that in mind you cannot assume that everything for sale at the grocery store qualifies as "food," let alone Clean-Eating, nutritious food. Next time you find yourself pushing your cart down the supermarket aisle, consider this as you make your grocery selections.

SUGAR IS THE ENEMY

One of the worst ingredients in food is also one of the tastiest, and most ubiquitous. I use the word "tasty" guardedly, since you will come to learn how delicious a crispy apple tastes if you stick with Clean

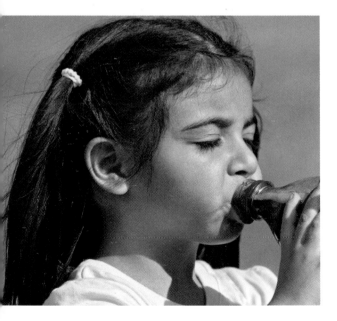

Eating. Far superior to a Twinkie! The more sugar and fake sugar you eat, the less you will be able to taste the natural goodness of a food, and the more excess fat you will have. Along with that excess fat come the inevitable diseases associated with carrying too much weight on the body – diabetes Types 1 and 2, metabolic syndrome X, pre-diabetes, stroke, heart disease, cancer, and high blood pressure. One of the quickest ways to start Eating Clean is to stop eating all refined and artificial sugars, except perhaps as part of a weekly treat.

FAKE SUGAR

What's worse, natural sugar or fake sugar? Both, because even sugar isn't natural unless it comes directly from fruit or dairy products. But we are a nation of soda drinkers, and the bigger the beverage the better. Beware! One soda alone can contain as much as 40 grams of sugar. If you or your child drinks more than that you need to be concerned. Actually you need to stop. So switching to diet soda or artificially flavored and sweetened so-called "water" drinks is better, right? WRONG! Fake sugars such as saccharin, aspartame, sorbitol and Splenda were originally intended for use by diabetics. But both real and fake sugars consumed in excess dramatically increase the risk of becoming overweight or obese. Does that surprise you? In fact, studies show that fake sugar is more likely to cause overweight than table sugar. Besides, do we really know what these products are doing in our body? They do not exist in

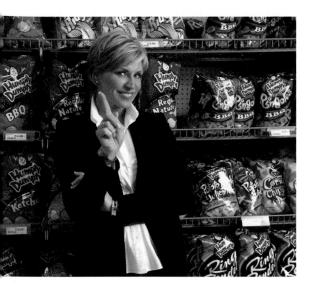

DELI-COUNTER DANGERS

All deli meats are processed in some way before they land at the deli counter. Much of the processing involves blending bits and pieces from a variety of animals, sick and healthy, and animal parts — skin, organs, fat and more. But processing also involves the use of chemicals to preserve the meat so it can languish in the deli case for countless days. These can include sodium nitrates and nitrites, among others; none of which contribute to health.

MORE WHITE STUFF

Some very brilliant person figured that stripping the brown out of grains made for a nicer-looking end product. Unfortunately, those brown bits contain much of the goodness of a plant, particularly fiber. Without fiber, the body has a terrible time digesting this refined stuff. Always search for unrefined whole grains and the usually brown, not white, complex carbohydrates from whole grains.

nature. There is all kinds of empirical evidence that artificial sugars cause serious health troubles. Why take the chance?

GREASY, FRIED FOODS

Fried foods often contain an abundance of unhealthy fats, especially the trans and saturated varieties. Trans and saturated fats are linked to a variety of diseases, particularly heart disease. Leave these foods in the store.

PREPACKAGED, PROCESSED FOODS

Although the convenience factor is tempting, the label should give you a clue. The long list of unpronounceable ingredients betrays what has happened to the food during processing. A big "NO THANKS!" to refined, over-processed foods.

SALT – GOOD OR BAD?

Many processed foods owe their long shelf life and "flavor" to salt. Salt today is a perversion of what it once was. Traditionally harvested from the sea, true salt contains 82 naturally occurring elements and minerals required by the body. Most free-running table salt today has been stripped of these components down to the basic sodium and chloride. Switch your regular table salt for sea salt right now and make it a point to look for excess sodium on food labels.

TOSCA'S TOP-10
INSTANT
KITCHEN MAKEOVERS

Substitute:

1 ★ **SEA SALT FOR REGULAR TABLE SALT**

2 ★ **AGAVE NECTAR FOR SUGAR**

3 ★ **UNREFINED WHOLE-WHEAT FLOUR FOR WHITE FLOUR**

4 ★ **BROWN RICE FOR WHITE RICE**

5 ★ **OATMEAL FOR SUGARY CEREALS**

6 ★ **WATER FOR JUICE AND POP**

7 ★ **75% OR MORE DARK CHOCOLATE FOR MILK CHOCOLATE**

8 ★ **OLIVE OIL FOR ORDINARY VEGETABLE OIL**

9 ★ **EGG WHITES FOR WHOLE EGGS**

10 ★ **NATURAL NUT BUTTERS FOR COMMERCIALLY PREPARED PEANUT BUTTER**

KNOWLEDGE IS EMPOWERING

The more you know about what lurks on the shelves of your grocery store and in the food you purchase and eat every day, the more empowered you will feel about making improved nutrition choices for your loved ones. It is not good enough to throw your hands up in the air and leave it to someone else to decide what is healthy. You can take your power back. Vote with your feet and your dollars. Purchase simple Clean-Eating foods that don't leave you guessing but do give you the power to alter the lives of those around you positively.

MISLED

In my mind there is absolutely no question that we have been and continue to be misled by giant food companies and the corporate suits leading them. They are in the business of creating "foods" that seduce us to eat them, while their bottom line is simply making money, the more the better. If you place your trust in these food giants *your* bottom line will be skewed, since in the deal you have traded your control of what goes in your family's bodies for

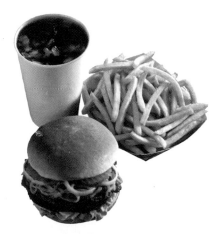

convenience. They win, you lose. McDonald's actually has a marketing plan which has been carefully devised with a mathematical formula to get customers in their door as many as 3.5 times per week. To that end they campaign constantly with advertising agendas to get the money out of your pockets and into theirs.

FAKE FOODS

Beware! The list of fakes and trickery is long and overwhelming. Children and parents today have been carefully enticed to eat a great deal of fake food. These are foods that are nutritionally suspect, calorie dense, and riddled with chemicals. In the rush to feed our families we stock our kitchen cupboards with food imposters and whiz to drive-thru windows to get our meals over with in order to rush on to the next item on the agenda.

Think of food imposters as those products that don't resemble any of the natural ingredients used to make them. I can't quite work out what natural food went into the making of a Twinkie. Foods like this confuse me. In fact I often feel confused in grocery stores – especially the cereal aisle. It is the longest aisle in virtually every grocery store I've ever seen. The sheer magnitude of cereal choices is too much to consider. I'll go into this in detail later on.

If you too are confused, on closer inspection you will come to realize, as I did, that most of these seductively packaged, super-fluffed and flavored victuals of wonder come from two products – corn and soybeans. As Michael Pollan wrote in *The Omnivore's Dilemma*, "…you would be hard pressed to find a late-model processed food that isn't made from corn or soybeans … the longer the ingredient label on food, the more fractions of corn and soybeans you will find in it. They supply the essential building blocks, and from those two plants (plus a handful of synthetic additives) a food scientist can construct just about any processed food he or she can dream up. (pg 91-92). In fact, even as you read these words, the same food scientists are sitting around creating the next must-have wonder food. Remember, processed food is manufactured for profit first and foremost. Nutritional value is normally far, far down on the list of priorities. Many of these companies seem to count on the fact that you won't ask questions.

IF YOU CAN'T READ IT DON'T EAT IT

I like the produce aisle, where there isn't a label in sight. This begins to relax me, because I don't have to make tough decisions about whether I want to feed my children such things as "sodium nitrates, sulfur, 2-methyl-3-(isopropylphenol)-propionaldehyde, alpha-heptyl-gamma-valerolactone …" Instead I can choose from a crunchy green apple, a fat sweet carrot and a ripe juicy melon, and in so doing ingest health rather than death. No ingredient lists here!

RECIPE CLEAN UP

You may have a wonderful recipe that has been passed from one family member to another. It would be a shame to lose out on the flavor and memories of a delicious dish that you treasure because you are cleaning up your diet. The good news is that you can easily make changes to the recipe that will clean up the fats, sugars and salt but still preserve the best things about it. Here is an example of one recipe a reader sent in for me to clean up:

LORI'S FAVORITE PASTA SALAD HER WAY

Yield: 3 cups • Prep Time: 10 min. • Cook Time: 15 min. • Cool Time: 2 hours

INGREDIENTS

2 cups / 480 ml bow-tie or spiral pasta, cooked and
    cooled

2 ripe tomatoes, diced

2 green onions, chopped

1 green pepper, chopped

2 stalks celery, chopped

DRESSING INGREDIENTS

⅔ cup / 160 ml white sugar

½ cup / 120 ml salad oil

⅓ cup / 80 ml ketchup

¼ cup / 60 ml white vinegar

Pepper and paprika to taste

PREPARATION

Mix pasta and vegetables in large bowl. Mix dressing ingredients in a shaker jar and pour over pasta and vegetables. Toss well to coat. Serve chilled.

NUTRITIONAL VALUE FOR HALF-CUP SERVING OF LORI'S SALAD:
Calories: 249 | Calories from Fat: 10 | Fat: 1g | Saturated Fat: 0.75g | Trans Fat: 0g |
Protein: 3g | Carbs: 46g | Dietary Fiber: 2g | Sodium: 500mg | Cholesterol: 0mg

Too much sugar is not good for you.

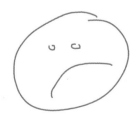

LORI'S FAVORITE PASTA SALAD ALL CLEANED UP

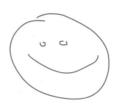

Yield: 3 cups • Prep Time: 10 min. • Cook Time: 15 min. • Cool Time: 2 hours

INGREDIENTS

2 cups / 480 ml brown rice, kamut, spelt, or other
whole-grain pasta noodles, cooked

All the vegetables can stay – we love veggies!

DRESSING INGREDIENTS

1 Tbsp / 15 ml agave nectar*

½ cup / 120 ml exotic oil**

⅓ cup / 80 ml Clean Ketchup (page 286)***

¼ cup / 60 ml white vinegar****

Pepper and paprika to taste

PREPARATION

Mix pasta and vegetables in large bowl. Mix dressing ingredients in a shaker jar and
pour over pasta and vegetables. Toss well to coat. Serve chilled.

NUTRITIONAL VALUE FOR HALF-CUP SERVING OF LORI'S SALAD ALL CLEANED UP:

Calories: 250 | Calories from Fat: 3.5 | Fat: 0.5g | Saturated Fat: 0g | Trans Fat: 0g |
Protein: 3g | Carbs: 43.5g | Dietary Fiber: 3g | Sodium: 80mg | Cholesterol: 0mg

HERE'S WHY:

* Two thirds of a cup is a lot of sugar, so leave that out and use one tablespoon / 15 ml of agave nectar instead. If you can't find that, then use honey. The flavor is delicious and the lower glycemic index is better for your health.

** I would not use regular salad oil. Here is your opportunity to use an exotic oil and introduce healthy essential fatty acids into your diet. Try avocado, walnut, rice bran, tomato seed, grapeseed, pumpkin or a classic olive oil.

***Rather than use commercial ketchup, which contains loads of sugar and sodium, make the version on page 286 of this book or use tomato paste as alternatives; the sugar content is much lower and the paste is chock full of healthy carotenoids – powerful cancer-fighting compounds.

****The white vinegar is fine, but experiment with rice vinegar or even white balsamic vinegar for an extra flavor punch.

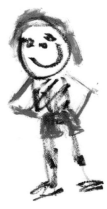

CHAPTER SIX

Habits of the Healthiest People

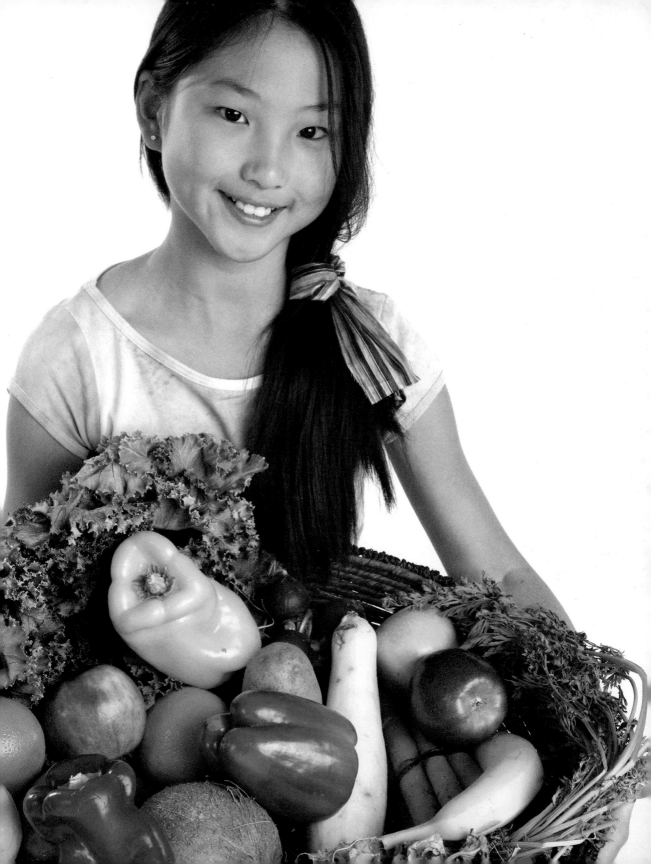

HABITS OF THE HEALTHIEST PEOPLE ON EARTH

A Western diet is full of ingredients quite foreign to other countries and cultures, and in many ways to our body as well. There is much to be gained by looking elsewhere for guidance as to the simple question of what to eat. A wonderful way to learn about other cultures is to sample their eating styles. It might surprise you to learn that the French eat plenty of food doused in butter and cream and chase it down with wine, without sacrificing health. Mexicans enjoy spicy foods like no other while traditional Inuit eat virtually no greens and plenty of animal meat and blubber and remain healthy.

Some of the healthiest nations on earth practice several very simple habits that could help North Americans escape the current path of health destruction they are on. Why not try to incorporate some of these healthy practices in your home today?

TEN HEALTHY PRACTICES TO GET YOU ON TRACK

❶ **Harvest or gather locally grown and wild foods.** In spring when the earth has warmed up sufficiently, I often see people out in meadows gathering something looking very much like weeds. It turns out I am not mistaken. These people are gathering purslane and wild dandelion greens at their tenderest and greenest moment, so they can be enjoyed as a healthy addition to the supper table. Why eat

weeds? Weeds, particularly dandelion, purslane and lambs' quarters, are among the most nutrient-dense foods on earth. In the bitterness that accompanies most wild plants lies the secret to their nutritional power – that bitterness houses the plants' defenses against pests and disease. Weeds and wild plants contain great quantities of phytochemicals, particularly omega-3 fatty acids.

Eating food that nature provides supports Clean Eating, since these foods are the most unprocessed, unrefined and pure offerings you could possibly find. Be sure to identify with 100-percent certainty any naturally growing wild foods before consuming them, since some plants and fungi can be toxic.

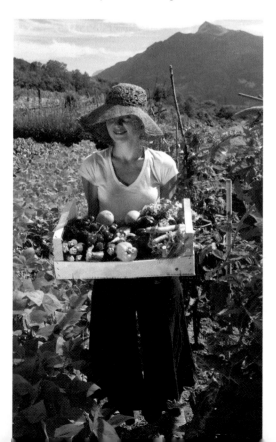

➡ **Purslane**

➡ **Wild leeks or ramps**

➡ **Lamb's quarters**

➡ **Wild garlic**

➡ **Common chickweed**

➡ **Berries** (check that they are safe before eating – they can be poisonous)

➡ **Dandelions**

➡ **Fiddleheads**

➡ **Wild arugula**

➡ **Cattail hearts**

➡ **Mushrooms** (Collect wild mushrooms only if you are very well educated in the difference between poisonous and safe fungus. Otherwise, purchase from a local mushroom expert.)

Mushrooms are funny looking vegetables.

❷ **Eat loads of richly colored foods.** The greater the variety of foods you consume, the greater the chance you will ingest a broad variety of nutrients. The darker the colors the better. White is not normally best when it comes to nutrition in plants. The deathly pallor of such foods usually means the goodness has been stripped out of them and they are of little or no use to you. Iceberg lettuce, white rice and white sugar come to mind. Look for beautiful black, mahogany, purple and other varieties of rice. Eat orange, red, purple, green and multi-colored peppers. Try purple or black potatoes, purple string beans and yellow tomatoes. Fill your plate with a kaleidoscope of color. Chances are these will be the ideal complex carbohydrates to partner with lean protein and that is the perfect Clean-Eating meal. Also remember that it takes kids at least 10 exposures to a new food before they begin to like it. Be patient with your little ones. They will come on board soon enough.

❸ **Sit down and relax while you eat.** Increasingly North Americans eat on the run, in a car, at a drive thru, in front of a television or anywhere but the kitchen or dining table. Sadly this lack of communal leisurely eating is adding to our significant list of eating problems in this nation. In countries including Japan, France, Italy, Spain and Greece, a meal is not a quickie deal. Diners eat for several hours at a time. A meal is an occasion even when the calendar doesn't say so. Spending time eating calmly and quietly in good company and in a pleasant atmosphere helps food digest better too. Excuse me now while I pour a glass of wine and converse with my loved ones.

❹ **Understand how much is on your plate.** Most of us have no concept of how much food is on our plates. We have been numbed by the Super-Size craze that has swept the continent. The most food on the plate for the least money is considered the best deal. I wonder how many of us will agree with that philosophy of eating when we wind up in a hospital facing severe health problems? We are short sighted on this topic. Concerned with getting value for our dollar, we forget that cheap calories cost us dearly in matters of health.

One study after another suggests the value of eating smaller portions, and that applies not just to control of weight, but also to the avoidance of chronic disease. So have a look at your hands. Use them to guide you

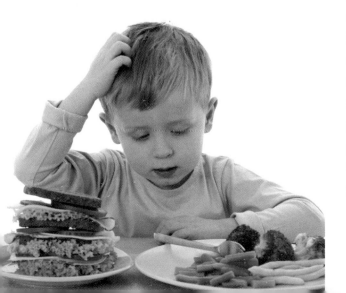

through this portion-size exercise. A serving of lean protein is the size of the palm of your hand. A serving of complex carbohydrates from whole grains fits into one hand lightly cupped, and finally a serving of complex carbohydrates from fruits or vegetables fits into two palms cupped together. Nothing could be simpler. Your body is created to give you perfect portion sizes, no matter how small or big you are.

Also remember that one of the most successful ways to lose weight is to eat less. Simply cutting down on the amount you eat each day will help you shed pounds.

❺ **Eat when you are hungry. Stop eating when you are almost full.** You are probably scratching your head wondering if I have lost my mind to write something so obvious, but a good deal of the trouble we are in now with respect to overweight is due to eating more than we need to simply because we don't listen to the body's own signals of hunger and satiety. So try this next time you are approaching mealtime. Wait until you are hungry. You will feel it because your stomach will be busy churning around and giving you hunger pangs. Now wait 30 minutes more. That's when you are ready to eat. Prepare Clean-Eating foods according to the portions described above, and sit down to eat that food. When you begin to feel full, that is the time to stop eating. You will discover as you get used to Eating Clean that these signals of hunger will appear in your stomach every three hours, and this is one of the reasons I suggest eating this often.

❻ Eat an array of unprocessed whole and natural foods. Fill your grocery cart with plenty of options from the produce department. Doing so will ensure you have loads of nutritious complex carbohydrates on hand, which serve the body far better than refined foods do. Clean Eating advocates just this kind of shopping. The more natural a food is, the better it is for you and your waistline. I avoid the dangerous, brightly colored aisles filled with sugary, floury, processed foods and stick to the produce, dairy, meats, nuts and grains sections.

❼ Jazz up food flavors with herbs and spices, vinegars and oils. The sheer abundance of flavor possibilities available when it comes to herbs, spices and vinegars makes cooking fun and far more satisfying than relying on a fast-food cook who depends primarily on grease and salt for flavor. The best news? These items are low in calories and taste wonderful. You can't call yourself a cook if you don't at least try to incorporate some of these wonderful flavor makers into your meals. Add some healthy oils, too. One of my favorite ways to have fresh herbs handy is to keep a container garden in my kitchen year-round. Fresh basil is never more than a snip away. Build a spice drawer filled with exotic nutmeg, cinnamon, turmeric, garlic, sea salt, paprika and whatever else your taste buds desire.

BRIAN'S STORY
A reader's testimonial

Dear Tosca,

It has been said that the most commonly thought about question in one's day is that surrounding dinner: i.e. what am I/ are we going to have for dinner? It is this question that brought me to your cookbook, The Eat-Clean Diet Cookbook. Like many, I want to eat healthy and still be both full and have something with a great flavor that would give me energy for a big night out. And that's when I came across the recipe Moroccan Chicken And Lentils, a simple yet beautiful dish bursting with both flavor and intrigue … a simple intrigue that soon had my mouth watering in anticipation, and in that moment I knew what we would be having for dinner that night. While I cooked it my family dropped by the kitchen in sheer anticipation of the meal to come as the aromatic and exotic spices and smells circled the house. I understood, the smell was intoxicating and the meal a true joy to make. This dish was amazing, with great portions for my family of both large and small eaters. Even surpassing my greatest expectations, this dish is healthy, satisfying, full of flavor, easy to make and full of the protein I needed for a big night out. And to look around the table and see my family engulfed in the food, and the look of joy on each face while doing so, was a great feeling. Thanks again Tosca, your cookbook is truly what real cooking is all about and I can't wait to see what you come up with next.

Sincerely,

Brian Beckett, 17-year-old avid eater

MANDY & DAN'S STORY

A reader's testimonial

"

Tosca,

Hi! This is Mandy Davis. My husband and I have struggled with our weight and feeling good about ourselves our whole lives. I have been in Weight Watchers since I was 13 years old. My husband was the skinny kid in school, but now he too wants to lean out. However, I was very active with sports in school, and I was a two-sport college athlete so I managed to keep my weight somewhat under control. We got married in December 2007 in the Dominican Republic. Dan is an active member in the US Army and he just got back from a year on tour in Iraq. We have made it our honeymooners' goal to eat clean and stay healthy together. We both enjoy working out and just need that extra boost to keep us in shape for our children.

Staying fit has not been easy for either one of us and there are health issues that sometimes hinder us. I almost lost my life in 2002 playing college volleyball and basketball. I was losing weight and feeling really hyper all the time, so that was really cool to me. But after I ran for a long time or played in a long game I lost feeling in my feet and legs. Finally my coach made me go to the doctor. Sitting on the doctor's table my heart rate was 140! Weird! My doc informed me that my heart was probably beating 220 times a minute when I played sports. That's why I was losing feeling in my feet and legs – the blood flow wasn't there. He did blood work and told me I could have hyperthyroidism and I will probably never play sports again. He said it was the most severe case at my young age of 21 that he had ever seen and I would have to have surgery immediately. This was the worst news I'd ever had. I had always been so athletic and it had helped me keep in shape and now it was going to be taken from me. Well I got the treatment and moved home for a semester so my doctor could keep an eye on me. Then I rehabbed myself and eventually went back to my college and played volleyball and basketball again. I had taken my health for granted and just assumed it would always be there. Since that point I have made a conscious effort to keep myself healthy from the inside out.

My husband loves lifting weights and is into working out like a bodybuilder. But he has a slow metabolism like I do, and struggles to keep fat off.

My near-death experience and my husband being in Iraq for a year have sure helped us put life into perspective. Sometimes we put our bodies' health last in life as if it isn't as important as our daily tasks. It took these extreme events for us to realize we need to take care of us. We have made it our goal to Eat Clean and start our new life together CLEAN. I am telling you this because maybe somewhere out there someone is searching just like we were. And maybe letting them know they are not alone will help. You have been a huge inspiration to us in our new life.

Mandy and Dan Davis
Elizabethtown, Kentucky

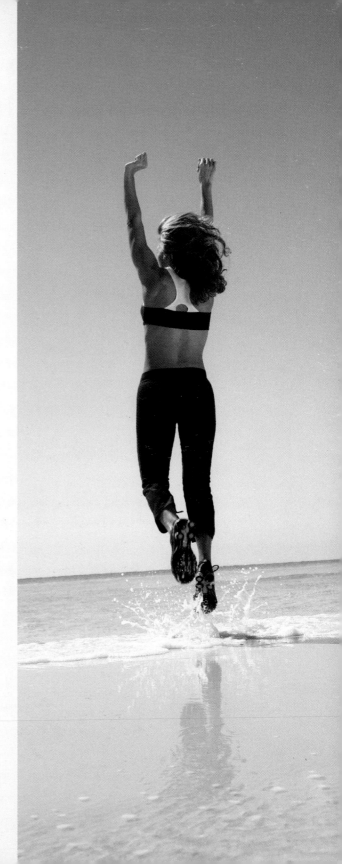

STRATEGIES TO ENSURE A
CLEAN-EATING ENVIRONMENT
★ BE A FOOD DETECTIVE ★

➤➤ **Take responsibility for what ends up in your grocery cart.**
  - Learn to read food labels.
  - Learn to distinguish between unhealthy saturated or trans fats and healthy unsaturated fats or essential fatty acids

➤➤ **Buy food that looks like food – that is, buy foods in their most natural wholesome state. I call these Clean-Eating foods.**
  - Fresh fruits, vegetables, and whole grains are perfect examples.
  - Remember these are your complex carbohydrates too.

➤➤ **Make it a habit to buy the fat-free or low-fat versions of foods, particularly dairy products, still keeping an eye on ingredient labels for hidden chemicals.**
  - You will likely be surprised if you read a cottage cheese or yogurt label. We think of these as healthy foods, but the food companies even manage to mess these foods up with mono and diglycerides, sugars and other food additives.

➤➤ **Avoid fast-food chains if at all possible.**
  - Most of the foods served from the kitchens of fast-food chains are loaded with trans and saturated fats, sugars, and chemical calories. Watch the movie *Super Size Me* if you need more than my words to convince you to avoid these ubiquitous sources of trouble. If you aren't prepared to ask questions about what is in your food then don't bother pulling up in the first place.

➤➤ **Pack a cooler or lunch bag and make Clean Eating portable.**
  - Chances are pretty high your child's school cafeteria menu is worse than you could ever have imagined. Visit the school at lunchtime yourself so you have it on good authority when your child complains about how bad it is. Your child's school is open to you, so schedule a lunch date with your child or another parent. Check out what's on the menu. It might shock you.

➤➤ **Be consistent with your food messages.**
  - If you Eat Clean as a part of your family's healthy lifestyle, do so even when it is a birthday or another time of celebration. Yes you can indulge a little but don't go completely overboard or you will be right back where you started.

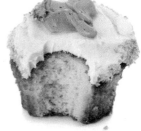

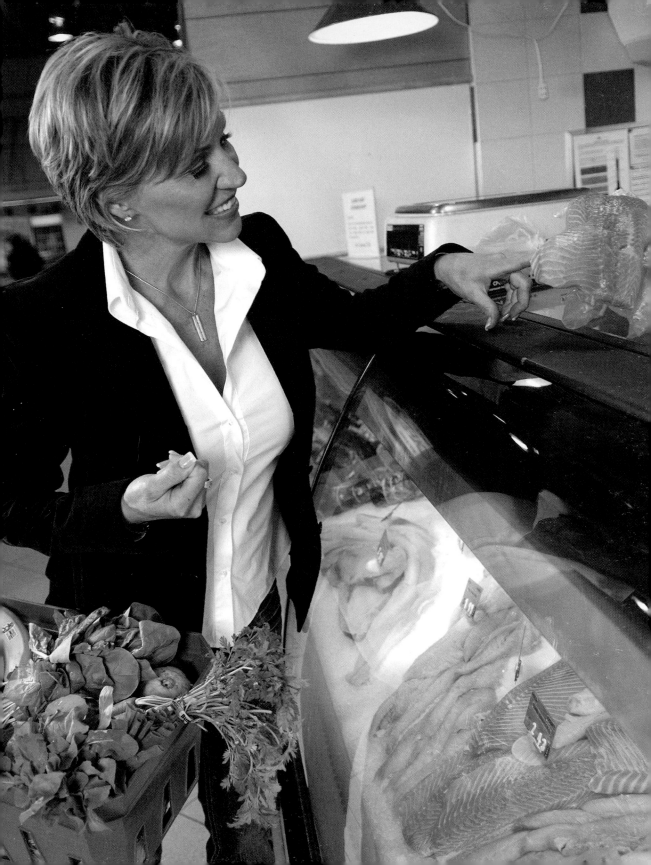

HOW TO READ A NUTRITION LABEL

It seems odd I know to have to include a paragraph about reading a label but if you have looked at one lately you might notice there are plenty of words you and I can't read. However, it is important to read them nonetheless. Here is my quick course on how to read a nutrition label. You can use it to help decide what you do and don't want to eat.

NUTRITION FACTS FOR OATMEAL

Directly under the words "Nutrition Facts" you will find the serving size. In the case of dry oatmeal, the suggested serving size is ⅓ cup, or **30 grams**.

Next you will find the number of calories in that serving size. In this case, 117 calories for that ⅓ cup dry oatmeal. If you eat more than a third of a cup you will also be consuming more calories.

Nutrition Facts

Serving Size 30 g   (Kilojoules 488)

Amount Per Serving

Calories   117

	%Daily Value
Total Fat 2.1 g	3%
Saturated Fat 0.4 g	2%
Cholesterol 0 mg	0%
Sodium 1 mg	0%
Total Carbohydrate 19.9 g	7%
Dietary Fiber 3.2 g	13%
Sugars 0 g	
Protein 5.1 g	
Calcium 16.2 mg Potassium 128.7 mg	

** Percent Daily Values are based on a 2,000 calorie diet. Your daily values maybe higher or lower depending on your calorie needs. These values are recommended by a government body. They are not CalorieKing.com recommendations.

Now we find the numbers for fat. Both saturated and trans fats are usually listed. You want to limit your daily intake of these largely unhealthy fats. Most grain-based foods contain small amounts of saturated fats, and oatmeal is not an exception. Don't worry about these small amounts of plant-based saturated fats.

Whole grains such as oatmeal are good sources of complex carbohydrates. Be sure to look carefully at carbohydrate amounts, since sugar is also listed in this category. Do keep in mind

 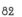

that the sugars listed here might be added sugars or they might be naturally occurring sugars. The ingredients will tell you the source. Some nutrition labels also list the vitamin content of the food. This is great because it helps us understand how much of these nutrients we are consuming.

Also under this category you will find the fiber content. Consuming adequate fiber helps keep bowels functioning properly and may reduce the risk of some diseases. A diet rich in fruits, vegetables and whole grains can reduce the risk of heart disease.

Protein is an important component of Clean Eating, so it helps to have it listed on the nutrition label. Oatmeal contains some protein but is better as a rich source of fiber and complex carbohydrate.

Printed along the right side of the label you will find daily percentage values for each nutrition fact. In general, 5% or less is considered low and 20% or higher is high.

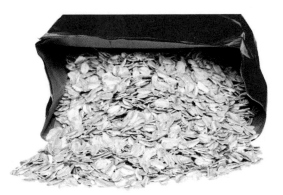

CLEAN-EATING SNACK OPTIONS

1 ❋ HOT AIR-POPPED POPCORN (WITHOUT THE BUTTER, GOLDEN TOPPING OR SALT)

2 ❋ RICE, SPELT OR KAMUT CAKES, SPREAD WITH NATURAL NUT BUTTER

3 ❋ KNOX GELATIN MADE WITH DILUTED FRUIT JUICE

4 ❋ SKIM-MILK SMOOTHIE

5 ❋ FRESH FRUIT

6 ❋ FRESH VEGETABLE CRUDITÉS

7 ❋ UNSWEETENED APPLESAUCE

8 ❋ PLAIN LOW-FAT YOGURT WITH FRESH FRUIT OR BERRIES

9 ❋ MELBA TOAST WITH HUMMUS

10 ❋ LOW-FAT COTTAGE CHEESE

11 ❋ KEFIR

12 ❋ DRIED FRUIT IN MODERATION

13 ❋ UNSALTED RAW NUTS IN MODERATION

14 ❋ UNSALTED RAW SEEDS IN MODERATION

15 ❋ NATURAL NUT BUTTERS

16 ❋ APPLESAUCE SPICE PROTEIN BARS
(Recipe page 309)

TAKING IT HOME

Once you have successfully made your grocery purchases and cleaned the junk from your cupboards you should already be feeling better. With no questionable, quasi-nutritious foods in your home the chances of keeping your family on a Clean-Eating path are far greater. Your shopping bags may be full of whole grains from a bulk food store, natural produce from an organic store, lean meats and fish from a butcher and canned goods from the grocery store. Wherever you shop, keep your choices as clean and natural as possible. You are now well on your way to a Clean-Eating kitchen.

THE ONE-INGREDIENT FOOD CHALLENGE

I want to issue you a challenge. Next time you go to the grocery store make a point of trying to purchase foods containing only one ingredient. To do this effectively, you will have to read the ingredient labels and this may be the first time you've done so. Look for as few ingredients as possible. One is best, but you may find many Clean foods with two or three ingredients. I would like you to create a list of as many foods as you can with the fewest amount of ingredients in them. Send your list to me at tosca@eatcleandiet.com. I will post the best lists on either of my websites, www.toscareno.com and www.eatcleandiet.com. Let's see how many we can come up with and I will then publish the 10 best lists in an upcoming issue of *Oxygen* in my "Raise the Bar" column. I will also send these folks all my *Oxygen* covers autographed! So get shopping.

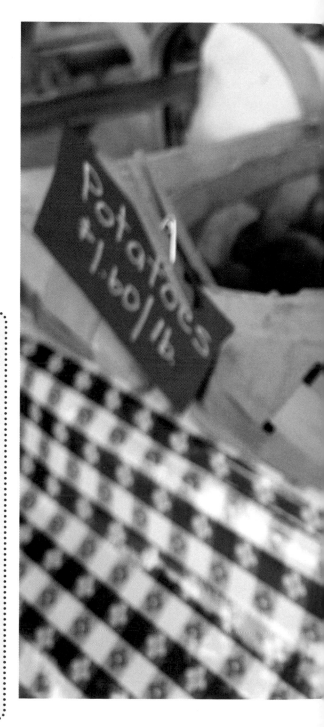

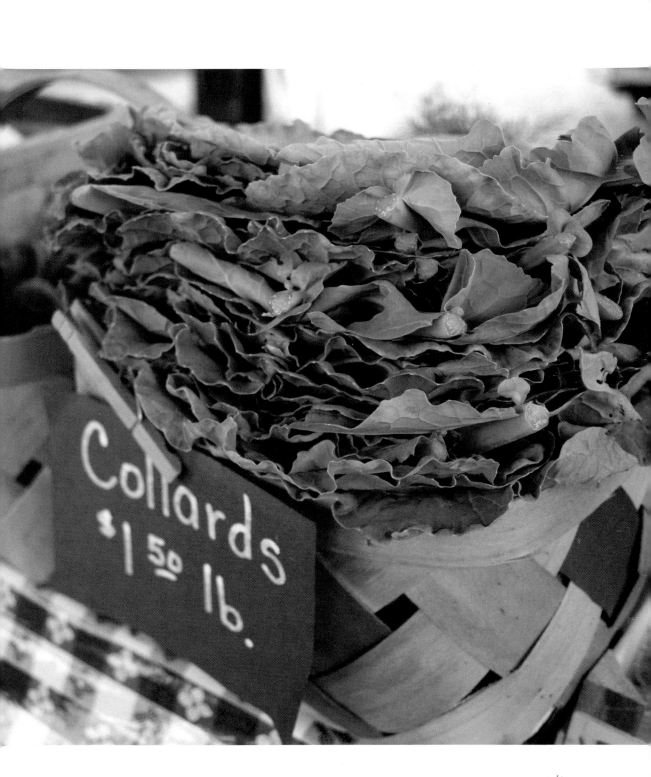

CHAPTER SEVEN

Breakfast and Chemical Soup

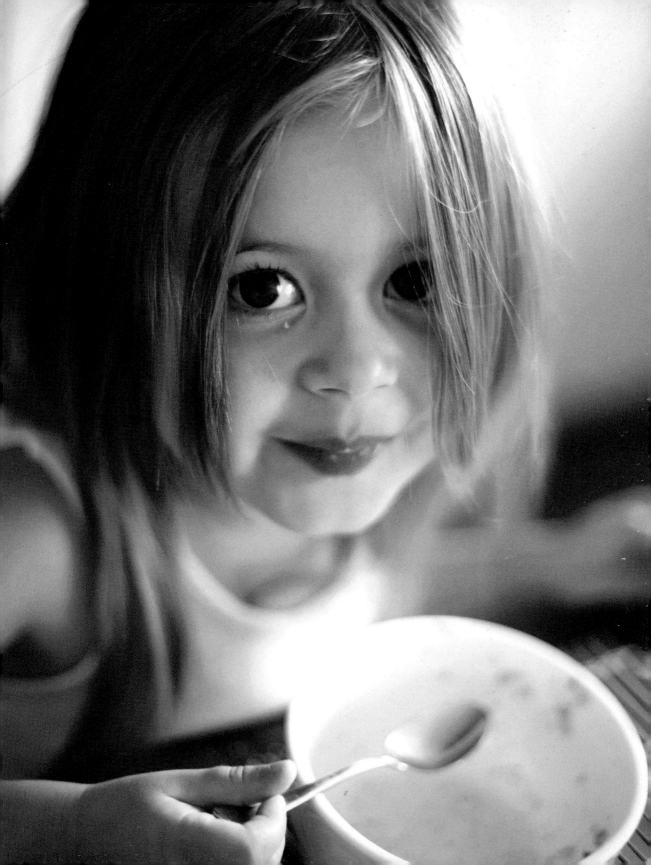

BREAKFAST, CHEMICAL SOUP AND MAKING IT ALL WORK

There isn't a meal more valuable to you and your family's day than breakfast. At the same time it is the meal most of us choose to skip. And when we don't skip it, we have developed many crazy ideas about what constitutes a good breakfast. I get the feeling we don't understand this meal much at all. In the west coast city of Portland, Oregon you can buy a doughnut made with bacon, peanut butter and cereal on top. In Las Vegas you can snake your way through buffet after buffet, each claiming to be the best and the biggest, serving everything from crab to cake and cookies for breakfast. Virtually every city has a diner or two known for dishing out breakfast fare just the way we like it – swimming in grease and butter. Oh sure, there is no lack of food for this starting meal but most of it contributes to the overweight epidemic gripping this country. The time has come to reconsider what we do or don't eat for breakfast.

Before I started Eating Clean I thought nothing of having a few strips of bacon alongside buttered toast, on top of which I smeared peanut butter if you can believe it. There was always cereal, which probably had too much sugar in it, and even my coffee was over the top with double cream. When I had leftover whipped cream I would put a dollop of that in my cup, too. Looking back I realize I just wasn't thinking about what I was eating. I suppose I was influenced by advertisements and TV commercials

along with magazine and newspaper articles. It was a haphazard way of gathering information about the most basic and yet the most complicated of human activities – eating.

I suspect many of you are in the same boat. Other than in a few Home Economics classes, we don't really get much education in this area unless we make a career out of food. Even then, a culinary student generally does not learn about the healthy or unhealthy aspects of food. He or she learns about

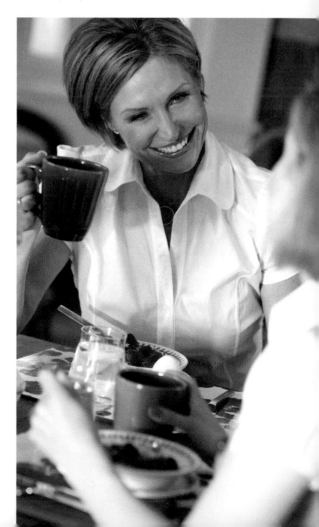

taste and texture. Blaming ourselves for this sketchy education does not help, either.

Some of us have a passionate interest in all aspects of nutrition. Nutritionists get it. They understand the most intimate details about food and digestion. Some of us have had to think about food in a different way because a family member has become ill and now needs to change what and how they eat. That's how

Eating breakfast is one of the most important things you can do. Making the change is easy.

WHAT DID YOU HAVE FOR BREAKFAST?

When conducting a seminar I often ask if people have had breakfast, and if so, what. Not once have I had a full house of hands going up saying they have eaten breakfast. A lot of you don't. Then I add my

Serving your children a Clean-Eating breakfast is one of the most important things you can do.

it happened in my house. My dad suffered a heart attack at the all-too-early age of 34. From then on our family became a heart-healthy house. Our breakfasts, formerly consisting of bacon, sugar and refined foods, changed dramatically. Suddenly it became all about whole grains, egg whites and fruit. Sometimes we need a shock to wake us up from the sleep we have been in. My dad's heart condition was exactly that.

I know some of you reading this are dealing with children who are either becoming sick or are already sick. So many diseases can be affected by what we eat, either positively or negatively: diabetes, hypertension, high cholesterol, cancer, irritable bowel syndrome and more. You as parents want to do the best for your children, and preventing disease is one of those goals. Serving your children a Clean-

hook: "Did you know the odds of being overweight or even obese are much greater if you don't eat breakfast?" A stunned silence settles in the room. Our calorie-counting culture has encouraged us to develop the Skipping Meals habit. Skipping a meal, and breakfast is the *most* skipped meal, certainly cuts out calories, but as we know, calorie counting does not give the whole picture. The habit of skipping breakfast is far more damaging than good for you.

IS THAT A KIT KAT BAR FOR BREAKFAST?

Cereal is confusing. It's a big one as far as corporate tricks go. Companies invest multiple millions of dollars yearly to seduce you and your kids to eat their particular brand of cereal. I feel like the cereal aisle is booby-trapped at entry point. At least when you are in the junk-food aisle you know it. Doritos

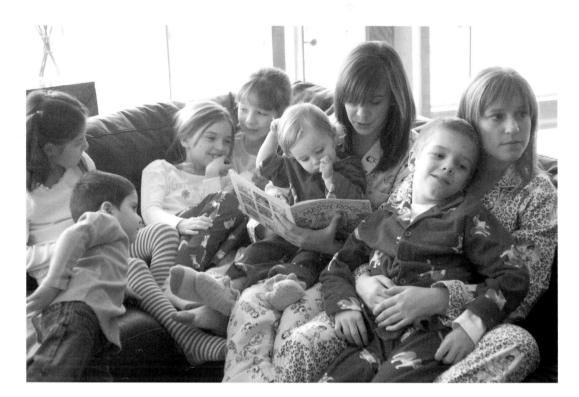

don't pretend to be healthy. Chips and candy don't either. Their manufacturers are not lying to you. Cereal is another matter entirely. On every level, even the junkiest of cereals is trying to present itself as a healthy food in the grain and breakfast aisle of the grocery store.

I often get a headache from everything going on in that aisle. Apparently there is a great deal of planned deception happening when you get to that very special place in the supermarket and I am not just talking about free toys hidden in your Frosted Flakes. Would it shock you to learn that the sugar content in a small serving of Froot Loops is about the

same as in a Kit Kat bar? I thought so. I have always believed that we as parents and consumers have no idea what is happening to us when we are bombarded with seductive advertising campaigns. Now we know for sure this is true.

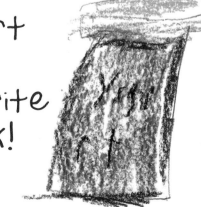

Yogurt is my favorite snack!

IS CEREAL CANDY? AND OTHER COMPLICATED QUESTIONS

**Keep in mind that these serving sizes are quite small. Most people – both kids and adults – pour 1 ½ to 2 cups into a cereal bowl.

NUTRIENT VALUE OF SOME CEREALS MARKETED TO KIDS

COCOA PUFFS
(1 oz or ¾ cup)

Calories: 110
Total fat: 1.5 g
Sat. fat: 0
Protein: 1 g
Sugar: 12 g
Fiber: 1 g
Sodium: 150 mg

CHOCOLATE LUCKY CHARMS
(1 oz or ¾ cup)

Calories: 110
Total fat: 1 g
Sat. fat: 0
Protein: 1 g
Sugar: 14 g
Fiber: 1 g
Sodium: 160 mg

OATMEAL CRISP TRIPLE BERRY
(1 oz or almost ½ cup)

Calories: 108
Total fat: 1.3 g
Sat. fat: .3 g
Protein: 2.6 g
Sugar 8.3 g
Fiber: 2.6 g
Sodium: 134 mg

FROOT LOOPS
(serving size 1 oz or 1 cup)

Calories: 120
Total fat: 1 g
Sat. fat: .5 g
Protein: 1 g
Sugar: 15 g
Fiber: 1 g
Sodium: 150 g

NUTRIENT VALUE OF SOME COMMON TYPES OF PACKAGED CANDY

SKITTLES
(1 oz, or ½ bag)

Calories: 125
Total fat: 1.5 g
Sat. fat: 1.5 g
Protein: 0 g
Sugar: 23 g
Fiber: 0 g
Sodium: 0 mg

KIT KAT BAR
(1 oz, or ⅔ bar)

Calories: 139
Total fat: 7.3 g
Sat. fat: 4.6 g
Protein: 2 g
Sugar: 14.5 g
Fiber: .3 g
Sodium: 20 mg

SNICKERS
(1 oz, or nearly ½ bar)

Calories: 135
Total fat: 6.8 g
Sat. fat: 2.4 g
Protein: 1.9 g
Sugar: 14.5 g
Fiber: .5 g
Sodium: 68 mg

JELLY BEANS
(1 oz, or 10 large)

Calories: 105
Total fat: 0 g
Sat. fat: 0 g
Protein: 0 g
Sugar: 19.5 g
Fiber: .1 g
Sodium: 14 mg

 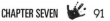

FOUR CENTS FOR FOUR DOLLARS

As Michael Pollan illuminates in his book *The Omnivores' Dilemma*, creating a superstar cereal is indeed an intense and highly secretive business. In a concrete structure called the Bell Institute, located in the American Midwest, 900 employees get paid to "create food," particularly cereal. This is the place, Pollan writes, where "four cents worth of commodity corn (or some equally cheap grain) is transformed into four dollars worth of processed food." Translation: that expensive sugary cereal made for less than a nickel has been scientifically created in such a way as to seduce your child and you, in that order, to purchase it. There is so much security around the creation of a new cereal that most people don't even know this place exists and you have to pass through many layers of security to get in. Unless employed there, most of us never do. Some places deep inside the Institute of Cereal Technology are verboten! No one is allowed to enter save a few highly paid

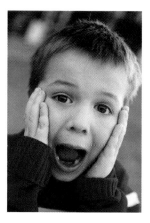

insiders with cereal secrets tucked up their sleeves. Now you may be able to develop a clearer picture of how badly these folks want your hard-earned buck, especially your cereal buck.

A LOOK AT "HEALTHIER" COLD CEREALS

KELLOGG'S RAISIN BRAN CRUNCH
(serving size 1 cup or 1.9 oz)

Calories: 190
Total fat: 1 g
Sat. fat: 0 g
Protein: 3 g
Sugar: 20 g
Fiber: 4 g
Sodium: 210 mg

KELLOGG'S ALMOND CRUNCH WITH RAISINS
(serving size 1 cup or 1.9 oz)

Calories: 198
Total fat: 2.6 g
Sat. fat: 0.4 g
Protein: 5 g
Sugar: 16 g
Fiber: 4.6 g
Sodium: 215 mg

KASHI GOLEAN CRUNCH*
(serving size 1 cup, or 1.9 oz)

Calories: 190
Total fat: 3 g
Sat. fat: 0 g
Protein: 9 g
Sugar: 13 g
Fiber: 8 g
Sodium: 95 mg

* Kashi GoLean Crunch does have 8 g of fiber and 9 g of protein.

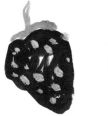
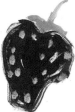

I CAN READ

Back in the grocery store, I ponder the colorful, giddily packaged cereal boxes and give up. I can see it would take me hours to decipher nutrition labels on the hundreds of cereals available in this minefield called The Cereal Aisle. I toss a few bags of oatmeal in my cart and push it back toward the produce aisle, where I feel comfortable. Just in case you are wondering what the ingredient label reads on my package of oatmeal, here are the details:

INGREDIENTS IN OATMEAL:
100% OATS

You can see why I chose oatmeal. I can actually read the label! I don't even need my glasses. I like the beautiful simplicity of that. I don't have time to read all that other garbage, so this is my choice every time I shop. Every time! Suddenly my headache is gone.

MORE ABOUT CEREAL

Cereals usually list a serving size as one cup, or 30 grams if you are under the metric system. I personally don't know any kids who use a measuring cup when serving themselves. I actually tried this experiment a few times: I had my daughters pour themselves a bowl of cereal straight out of the box (Ezekiel or Kashi). Each time, without fail, the serving measured 1½ cups. Then I checked out what my husband served himself. He always dumped about two cups into his bowl. I had suspected that because I

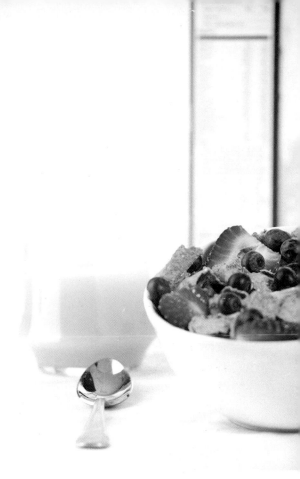

would finish my cereal about 10 minutes before he did. Apparently serving sizes don't mean anything unless you are willing to measure.

When kids fail to measure the suggested one-cup serving size of cereal established on the box, the nutritional content will be off as well. Rather than consuming the sugar content in one cup of Froot Loops, a child might end up eating twice that much. The same goes for Lucky Charms. One and a half cups of Lucky Charms contains the sugar of an entire package of Reese's Peanut Butter Cups. Most of us don't take that into consideration.

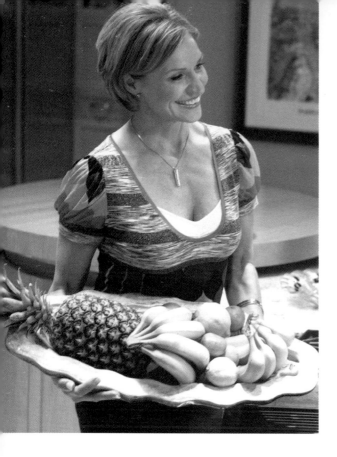

Now, you might be willing to accept all this — or even feel a little proud since you already know neither of these cereals have redeeming qualities and have not been allowing them into your house, but the story worsens. Consider Oatmeal Crisp. This cereal sounds healthy but contains a scary secret. What could be wrong with oatmeal? This particular version of "oatmeal" has been created in such a sugary sweet way as to contain as much of that white poison as an entire Snickers bar. But you thought you were buying oatmeal! Not so.

This is where I start to get worried. If you don't spend a minute and consider this information but instead simply read a box that says: "healthy," "good for you" or even contains a word filled with natural, healthy images, such as "muesli," you will fall right into the hands of the food manufacturers. Cereals in particular are riddled with little marketing tricks to convince you, the hurried shopper and harried parent, to buy them. This is where you, as a consumer and often the food-decision maker in your family, get to vote with your dollars. Don't rely on the box's marketing copy to tell the truth about what's good for you and your family. Read the nutrition label. Be skeptical. Spend your money on whole food, not garbage foods masquerading as healthy. Become an independent thinker. Let food manufacturers know who's in charge of your family's food choices by making an informed selection.

IS ANYBODY LISTENING?

Kellogg's, one of the nation's biggest cereal producers, has made an effort to address this cereal maze, at least in part. This food giant has decided not to promote foods to an audience expected to be at least 50 percent under the age of 12 unless it meets a set of self-determined criteria. These criteria include that a serving size must contain no more than 200 calories, no trans fats and not more than 2 grams of saturated fat. They insist on no more than 230 milligrams of sodium and no more than 12 grams of sugar per serving (but exclude Eggo waffles, which have a higher sodium content).

FOOD LABELING – A 21st CENTURY REQUIREMENT

The Nutrition Labeling and Education Act (NLEA) became law in 1990 but the laws were not enforced until 1994. Food manufacturers were already identifying sodium and potassium content in food, but other ingredients were listed only voluntarily as of 1974. Today companies are required to list every ingredient!

As always, there are plenty of exemptions. Food served in an airplane or hospital cafeteria does not have to carry a nutrition label. The same applies for food sold on the street, at a mall cookie counter or out of a vending machine. Any foods prepared onsite, as in a bakery, deli or candy store, do not have to comply with NLEA laws, either. Other exemptions include: food shipped in bulk that is not sold to the consumer that way, medical foods, particularly foods given to patients with certain diseases, plain coffee and tea, spices, and other foods that have little nutrient value. Although produce is exempt at this point, the day is approaching when fruits, vegetables, fish, poultry and raw meat will be required to list nutrition facts.

The following businesses can apply for exemption from labeling laws: Small businesses with fewer than 100 employees if they sell fewer than 100,000 units annually, retailers with annual gross sales in the United States of less than $500,000 or with annual gross sales of food to consumers in the United States of less than $50,000. There are many places where you, the consumer, are not fully informed or protected through food-labeling laws. The onus is on you to get smart about what goes in your own mouth and those of your loved ones.

www.cfsan.fda.gov/~dms/fdnewlab.html

NOTE: As of this printing New York City's health department has introduced a mandatory calorie labelling law on all foods in restaurants with over 14 chains nationwide. Other cities seem to be following suit, including San Francisco.

WHAT DOES THAT MEAN?

Ingredients on food labels often read like a chemistry experiment. This is the list of preservatives and other chemicals poured into your processed food. Chemicals and preservatives arrived on the food scene when people clamored for foods that required spending less time in the kitchen and more time doing something else. (I think we have given ourselves twice the time to do four times as much, but that is just my opinion.) Convenience foods are convenient because they are right there ready to use, either on the supermarket shelves or in your cupboards. The trade-off is, of course, that you get both the food and its array of evil dancing partners.

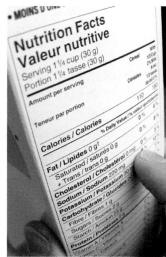

ANGELA'S STORY

A reader's testimonial

"

Hello Tosca,

I just wanted to say I absolutely love what you are doing to help people better themselves. I have been on this fitness mission. I tell everyone about eating clean and my friends are calling me the Eat-Clean Queen. I am a Natural Foods Chef and trainer.

My son is healthy and fit, and his friends are all little athletes BUT most of them are WAY overweight. I think, "How can this be? They run around outside all the time." I think it's all the junk we feed our babies.

My daughter has a bad case of food-allergy-related eczema. Once I started feeding her only Clean foods her skin really started to get much better! I was trained in holistic medicine. I had planned to become a naturopathic doctor, but my family had to come first. Natural medicine is still very much a part of my life. I want more than anything to reach out and help these kids learn about eating Clean. Teaching kids about eating clean, getting exercise and living a greener lifestyle is vital. My school is called Greenwood Learning Academy, and I will be caring for and educating our youth and families. I plan to serve Clean foods only. I will educate these kids about weight training and keeping our environment and homes clean of toxins – a major factor in contamination of our foods and homes.

The American family has come to the point of destruction. We are time strapped. We will eat anything and pop anything into the microwave just because it is labeled "dinner." We are committing suicide with food. Period. I have never seen so many fat, unhealthy, depressed and stressed-out people ever. And it's sad because people seem to want very badly to do better but just don't have the time or the know-how. I hope by starting this learning center I can educate these kids and hopefully they will grow up with the tools and knowledge to do better for themselves. I want to thank you, Tosca, for doing all you do. I just wanted to let you know how you've touched my life in the greatest way. Oh yes! I lost 65 pounds thanks to you.

"

Keep the books coming. We love them.
Angela

CHEMICAL SOUP

The entire human race (along with all other living things) is currently involved in a chemistry experiment the likes of which has never been seen before. Chemicals, pollutants, drugs and hormones sift over our heads and down into the ecosystem, settling on us like a toxic cloud, contaminating what was once pristine. It is difficult to escape, much less ignore. There are signs this chemical experiment is going awry. Cancer was once a disease of the elderly and infirm. Today cancer is the disease of everyone. Sadly, even babies are being born with this wretched disease. No one is exempt. There are so many plastics and hormones in the food chain that hunters are noticing a frightening trend. The animals they fell are increasingly found to be hermaphroditic – that is, they carry both male and female sex organs. This discovery is paralleled in fish. The day has come that this abnormality is now also found in humans.

When you think of those guys over in the Bell Institute creating foods and cereals like crazy, think of what their science involves. Sure they conjure up a

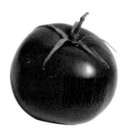

Cereal Superstar, but in order for us to enjoy it weeks or months later, chemical preservatives must be added. This is part of that chemistry experiment we are all involved in. We have no idea what some of these molecules will do to us long term. That is why I am always so skeptical of what I eat. Perhaps my brain is just too small or I have limited patience to deal with this stuff, but I prefer to know what I am eating, how to pronounce its ingredients and from whence it came. Clean Eating simplifies this for me, and also for you.

PRESERVATIVES – THE ONES YOU WILL COME ACROSS MOST OFTEN

The following is a list of some of the most commonly used preservatives. Knowing what these are and a little about what they do in your processed foods will help you identify what is on your food ingredient list and whether or not you want to eat it.

NITRATES

Nitrates inhibit the growth of the bacterial spores that cause botulism, or food poisoning. In severe cases botulism can cause death. Nitrates are commonly used in meats, especially processed meats, to help enrich the color. However, nitrates react with amino acids, which our body is full of, and create new

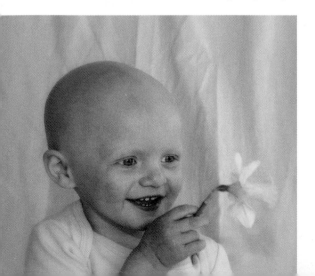

 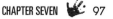

molecules called nitrosamines, which are known to cause cancer. Many food companies see the risk of death from food poisoning as the greater worry, and that is why nitrates in small amounts are allowed.

BUTYLATED HYDROXYANISOLE (BHA)

I often see this ingredient on cereal boxes, since it is commonly used as a dry food preservative. It is also used in foods that have a high fat or oil content. BHA helps to prevent rancidity, which is what happens to fatty foods when they come into contact with oxygen. It is thought that the increased incidence of hyperactivity, skin rashes and asthma in children is partially a result of the increased use of BHA in processed foods.

SULFITES

Sulfites, including sodium and potassium bisulfite and metabisulfite as well as sulfur dioxide, inhibit bacterial growth. Such chemicals are often used to treat light-colored fruits and vegetables to preserve them. They are also used to bleach flour and food starch. These chemicals can cause breathing problems, stomachaches, hives, and anaphylactic shock in the severest cases.

BENZOATES

The list of benzoates is long and includes sodium and potassium benzoate, calcium benzoate, benzoic acid, propylparaben and methylparaben. Benzoates kill bacteria, yeast and fungi. The benzoates appear as preservatives in acidic foods. When sodium benzoate is combined with vitamin C, the result is a molecule called benzene, which is carcinogenic. By itself sodium benzoate is not cancer causing, although it's considered toxic by many and is highly regulated in some countries.

OUR FOODS ARE FULL OF CHEMICALS

Preservatives are not the only dirty players in food. They appear not only because they have been deliberately added to the food during processing and refining but through a variety of other ways. Think about where your spinach grows. Pesticides, fertilizers, additives, preservatives and even coloring agents are sprayed directly onto crops right from the get go. Many food crops are contaminated when they come into accidental contact with untreated

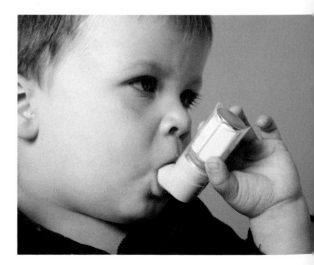

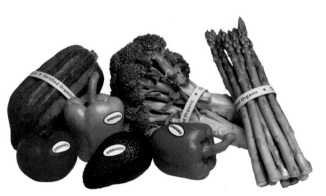

animal or human waste and environmental pollution. The meat you buy, if it is not organic or naturally raised, will have been given hefty doses of antibiotics, other drugs, and growth hormones. If your broccoli has been languishing in plastic wrap, then it will have had a helping of plastic chemicals leaching into its bumpy green head.

It is important for you to know where these chemicals can lurk and how they got there. Now you can figure out whether the food you are purchasing is healthy for you and your family or not. The list of our most-contaminated foods will give you the heads up on which to avoid, or at least handle differently before you eat them.

TIP Unsure about pesticides and chemicals? I suggest looking for organic fruits and vegetables.

CONTAMINATED FOODS ➡ CONTAMINANT(S)

CONTAMINATED FOODS	CONTAMINANT(S)
BUTTER	organochlorines stored in fat
RED APPLES	pesticides stored in skin
ZUCCHINI	pesticides stored in skin & flesh
CREAM CHEESE	organochlorines stored in fat
FRESH STRAWBERRIES	pesticides stored in skin and flesh
SALMON	pollutants stored in fat
FRESH SPINACH	pollutants, pesticides stored on leaves
RAISINS	pesticides stored in skin of grapes
GREEN BELL PEPPERS	pesticides, pollutants stored in skin
COLLARD GREENS	pesticides, pollutants stored on leaves
US PROCESSED CHEESE	pesticides, hormones stored in fat
PEANUT BUTTER	pesticides, pollutants stored in skin of nut
TUNA	mercury stored in fat and flesh

According to *The Eat-Clean Diet for Family and Kids* survey we have cause to be concerned with this list of dirty foods. Processed cheese in the form of cheese strings accounts for 50 percent of the average child's dairy intake each day, presumably because it is a highly portable food. Fattier foods – and cheese is 50 percent or more fat – are more highly contaminated because toxins are stored in fat (including your body fat). The same applies to salmon, which is an ideal Clean-Eating food, but a contaminated one at the same time. Our waters are increasingly polluted. Salmon is higher up on the food chain so these fish concentrate chemicals in their bodies from their lower-on-the-food-chain food sources and as a result of their fatty flesh. You may be able to avoid unwittingly consuming chemically charged fish by looking for products that are farmed carefully and organically, and by eating wild fish, especially those lower on the food chain. You can avoid some of the chemical contamination in an apple by peeling it, since the skin tends to retain pollutants while the flesh does not.

> Fattier foods – and cheese is 50 percent or more fat – are contaminated because toxins are stored in fat (including your body fat).

GOING ORGANIC AND NATURAL

I realize even as I write this that selecting only organic foods for your family may not be within your budget. Organic, traditionally grown foods still carry a hefty price tag compared to conventionally grown foods (foods grown using pesticides, herbicides and fertilizers). However, I do notice a trend toward traditionally grown foods. Slowly the consumer is becoming wiser and choosing organic. Increasingly these foods are of comparable cost to conventionally grown options. For example, at my local grocer I can buy conventional bananas for 59 cents per pound. In the same produce section I can purchase organic bananas for 69 cents per pound. That is a price difference I am willing to absorb, especially when I take into consideration my family's long-term health.

VISIT A LOCAL FARMERS' MARKET

Another way to keep the cost of organic purchases down is to visit a local farmers' market. Many towns hold markets as soon as the weather improves and

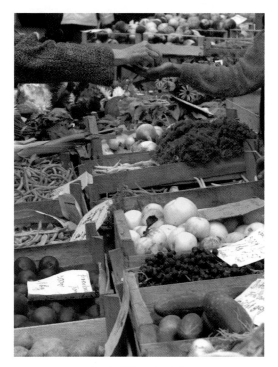

crops start coming in. When I think of the nature of small town America or Canada, I feel a strong connection to the many little places that dot our map and our culture. Having moved many times in my life – more than 15 – I have had to be a self-starter, making new friends wherever I could and as quickly as I could. Finding yourself in a new place with no familiar faces in the crowd can be challenging for anyone. No matter what you eat! I have often begun the process of joining the new community I have moved to by visiting the local farmer's market.

Wherever there are groceries and food items there are people, because they are all eating too – that is not exactly rocket science, I know, but you get my meaning. I made a point of searching out farmers' markets and local co-ops so I could not only buy the freshest foods but also mingle with town residents. I'd say hanging out over food is a fairly simple thing to do. What makes it more interesting is to visit with the people who grow some of that food. At farmers' markets you can chat with the person who actually grew the onions and tomatoes you are about to put into your tomato sauce. These grassroots places are where I learned to love bison and venison, cook with juniper berries and make foods sizzle with homemade raspberry vinegar. With every town I moved to I got down to the business of locating the nearest farmers' market and heading there as soon as I could. Whether it was in Ardrossan, Alberta; Caledon, Milton, Kingston, Belleville or London, Ontario; Chester or Morristown, New Jersey; or the Delftse Maart in Holland, I went with the dual purpose of immersing myself in local foods and making connections with the people of those diverse towns.

FIND A LOCAL BUTCHER

It seems easier to make a visit to a local grower to find fresh produce. When the harvest is in you can drive by virtually anyone's house in the country and see zucchini, tomatoes and squash for sale purchased on the honor system. But buying meat from a local grower? Really? This is probably more feasible than you think. I happened on a farmer at a local market who believed in letting his animals roam his meadows eating only grass and whatever else his four-footed creatures desired. Once I had made the connection with him, I was allowed to visit his farm during the winter to access his gorgeous, lean meats. Here I could purchase venison, bison and elk. I ordered the Thanksgiving and Christmas turkeys from him, too.

You will also find buying direct from the farmer to be considerably less expensive than buying from a store. And you won't believe what a difference it makes in the flavor of the meat when an animal is allowed to graze on nature's superior convenience food: grass. Vegetarian or not, you have to agree, when animals are allowed to roam freely and eat natural foods packed with the goodness of sunshine and earth, the end result will always be superior. For an amazing account of the value of raising animals in this humane way, read Michael Pollan's *The Omnivore's Dilemma*. You won't be able to put it down.

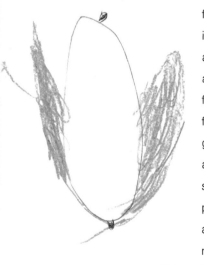

If you can't easily visit a farm then go to your local butcher and ask for exotic, grass-fed meat. If you become a regular customer the butcher will happily meet your request and stock his coolers with what you want. The old adage is true, "If you don't ask, you don't get."

MAKING YOUR OWN CONNECTIONS

In the same way you can make your own set of connections with local growers and bring home some of their most-treasured produce. I still recall a little farm I found on an old sideroad near Chester, N.J. Here I found purple beans (which I had previously thought were always green), tiny succulent blueberries, golden raspberries and yellow cauliflower. I felt I had found buried treasure for my family when I could bring these fresh and somehow still-living foods home. I went back time after time to purchase farm-fresh eggs from the farmer's free-range hens and made a wonderful discovery one day when the farmer's wife offered me a sample of her homemade goat cheese. I had never tasted anything so good.

These are the kinds of experiences you too can bring into your own kitchen repertoire. Somehow the foods found in these towns and villages helped me to connect more strongly with the food my family and I would ultimately eat. It is still enormously important to me to continue making connections like these. Try to visit a local farmers' market near you on an upcoming Saturday. Have your first cup of steaming coffee at the market while you hover over racks of freshly baked breads, pasta noodles or one of the many other delights you will find there. I highly recommend it.

CLEAN EATING IS
GREEN EATING!

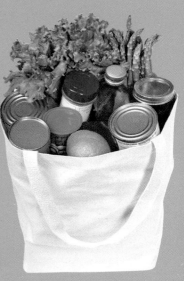

THE GREEN MOVEMENT

It's hard to miss the Green Movement happening all across this polluted planet. Plastic shopping bags are being banned in many states and have been replaced with reusable shopping bags. My mom and all of her many Dutch relatives used string shopping bags at least 60 years ago. Glad we are finally catching up. Earth Day and Earth Hour are events the global community can participate in and make a small but important contribution to our planet's clean up and green up. But did you know that if you Eat Clean you also Eat Green?

CLEAN EATING IS RESPONSIBLE EATING

Yes! By making more informed food choices you are doing your part to improve the health of this planet. The foods we eat every day have an enormous impact, not only on our health, but also on the world in which we live. By reviewing your diet and making Clean-Eating choices you are cutting unhealthy fats, sodium, refined foods, sugar and chemicals from your diet, and you also lessen the negative impact on the environment. Clean Eating promotes sustainability. The changes you make to your body when reaching for clean foods also clean up our water, air and soil.

Purchase food from local growers, particularly when foods are in season. By reaching for a berry grown in local soil rather than one grown 3,000 miles away, you lessen the carbon footprint and you also receive the most nutrition.

Have you noticed how little packaging there is with produce and whole foods? By eating more whole foods and rejecting processed foods you are at the same time eliminating excess packaging, which helps to keep garbage out of landfills. Staying away from fast-food and take-out establishments also helps reduce the amount of garbage you produce.

It is a wonderful feeling to Eat Clean, Eat Green, and make a positive contribution to the environment. If enough of us vote with our dollars to steer clear of irresponsibly produced foods, the effect will get the attention of food companies and hopefully the government. Do your bit. Eat Clean. Eat Green.

CHAPTER EIGHT

Your Clean-Eating Kitchen

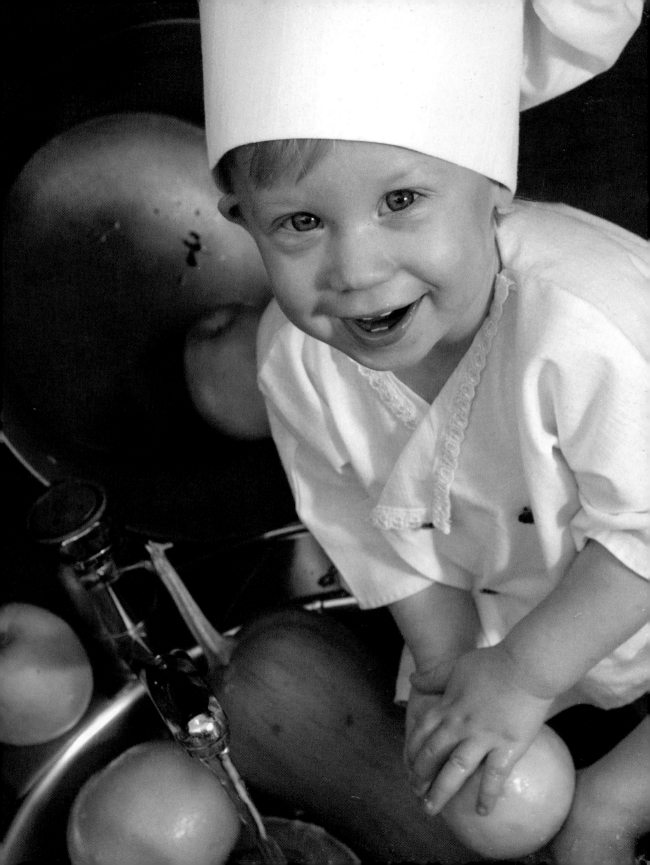

ANYONE CAN DO IT

Now that you have carried your groceries home, another aspect of your Clean-Eating transformation challenge begins. It will be up to you to turn these basic ingredients into food. Although that may sound daunting I want to assure you that you don't need to have studied at Cordon Bleu culinary arts school to create healthful, delicious food. I am a cook but not a chef, so I would never expect you to have fancy skills under your belt in order to Eat Clean. All you need is the most basic cooking knowledge and you will soon be preparing food your family will be dying to eat.

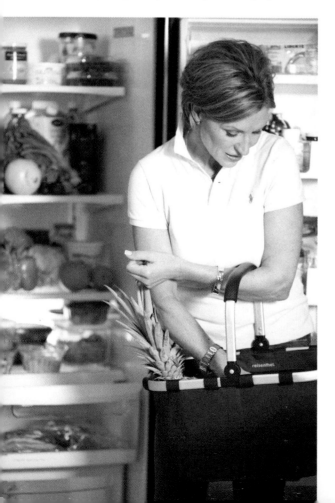

UNPACK THE GROCERIES

It is a good idea to clean and store all fresh produce carefully in the refrigerator. I often chop up some of the raw vegetables into crudités so they are ready in a pinch for hungry snackers. Another helpful hint is to store any perishables in clear glass containers in the fridge so you can readily see what's inside. I do this with flour, which can go rancid, flax seeds, nuts and other seeds. I keep other whole grains in airtight containers. Once they have been opened I store them in the refrigerator. Meats are unpacked and sent to the freezer until they are needed. The unpacking continues until everything is in its rightful place.

One of the most practical tips I can pass on to you is to always have plenty of a variety of staple foods in your cupboards, freezer and fridge. This way a meal can be prepared no matter how little time you have. Being prepared is an important part of your success with Clean Eating.

I often chop up some of the raw vegetables into crudités so they are ready in a pinch for hungry snackers.

⭐ WHOLE GRAINS

- ☐ Assorted rice in deep colors, including black, wehani, jasmine, brown, mahogany, and wild
- ☐ Wheat germ
- ☐ Oatmeal
- ☐ Oat bran
- ☐ Cream of wheat
- ☐ Quinoa
- ☐ Wheat, kamut and spelt berries
- ☐ Buckwheat
- ☐ Millet
- ☐ Whole-grain couscous
- ☐ Whole-grain pasta – a variety

⭐ NUTS AND SEEDS

- ☐ Raw unsalted nuts, including almonds, walnuts, cashews, brazils and pistachios
- ☐ Raw unsalted sunflower, sesame and flax seeds
- ☐ All-natural nut butters
- ☐ Tahini (to make hummus)

⭐ DRY CEREALS

- ☐ Muesli (check for sugars)
- ☐ Kashi cereals (check for sugars)
- ☐ Shredded wheat
- ☐ Ancient grains
- ☐ Ezekiel cereals

⭐ DRIED FRUITS (unsulfured is best)

- ☐ Apricots
- ☐ Raisins
- ☐ Dried apples
- ☐ Prunes
- ☐ Cranberries
- ☐ Cherries
- ☐ Figs
- ☐ Dates

Yummy!

⭐ CONDIMENTS

- ☐ Mustard
- ☐ Salsa
- ☐ Low-sodium soy sauce
- ☐ Tamari

⭐ OILS

- ☐ Extra virgin olive oil
- ☐ Grapeseed oil
- ☐ Safflower oil
- ☐ Pumpkin oil
- ☐ Other exotic oils including avocado, rice bran oil and other nut oils

⭐ PANTRY ITEMS

- ☐ Yams
- ☐ Sweet potatoes
- ☐ Onions
- ☐ Garlic
- ☐ Squash
- ☐ Turnip

 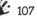

TIP •••••• *Throw some grapes in the freezer — frozen grapes are a refreshing snack during the hot summer months. Bananas, peeled, wrapped in plastic wrap and frozen are great too!*

⭐ DRY GOODS

- ☐ Whole-wheat flour
- ☐ Spelt or kamut flour
- ☐ Baking soda
- ☐ Baking powder
- ☐ Vanilla
- ☐ Sea salt
- ☐ Black pepper
- ☐ Dark chocolate
- ☐ Cocoa powder
- ☐ Tea
- ☐ Coffee
- ☐ Bouillon cubes
- ☐ Herbs and spices

⭐ CANNED GOODS

- ☐ Beans – *white, kidney, navy, pinto, lentils, black, lima, black-eyed peas, chick peas, and others you enjoy*
- ☐ Unsweetened applesauce
- ☐ Tomatoes – *canned, crushed, paste and sauce*
- ☐ Tuna – *water packed*
- ☐ Salmon – *water packed*

- ☐ Low-fat ready-made soups (check ingredients)
- ☐ Stock – *low-sodium chicken, beef or vegetable (check ingredients – organic is best)*
- ☐ Almond or soy milk, if desired

⭐ FREEZER

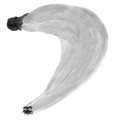

- ☐ Whole-grain wraps
- ☐ Brown-rice wraps
- ☐ Ezekiel bread
- ☐ Homemade granola bars
- ☐ Flash-frozen fruit and berries
- ☐ Frozen vegetables
- ☐ Pork tenderloins
- ☐ Chicken breasts
- ☐ Turkey breasts
- ☐ Ground turkey
- ☐ Exotic game meats if available
- ☐ Salmon
- ☐ Tilapia
- ☐ Jumbo shrimp

⭐ REFRIGERATOR

- ☐ Almond or soy milk, if desired
- ☐ Skim milk
- ☐ Tofu – *silken and firm*
- ☐ Kefir
- ☐ Plain yogurt
- ☐ Eggs
- ☐ Fresh berries when in season
- ☐ Leafy greens, including spinach, kale, romaine, sprouts

- ☐ Cooked chicken breasts
- ☐ Fresh fruits
- ☐ Fresh vegetables
- ☐ Lemon and lime juice
- ☐ Lemons and limes
- ☐ Olive oil-based margarine
- ☐ Plenty of leftovers!

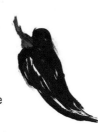

IDENTIFYING THE LEANEST CUTS OF MEAT

Beef and other meats are not what they used to be. It is not a bad idea to take a closer look at meat and the fat content associated with various cuts. See if you can make some simple changes in your shop-

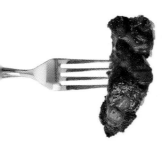

ping habits by getting familiar with terms such as "lean" and what that really means. Also make a point of getting to know the terms "game" and "exotic" meats.

Instead of beef, try game meat, which has the lowest amount of saturated and total fat.

BISON – A 3 oz serving, roasted, provides only 2 grams of fat and is a great source of protein, providing 28 grams. It also offers plenty of iron.

Other good options:

VENISON – 26 g protein

ELK – 26 g protein

POULTRY – white meat from chicken or turkey without the skin contains just 3 grams of fat and 27 grams of protein per 3 oz serving. Stores sell ground chicken or turkey that can be as high in fat as ground beef because they grind dark meat, which contains more fat, along with skin and fat in the mix. Choose ground breast meat.

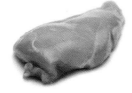

BEEF – choose roast or loin cuts. Per 3 oz serving "select," broiled:

- Eye of round roast contains 4 grams of fat and 26 grams of protein.
- Top round roast contains 5 grams of fat and 28 grams protein.
- Bottom round roast contains 5 grams of fat and 24 grams of protein.
- Top sirloin steak contains 4 grams of fat and 26 grams of protein.

VEAL – per 3 oz portion, separated, lean only, roasted:

- Leg top round contains 3 grams of fat and 24 grams of protein.
- Sirloin contains 5 grams of fat and 22 grams of protein.

 PORK – Per 3 oz portion, separated, lean only, roasted:

- Tenderloin contains 3 grams of fat and 22 grams of protein.
- Top loin chop contains 4 grams of fat and 23 grams of protein.
- Sirloin roast contains of 7 grams of fat and 25 grams of protein.

 LAMB – per 3 oz portion, broiled, separated, lean only, cut to ½" fat:

- Shank contains 6 grams of fat and 26 grams of protein
- Chops contain 7 grams of fat and 23 grams of protein (cut to ⅛" fat)

TIP Take your children to the grocery store with you. This way you can teach them about healthy foods.

 SALMON – per 5 oz:
- Pink salmon contains 5 grams of healthy fat and 36 grams of protein.
- Atlantic salmon contains 9 grams of healthy fat[1,2]

Choose ground beef with 90 percent or more lean meat. When reading labels look for "**select**," which is the leanest cut at 7 percent fat by weight. This is a better choice than "**prime**," which is heavily marbled (fat distributed in the lean) and high in unhealthy saturated fats.[3]

Extra lean: this means a 100 g or 3 ⅓ oz serving of meat, poultry, seafood or game meat contains less than 5 g of fat, less than 2 g of saturated fat and less than 95 mg of cholesterol.[4]

MENU PLANNING

At this point in most books that discuss diet the reader is usually prompted to plan a menu for the week. I don't know about you but I find this hard to do even if it is good advice. So here is what I do. When I can, I plan a few meals around a main protein source. If it is chili night, which it often is on Friday (see the recipe for Friday Night Chili on page 290), I will base at least two meals on this dish. The first will be a big steaming bowl served with a piece of crusty whole-grain bread. The next meal will be the same chili served over brown rice with a salad on the side. Leftovers will do nicely for a few smaller meals in my family's lunches.

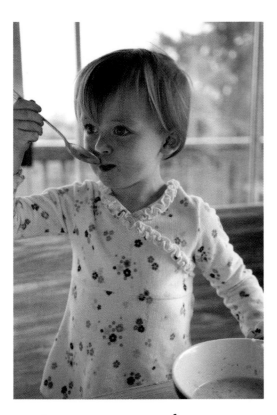

I like soup 'cause
it's fun to eat!

I do the same with turkey breasts. I like to buy two of these and will roast them both at the same time. While the oven is hot I will also roast a big squash, a few heads of garlic and other vegetables to round out the meal. I don't like to spend too much time fussing over foods, so I am a bit of a lazy cook. I like to make a lot of one thing and then use it to spin other meals over the next two days. When most of the meat has been removed from the bones of the turkey breast I

then pop the bones into a soup pot and begin creating yet another meal, soup! Soup is a regular meal offering at our house because it is a satisfying dish that stands up to busy schedules, which everyone in our household has.

If you are good at menu planning then go ahead and plan away. Any method will work as long as you are preparing Clean foods and serving several smaller meals each day.

PLANNED LEFTOVERS

Probably my biggest piece of advice for you is to make Planned Leftovers. I never cook just enough to satisfy one meal. I always, always make extras because these extras work well for the many meals you need for Clean Eating. When leftovers are handy no one is munching on empty foods. When leftovers are handy, you are liberated from the stove, and that is a very good thing.

The way I make Planned Leftovers is to scale up a recipe. If a recipe calls for one cup of cooked rice I will prepare two. It takes about the same time to cook and then I can use the extra rice as a base for another dish or to use with lunches. Instead of boiling one or two eggs I always boil the entire dozen. They keep well anyway, and I know for sure if I make extra someone will eat them. They pack well in coolers and lunch pails, too. When I am grilling meat I prepare extra. Never do I cook just one or two chicken breasts, but usually six at a time. The beauty of that is I can use the grilled meat for dinner served with cooked rice and steamed vegetables one night and the next night I can use the leftover grilled chicken in a wrap, a stir-fry, stew, omelet, or some other dish.

Working Planned Leftovers into your cooking cuts way down on time spent in the kitchen. Some days you simply have less time or energy to fuss with food. Busy schedules do that to you. Rather than pass through a fast-food joint on the way home from soccer practice, I depend on leftovers. They keep my family and me consistently Eating Clean.

CLEAN UP YOUR COOKING METHODS

Cooking requires you to prepare food by applying heat, but it helps to know which cooking methods work best with Clean Eating. Heat can be applied to food in any number of ways, some of which contribute to the overweight epidemic in North America. Your cooking technique could make an important difference to you and your family's waistline, and even your health. By now most of us already know that deep-fried foods should be avoided and that grilling is a good thing, as Martha Stewart would say.

Frying foods in a vat of recycled oil the way most fast-food French fries are prepared is hardly appetizing, but the worst bit of news is that frying in

TIP Life is busy! If you find yourself running from school to soccer practice, try to encourage your kids to pre-pack their dinner and snacks in the morning along with lunch. If time does not permit, opt for pre-made sushi, salad, or a wrap at your grocery store. A burger and fries at your local greasy fast-food joint is simply not an option!

this manner adds hundreds of unwanted chemicals and calories to food. Virtually all of the heat needed to cook a French fry, for example, comes from fat. There are ways to cook food that don't involve extra fat. Think of stir-frying, steaming, roasting and baking as healthy alternatives.

Other cooking methods involve heat from an oven, grill, fire or barbecue. Heat can be dry or moist, depending on the method chosen. The oven is a dry heat source, as is a grill. A food such as a roasting chicken is placed in the oven and roasted with very little additional liquid. You can also cook with moist heat, which is how food is cooked when it is braised or placed in a slow cooker.

Refer to this handy guide to help you sort out which is the best way to cook lean protein in your smashing new Clean-Eating kitchen.

CLEAN-EATING COOKING
REFERENCE GUIDE

BAKING › a hot oven is used to cook food by surrounding it with heat. The heat source is dry.

ROASTING › a heat source such as an oven or fire is used to cook a food contained in a pan or other container. The food is surrounded by heat. Fat drips out into the pan.

GRILLING › involves direct exposure to a heat source. Food sits upon a hot grill. Includes a barbecue or fire. Fat drips away from the food.

BROILING › a method of sealing juices into a food by exposing it to a direct source of heat. Fat drips away from food into a broiling pan.

SAUTÉEING › food is cooked over a direct heat source in a pan with little to no fat.

STEAMING › involves setting food in special steaming basket over a source of boiling water or liquid and letting the hot steam cook the food.

BRAISING › involves browning a food (usually in fat) first, and then finishing the cooking process in a small layer of liquid

POACHING › involves cooking the food entirely in water or other liquid.

STEWING › involves cooking different foods together over long periods of time with a great deal of stock or other liquid.

CONVECTION-OVEN COOKING › some ovens are equipped with a special fan that continually circulates hot air around the cooking food.

MICROWAVING › involves cooking food by exposing it to high frequency electro-magnetic waves.*

*Many people are taking exception to using this method of cooking today. Researches Blanc and Hertel found that microwaving food **changes** the food's nutrients. Notably, these two found that when people ate microwaved food their hemoglobin levels (red blood cell counts) decreased. The more microwaved food a person eats, the worse the problem. Cholesterol levels have also been found increased in people who eat microwaved food. In some countries, including Russia, microwave ovens have been banned. Find out more yourself by searching on the Internet.*

CLEAN-EATING BAKING TIPS

KEEP UNHEALTHY FAT OUT OF YOUR KITCHEN!

Thankfully there are many ways to keep unhealthy trans and saturated fats out of the kitchen. Keep this list of tips handy when trying to clean up favorite family recipes. You will discover wonderful new flavors this way while keeping your family on the Clean-Eating track.

FAT REPLACEMENT GUIDE FOR BAKING

→ Replace shortening or oils with any of these: the same quantity of pureed fruit + $\frac{1}{3}$ quantity healthy oil*. Example: if a recipe calls for $\frac{1}{3}$ cup shortening or lard, use $\frac{1}{3}$ cup unsweetened applesauce + 2 tablespoons healthy oil (*see page 116).

→ Replace butter or oil with mashed or puréed fruit or vegetables, including bananas, dates, apple butter or unsweetened applesauce. Try unsweetened mashed pumpkin, sweet potato, squash, or even leftover cooked hot cereal, including corn meal, oatmeal or Cream of Wheat.

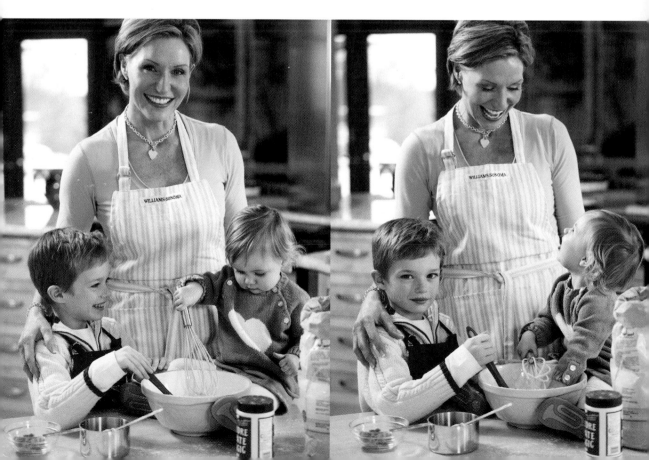

→ When a recipe calls for chocolate use unsweetened dark chocolate or cocoa – 75% or darker is best.

→ Use egg whites in place of whole eggs. Example: substitute two egg whites for every whole egg.

→ Some recipes depend on a little fat from the yolk of an egg so if the recipe calls for several eggs, reserve one or two yolks. Example: replace three whole eggs with one whole egg and four egg whites.

→ Piecrust is usually made of lard or some kind of animal shortening. Use cookie crumbs or cereal crusts such as oatmeal instead.

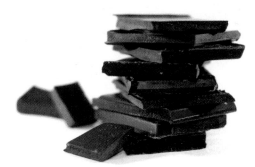

→ Replace heavy cream with skim milk – use flour or cornstarch to thicken.

→ Replace roasted, salted nuts with healthier unsalted and raw almonds, walnuts or peanuts.

→ In recipes that call for refined flours, replace half the flour with enriched, unprocessed, unbleached flours, and use whole-wheat flour for the remaining quantity.

→ Use buttermilk or low-fat, plain yogurt to replace some of the oil in a recipe. If you don't have buttermilk at home, sour one cup of regular skim milk with one tablespoon of lemon juice. You will have to increase any lost volume (airiness or lightness of a baked good) by increasing the amount of baking powder you use by ¼ teaspoon.

→ Consider using my recipe for Yogurt Cheese (see page 255) as a substitute for butter in recipes, too. It is delicious and super easy to make. It is even a perfect base for icing! Who knew?

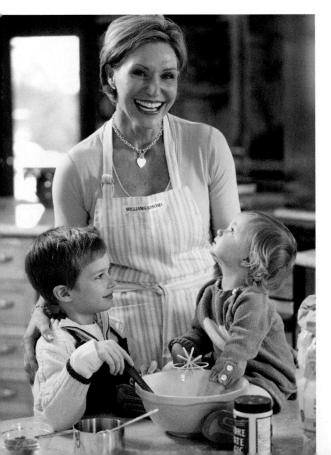

WHAT ARE HEALTHY OILS OR FATS?

Occasionally you will need to depend on fat for cooking. That doesn't mean using bacon drippings from a tin can. Use healthier fats. Coconut oil is one hot customer. It is easily digestible and has a high smoke point, so cooking does not make this healthy fat turn into unhealthy free radicals upon heating. Olive oil is another ideal healthy fat perfect for cooking and baking.

Consider yourself newly informed. To the right is the list you have been looking for when wanting to whip up something delicious in the kitchen. This guide for cooking and baking with healthy fats will help you keep it lean and clean in your kitchen.

YOGURT CHEESE IS A MUST IN YOUR CLEAN-EATING KITCHEN

Yogurt cheese has become a staple in my kitchen for many reasons. It is simple to make and takes no special skill. The wonderful creamy cheese marries beautifully with so many sweet or savory ingredients and it is the perfect base for creating decadent dishes that might otherwise be far too fatty for a Clean-Eating palate. Using yogurt cheese will help you clean up various dishes you may already love. You can even "thin out" your favorite ice cream by mixing equal parts of yogurt cheese and ice cream. The wonderful creamy consistency of yogurt cheese

OIL SMOKE POINTS

OILS	FAHRENHEIT	CELCIUS
Flaxseed Oil	225	107
Pumpkinseed Oil	225	107
Hempseed Oil	330	166
Butterfat	350	177
Coconut Oil	350	177
Sesame Oil	350	177
Lard	370	182
Canola Oil	400	204
Walnut Oil	400	204
Extra Virgin Olive Oil	420	160
Cottonseed Oil	420	216
Almond Oil	425	218
Hazelnut Oil	430	221
Sunflower Oil	440	227
Olive Oil	440	227
Peanut Oil	440	227
Corn Oil	450	232
Palm Oil	450	232
Safflower Oil	450	232
Rice Bran Oil	490	254
Soybean Oil	495	257
Avocado Oil	520	271

mimics that of many sinfully delicious desserts such as cheesecake. Yogurt cheese is so good it already seems a treat on its own. See recipe for Yogurt Cheese on page 255.

SOME IDEAS FOR USING
YOGURT CHEESE

❖ YOGURT CHEESE RATHER THAN CREAM CHEESE

A bagel with cream cheese is a decidedly fatty breakfast option. Eighty-eight percent of the calories in cream cheese come from fat, and most of that fat is saturated. Substitute yogurt cheese for the cream cheese and opt for a multi-grain bagel or, even better, switch to toasted Ezekiel bread.

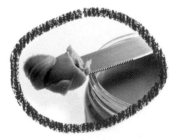

❖ LIGHTEN UP NUT BUTTERS

Mix equal parts of yogurt cheese and your favorite nut butter to reduce fat and sugar content. The yogurt cheese takes on the flavor of the nut butter. Remember to keep any extra in the refrigerator and use within a few days, since yogurt cheese is a dairy product and will go bad if not stored properly.

❖ CLEAN-EATING WHIPPED CREAM

Bet you did not think you could have whipped cream on a Clean-Eating nutrition plan! Prepare yogurt cheese and add a pinch of cinnamon and a dash of vanilla. Use an electric mixer to blend and voilà! Delicious Clean-Eating whipped cream! Again, store leftovers in the fridge.

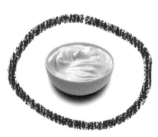

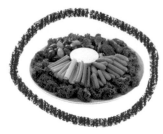

❖ TOPPING FOR BAKED POTATOES OR DIP FOR CRUDITÉS

Sour cream contains so much fat it is appropriate only for a treat if you are Eating Clean. Mix your favorite herbs, especially chopped chives, into yogurt cheese and enjoy the same indulgent texture and flavor as sour cream with far less fat and fewer calories. Use yogurt cheese as a base for making a delicious crudité dip as well. Combine any fresh or dried herbs and a dash of garlic with yogurt cheese and serve.

❖ MAYONNAISE ALTERNATIVE

Combine one half-cup yogurt cheese with a splash of vinegar and mix. This is your mayonnaise alternative, minus the heavy fat content.

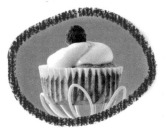

❖ FROSTINGS AND ICINGS

A recipe for yogurt cheese frosting can be found on page 193 in this book. Use yogurt cheese as the base for any of your favorite baked goods or spreads to cut out virtually all the fat and a lot of sugar. Add chocolate, lemon or other favorite flavors to get just the right taste!

IT'S A WRAP!

There it is! A way to clean up your kitchen and the eating habits of your family. It won't be long before your family sees and experiences results. This is the only way to eat that both guarantees optimal health and a slim physique. The two go hand in hand. I can't wait to hear your success story.

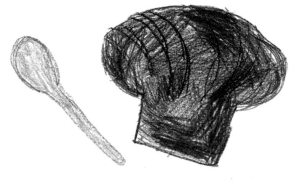

References:

1. www.med.umich.edu/umim/clinical/pyramid/meats.htm 2. www.nutritiondata.com 3. www.cnn.com/HEALTH/library/NU/00202.html
4. www.deliciousdecisions.org/cb/hhc_easy_meat.html

BARBARA'S FAMILY'S STORY

A reader's testimonial

"Well it is about time someone finally told me how to eat. You would think after all these years of living I might have had a clue but my family eating habits are questionable. I grew up eating everything fried and swimming in sauce. That was the way my mom cooked. Her food was good but now I am fighting a huge weight problem and it is trickling down to my kids. My mom died of heart disease way too young and my dad had diabetes until he too passed. I don't get much support from my husband and he pretty much eats anything he wants. I was getting scared I would lose what matters most to me – my family!

So here you come along with a book that is as simple as it gets and suddenly everything about eating makes sense. I started following your ideas and am proud to say I am a Clean Eater. What I noticed besides losing weight – my pants are loose on me after only a few weeks of this – is that I have energy like crazy.

My youngest son could never go to the bathroom properly and now even that is a breeze. I couldn't stand to hear him crying before but that is in the past. I put flax seed in his cereal and just about everything else too. He loves it! I think I love it more. My teenage daughter had bad skin. I guess I must have plugged her up with bad food. Now that she is eating your clean food she no longer has problems with her skin either, and she has lost that roll on her waist that was pretty much scaring me.

This is a long letter but I had to tell you everything because I feel hopeful that we can be a healthy family thanks to clean eating. I will never eat another way again!"

Sincerely,
Barbara Johnson

CHAPTER NINE

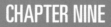

Eating Out

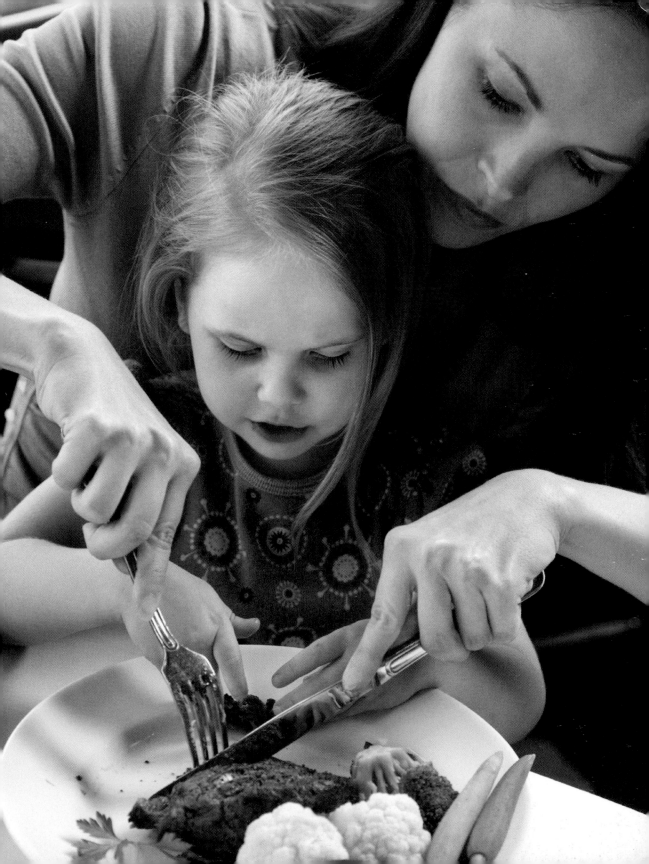

EATING OUT AND EATING CLEAN

There is no reason to abandon Clean-Eating efforts the minute you open a restaurant door, and forgoing eating out is not feasible either. Life today often necessitates eating away from home, and dining out is also a popular way to celebrate happy occasions. Although I make every effort to prepare healthy meals for my family there are times when I just have to depend on other cooks and chefs. My daughter's late volleyball game; dance classes and recitals in distant towns; travel for business … these are just some of my reasons for not putting dinner on my own table.

North Americans dine out a lot. The Mastercard, Dining Out survey found that 46 cents of every food dollar is spent on food eaten outside of the home. Another way to look at it is Americans consume one-third of their daily nutritional requirements outside of the home. *(Source: KidShape, Naomi Neufeld, pg. 127)* It is doubtful we will give up the habit of eating out any time soon. However, just because you have to depend on someone else's kitchen for meals does not mean you have to give up the healthy eating habits you are accustomed to at home.

It is a good idea to plan for dining-out occasions with Clean-Eating strategies. You can cope with just about anything life throws at you as long as you have the skills to do so. Parents, this means you are in charge of staying the course. You need to remain firm about insisting on healthy nutrition for you and your children even while you are gathered around the table at Applebee's. Therefore, parents, you must lead by example. Children imitate their parents' behavior, good or bad, and they will be watching what you order when dinner is not at home. This is the ideal opportunity to model Clean Eating.

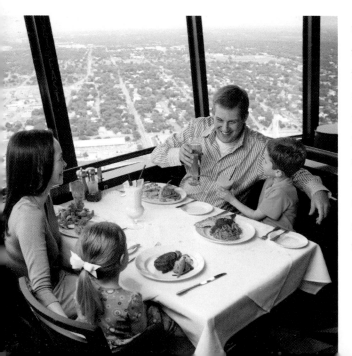

When I eat out with my family I am usually the first to order, since I can scan a menu pretty easily and figure out which dishes will be good Clean-Eating choices. I make sure to ask for my fish grilled and my veggies steamed, no butter, and hold the mashed potatoes. It doesn't take long for my family to pick up on my lead. We have been Eating Clean for so long we are all pros at ordering out. It's grilled tenderloin and steamed vegetables for them, too. When everyone at the table eats the same way, it is easy to stick to healthier eating principles.

Keep in mind that eating out does not have to be a "splurge" situation. It's easy to develop this attitude: "If I eat well at home why can't I splurge a little when I eat out?" This wouldn't be a problem if indeed you rarely ate out, but as the statistics show, we are not occasional restaurant-goers, and that is in large part why we have gotten so obese and sick in the last decade.

EATING OUT STRATEGIES

Many strategies will help you be a successful Clean Eater while dining out, and they are simpler than you think. Knowing how to order and which restaurant to visit gives you the power to remain in control of your healthy eating habits. Now that I have become familiar with the restaurants near where I live, selecting one is simple. One of my favorites is a little place called "Juniper." Here the chef Daniel and his partner Nadia prepare dishes from locally grown ingredients, gathered foods and foods grown in their own garden. Meat and fish come from local farms. I feel as if I am eating the perfect Clean foods every time we go. Their version of venison topped with wild blueberries tastes unbelievably delicious. I order it often. Nadia has created her own falafel that is both healthy and low in fat and it always leaves me wanting more. It's a good idea to become familiar with a restaurant and make a point of understanding what goes on in their kitchen so you feel comfortable ordering foods that will keep you on the Clean-Eating track.

- ✪ **Use the Internet to review the menu of restaurants before you go. Most post their menu online nowadays.**
- ✪ **Call ahead to learn if the restaurant is willing to work with dietary concerns.**
- ✪ **Look at the reviews.**
- ✪ **Look for heart-healthy restaurants**

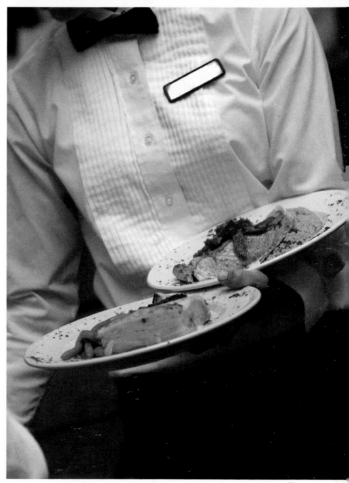

HOW TO DEAL WITH
FAST FOOD

Fast-food restaurants make a career out of serving up fatty, greasy, fried foods full of chemicals, unhealthy ingredients and excessive calories. Knowing how to navigate your way through fast-food menu items will make ordering Clean food much easier. The following strategies will keep you Eating Clean.

1 **Look for and order meats without breading or coatings and avoid fried options.**

2 Grilled, baked, or broiled options are best.

3 Steer clear of fatty condiment additions such as mayonnaise, sour cream, "special sauce," butter, and dressings.

4 Drink water or low-fat versions of milk rather than sodas, fruit beverages or whole-fat milk.

5 Eat your salad dry or spritzed with citrus juices such as lemon, lime, orange or grapefruit, or balsamic or other vinegars and a small amount of heart-healthy oils if you wish.

6 Try healthy "burger" options such as grilled chicken, bison, turkey, fish or Clean vegetarian.

7 Avoid the fatty accoutrements that often come with salads, such as croutons, whole eggs, bacon bits, cheese, and deep-fried tortillas.

8 Ditch the fries and choose a baked potato – stick with Clean Eating by topping it with plain nonfat yogurt or cottage cheese, salsa, beans, or other steamed vegetables rather than sour cream, bacon or cheese.

CLEAN EATING-OUT STRATEGIES

Here are a few strategies I use to help me Eat Clean while eating out.

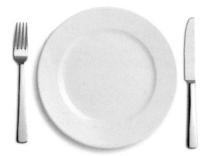

◆ Use the Internet to review menus before visiting a restaurant. Most eating establishments post food offerings online, and checking the menu before you go will give you some idea which Clean Foods are offered. If there aren't any, you can easily look for an alternative restaurant that supports your healthy eating habits.

◆ Balance your menu choices so your meal contains lean proteins and complex carbohydrates from fresh produce as well as whole grains. French fries and a hot dog with ketchup don't qualify!

◆ You may also call ahead and chat with someone at the restaurant to determine whether the cooking staff is willing to make changes to menu offerings in keeping with your dietary concerns. You may be pleasantly surprised to discover how many restaurants will work with you. Independently owned restaurants are definitely more willing and able to help you. Most of the food at chain restaurants is pre-made.

◆ Check newspaper and online reviews for the public's opinion of eateries as well. I often do this to learn information not made available through other means. In Santa Monica is a restaurant called "The Firehouse", and I discovered that the entire menu is Clean Eating from a fan who read about it in a newspaper review. I invite you to send me your Clean Eating restaurant favorites too!

◆ Restaurants also carry "Heart Healthy" accreditations to help people select a restaurant suited to their lower-fat dietary restrictions. You will find "Heart Healthy" eating establishments support Clean Eating, for the most part.

◆ Watch portion sizes and consider the fact that servings have increased greatly over the last 20 or 30 years. Would that salad serve you and someone else? Is an appetizer enough for a meal?

◆ Rather than quench thirst with sugar-loaded sodas or juices, drink water or skim milk. This way you will avoid empty calories, the sugar high and the chemical load you would otherwise get from colas and energy drinks. Avoiding alcohol will not only save you the sugar calories, but drinking alcohol lowers your resistance, making it more likely that you will eat things you would otherwise avoid.

WHAT TO EAT

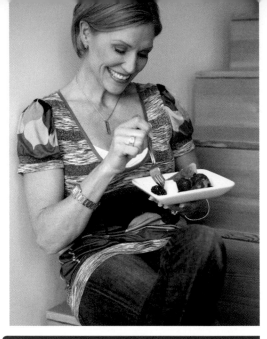

STARTERS

- Broth-based soups.
- Shrimp cocktail.
- Smoked salmon.
- Crudités with hummus or other Clean-Eating spreads.
- Salad.
- Fresh spring rolls (not fried), stuffed with shredded vegetables.

ENTRÉES

- Meats prepared by grilling, baking, roasting, steaming, broiling or barbecuing.
- Vegetarian items created with low-fat milk products, TVP, soy, quinoa, and whole grains. Make sure these are not fried.

VEGGIES AND SIDES

- Prepared by steaming, grilling, stewing, stir-frying, roasting, boiling, or simply eaten raw.

SALADS

- Filled with leafy greens and raw vegetables but no fatty dressings.

BREAD

- Limit bread consumption and try to stick to whole-grain varieties, flatbreads or lavash.

FATS

- Look for healthy fats from exotic oils including olive oil, pumpkin and so on.

DESSERTS

- Fresh fruit is best. If you decide to treat yourself to a rich dessert, try sharing with others and have just a bite or two. You'll probably find it just as satisfying.

BEVERAGES

- Water, coffee, tea, and juices mixed with water or sparkling water.

TIP Choose healthy restaurants when your family plans a dinner outing. Stay away from fast-food chains and research organic, local restaurants.

PIZZA PIE POSSIBILITIES

CLEANING UP NORTH AMERICA'S FAVORITE TAKE-OUT TREAT ONE TOPPING AT A TIME

EAT-CLEAN CRUST

⭐ Choose a whole-wheat, thin crust.

HEALTH-SAVVY PIZZA SAUCE

⭐ Choose a red sauce or pesto sauce.

CLEANER CHEESY CHOICES

⭐ Low-fat mozzarella

⭐ Low-fat feta cheese

⭐ Goat cheese

⭐ Hard parmesan

PERFECT PROTEINS

⭐ Grilled chicken breast, cut into strips

⭐ Grilled turkey breast, cut into strips

⭐ Marinated grilled tofu, cut into cubes

VIBRANT VEGGIES

⭐ Eggplant

⭐ Zucchini

⭐ Mushrooms

⭐ Red, green, yellow or orange peppers

⭐ Sweet onions - caramelized onions are delicious

⭐ Black olives

⭐ Sundried tomatoes

⭐ Artichokes

⭐ Spinach

⭐ Broccoli florets

⭐ Fresh tomatoes

⭐ Fresh basil

I love making my own pizza because I know exactly what's in it. See page 247 for Homemade Pizza for Clean Eaters.

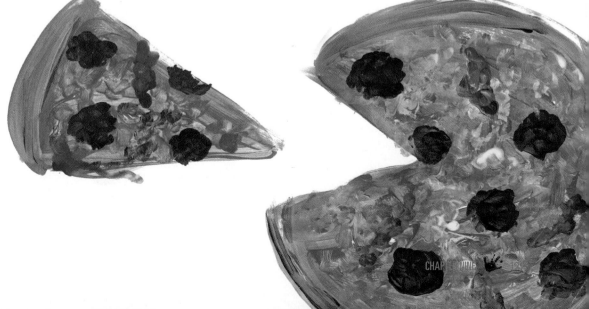

MORE CLEAN ORDERING

The right skills will help you recognize food for what it is or is not. In my first Eat-Clean book, *The Eat-Clean Diet*, I provided several simple tips to help you make menu selections. Here is that list with extra strategies to keep you Eating Clean.

➤➤ While waiting for your food to be served, the breadbasket stares you right in the eye. I often ask the waiter not to bring it at all, or I will choose a flatbread or whole-grain crunchy offering. If a healthy spread or olive oil for dipping is not provided I eat my selection plain. In general, the breadbasket is not the place I choose to indulge.

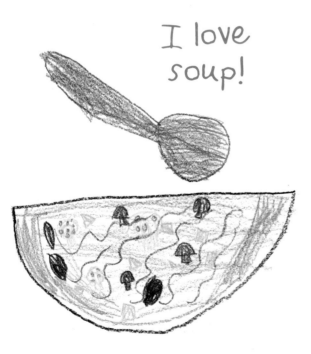

I love soup!

➤➤ Substitute raw or steamed vegetables, including salad greens or sliced tomato, for buttered veggies or French fries.

➤➤ Drink plenty of water with your meal rather than alcohol, and have black coffee or tea as beverage options. Children will enjoy water in time. Add lots of ice and slices of limes and lemons to make it more interesting for them.

➤➤ Proteins in your meal can be grilled, baked, broiled, steamed or poached to reduce unnecessary fat.

➤➤ Scan the appetizer list for Clean-Eating options. An appetizer might be all you or your child needs as a dinner entrée. Servings are so big today that having a starter for your main course is a good idea.

➤➤ If you do end up with a larger-than-life entrée, consider sharing the dish or asking for a doggie bag right away. I often do this for my daughters, who love to take my restaurant leftovers for lunch the next day.

➤➤ Some soups come with a dollop of sour cream or fried tortilla strips and even loads of cheese on top. Ask for these to be left off if possible. If not, remove them yourself once your soup has arrived.

➤➤ Have sushi or sashimi as an ideal Clean-Eating, eating-out meal.

➤ Ask that all sauces and dressings be served on the side. You can also ask that vegetables be served steamed and not doused with butter.

➤ In general you will find most restaurants are quite willing to help you deliver your meal to you the way you want it.

RESTAURANT FOOD FACTS YOU NEED TO KNOW

ITALIAN FOOD

I love Italian food as much for the fun of eating slurpy noodles as for the social, joyful atmosphere of this fun-loving culture. Italians love to eat! But how can we keep it clean and eat Italian at the same time? My beautiful Italian friend Franca has worked miracles with her body (and her family) by incorporating Clean-Eating principles into her diet. Her family comes from southern Italy. Before Franca discovered Clean Eating she ate Italian foods slathered with cheese, cream and butter. She also weighed more than she wanted to. Now fresh foods appear at every meal and she loves to serve vegetables along with noodles in every shape and color.

Fine tune your Italian cravings by avoiding dishes heavily doused in fatty cheese, butter and sauces. Tomato sauce is an ideal Clean-Eating food if you leave out sugar and fatty meats that often creep into this ubiquitous sauce. Hide plenty of vegetables

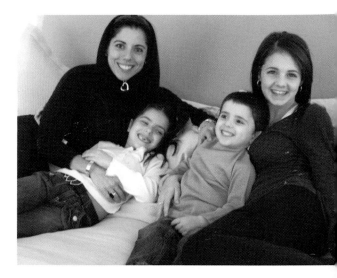

in your own homemade spaghetti sauce. A hearty sauce can easily accommodate a few grated carrots or a sweet potato and none of your kids would be the wiser – but they would be healthier. One of my favorite Italian salads is Tricolore, made with juicy, ripe tomatoes and boconcini cheese (a small amount) sprinkled lavishly with fresh basil and a little extra virgin olive oil. Delish!

TIP Teach your children the benefits of eating six small meals a day. When you set the Clean-Eating example in your household, your children will maintain this lifestyle as they grow up.

CHINESE FOOD

I was surprised to discover how much fat is in Chinese food. I had always thought of Chinese food as low in fat because of the appearance of so many vegetables in its dishes. But even that fortune cookie at the end of your meal packs a surprising amount of fat. Many of us, myself included, opt for Chinese food when eating out because we feel it

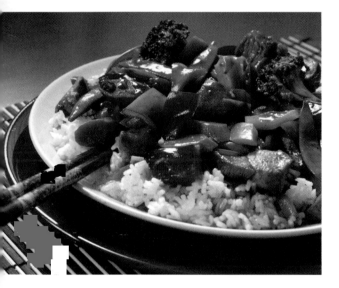

is "healthier" for us. Not so! It pays to check out the menu of your favorite eatery in advance so you know which dishes to choose before you get there.

Stick to steamed vegetables, dishes based on lean chicken, beef or beans, especially stir-fries, and opt for steamed brown rice if you can get it. Need I say that you should never choose fried rice? Savvy Asian eateries now serve low-sodium soy and tamari sauce.

If you can have your dish served without that glistening coating of sauce (whatever it is), then do so.

MEXICAN FOOD

It's difficult to name a Mexican dish that does not come fried or loaded with cheese – at least the American-Mexican food. Most of what we think of Mexican food does not qualify as Clean-Eating fare, but you can make healthier choices by omitting cheese, fried options and heavy sauces. Instead reach for zesty vegetable and/or fruit salsas and sliced tomatoes. Most of these include a variety of chopped vegetables, fruits and herbs along with spices that add delicious Clean-Eating flavor to virtually any dish. I make salsas all the time because they keep well and help make my cooking taste better. A few of my favorites include mango, grapefruit and tomato salsa. They are just delicious! Round out your meal with grilled fish or chicken.

FAST FOOD AND WHAT YOU GET

Following is some information about a few of the most popular or well-known fast-food restaurants. The charts lay out the most-ordered food item and how many calories you are getting, as well as how much fat, including the unhealthy saturated and trans fats. You can also find out how much sodium is in each of the menu items. Get ready for a shock! Now you know what you are paying for when you order Fat Food.

McDonald's	BIG MAC	MCNUGGETS* (6 PIECE)
TOTAL CALORIES	540	250
CALORIES FROM FAT	260	130
TOTAL FAT (G)	29	15
SATURATED FAT (G)	10	3
TRANS FAT (G)	1.5	1.5
SODIUM (MG)	1040	670

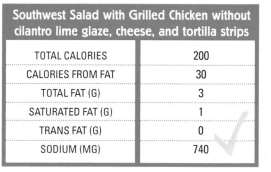

* Totals without sauce
* With Sweet and Sour Sauce add 50 calories, 10 g of sugar, and 150 mg of sodium

CLEANER OPTIONS

Asian Salad with Grilled Chicken without almonds and orange glaze	
TOTAL CALORIES	200
CALORIES FROM FAT	35
TOTAL FAT (G)	4
SATURATED FAT (G)	1
TRANS FAT (G)	0
SODIUM (MG)	740

Southwest Salad with Grilled Chicken without cilantro lime glaze, cheese, and tortilla strips	
TOTAL CALORIES	200
CALORIES FROM FAT	30
TOTAL FAT (G)	3
SATURATED FAT (G)	1
TRANS FAT (G)	0
SODIUM (MG)	740

Premium Grilled Chicken Classic Sandwich with whole wheat bun and without mayo	
TOTAL CALORIES	370
CALORIES FROM FAT	40
TOTAL FAT (G)	4.5
SATURATED FAT (G)	1
TRANS FAT (G)	0
SODIUM (MG)	1110*

*Sodium is high in this dish.

Fast-food burgers hurt my stomach.

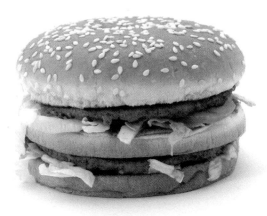

Wendy's

	JR. BACON CHEESEBURGER	CRISPY CHICKEN SANDWICH
TOTAL CALORIES	310	340
CALORIES FROM FAT	140	120
TOTAL FAT (G)	16	14
SATURATED FAT (G)	6	2.5
TRANS FAT (G)	0.5	0
SODIUM (MG)	690	810

CLEANER OPTIONS

Mandarin Chicken Salad without roasted almonds, crispy noodles, or dressing		Chicken Caesar Salad without dressing, croutons, or parmesan cheese	
TOTAL CALORIES	170	TOTAL CALORIES	160
CALORIES FROM FAT	20	CALORIES FROM FAT	40
TOTAL FAT (G)	2.5	TOTAL FAT (G)	5
SATURATED FAT (G)	0.5	SATURATED FAT (G)	1.5
TRANS FAT (G)	0	TRANS FAT (G)	0
SODIUM (MG)	520	SODIUM (MG)	575

Burger King

	WHOPPER WITH CHEESE	TENDERCRISP CHICKEN SANDWICH
TOTAL CALORIES	760	790
CALORIES FROM FAT	423	396
TOTAL FAT (G)	47	44
SATURATED FAT (G)	16	8
TRANS FAT (G)	1.5	4
SODIUM (MG)	1450	1640

CLEANER OPTIONS

TenderGrill Chicken Garden Salad without croutons, dressing, or cheese	
TOTAL CALORIES	180
CALORIES FROM FAT	35
TOTAL FAT (G)	4
SATURATED FAT (G)	1
TRANS FAT (G)	0
SODIUM (MG)	610

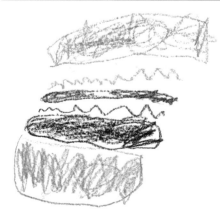

Taco Bell

Taco Bell	BEEF TACO SUPREME	BURRITO SUPREME – BEEF
TOTAL CALORIES	250	420
CALORIES FROM FAT	117	153
TOTAL FAT (G)	13	17
SATURATED FAT (G)	6	8
TRANS FAT (G)	0.5	1
SODIUM (MG)	650	1340

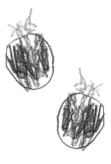

CLEANER OPTIONS

Chicken Ranchero Taco, Fresco Style without cheese, salsa, or avocado dressing	
TOTAL CALORIES	170
CALORIES FROM FAT	36
TOTAL FAT (G)	4
SATURATED FAT (G)	1.5
TRANS FAT (G)	0
SODIUM (MG)	730

* Taco Bell offers a Fresco Menu, for which all items contain less than 8 g of fat.

Hardee's

Hardee's	PHILLY CHEESE STEAK THICK BURGER
TOTAL CALORIES	930
CALORIES FROM FAT	570
TOTAL FAT (G)	63
SATURATED FAT (G)	24
TRANS FAT (G)	0
SODIUM (MG)	1750

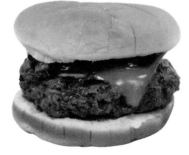

CLEANER OPTIONS

Charbroiled BBQ Chicken Sandwich without BBQ sauce	
TOTAL CALORIES	295
CALORIES FROM FAT	36
TOTAL FAT (G)	4
SATURATED FAT (G)	1
TRANS FAT (G)	0
SODIUM (MG)	822

TIP Teach your children how to make healthy menu choices — tell them to try a baked potato or salad instead of fries.

Sonic

	SONIC CHEESE-BURGER W/ MAYO	EXTRA-LONG CHILI CHEESE CONEY
TOTAL CALORIES	700	600
CALORIES FROM FAT	378	297
TOTAL FAT (G)	42	33
SATURATED FAT (G)	14	11
TRANS FAT (G)	2	1
SODIUM (MG)	1020	1700

CLEANER OPTIONS

Grilled Chicken Sandwich without Honey Mustard sauce	
TOTAL CALORIES	250
CALORIES FROM FAT	45
TOTAL FAT (G)	5
SATURATED FAT (G)	1.5
TRANS FAT (G)	0
SODIUM (MG)	800

Grilled Chicken Wrap without Ranch Dressing	
TOTAL CALORIES	303
CALORIES FROM FAT	36
TOTAL FAT (G)	4
SATURATED FAT (G)	1.5
TRANS FAT (G)	0
SODIUM (MG)	1047

Subway

	6" CHICKEN AND BACON RANCH SANDWICH	6" MEATBALL SANDWICH
TOTAL CALORIES	510	560
CALORIES FROM FAT	220	210
TOTAL FAT (G)	25	24
SATURATED FAT (G)	8	10
TRANS FAT (G)	0.5	1
SODIUM (MG)	1230	1580

CLEANER OPTIONS

6" Oven-Roasted Chicken Breast with no sauce, but include lettuce, tomatoes, pickles, onions, green peppers and olives	
TOTAL CALORIES	300
CALORIES FROM FAT	45
TOTAL FAT (G)	5
SATURATED FAT (G)	1.5
TRANS FAT (G)	0.2
SODIUM (MG)	780

Chick-fil-A	CHICKEN SANDWICH	CHICK-N-STRIPS
TOTAL CALORIES	410	310
CALORIES FROM FAT	150	140
TOTAL FAT (G)	16	15
SATURATED FAT (G)	3.5	3
TRANS FAT (G)	0	0
SODIUM (MG)	1300	890

CLEANER OPTIONS

Chargrilled Chicken Garden Salad without croutons, dressing		Chargrilled Chicken Sandwich without BBQ sauce	
TOTAL CALORIES	110	TOTAL CALORIES	270
CALORIES FROM FAT	35	CALORIES FROM FAT	30
TOTAL FAT (G)	3.5	TOTAL FAT (G)	2.5
SATURATED FAT (G)	2.5	SATURATED FAT (G)	1
TRANS FAT (G)	0	TRANS FAT (G)	0
SODIUM (MG)	480	SODIUM (MG)	940

Jack-in-the-Box	BACON ULTIMATE CHEESEBURGER	JACK'S SPICY CHICKEN WITH CHEESE
TOTAL CALORIES	1090	700
CALORIES FROM FAT	700	330
TOTAL FAT (G)	77	37
SATURATED FAT (G)	30	10
TRANS FAT (G)	3	3
SODIUM (MG)	2040	1410

CLEANER OPTIONS

Asian Grilled Chicken Salad without dressing		Chicken Strips – Grilled (4)	
TOTAL CALORIES	162	TOTAL CALORIES	180
CALORIES FROM FAT	15	CALORIES FROM FAT	20
TOTAL FAT (G)	1.5	TOTAL FAT (G)	2
SATURATED FAT (G)	0.5	SATURATED FAT (G)	0.5
TRANS FAT (G)	0	TRANS FAT (G)	0
SODIUM (MG)	376	SODIUM (MG)	700

In most surveys **Wendy's** is chosen as the most popular fast-food restaurant. Here is the difference between a regular meal and a Clean meal:

McDonald's is the most widely known fast-food place, with their golden arches being a cultural symbol. Here is the difference between a regular meal and a clean meal:

REGULAR MEAL

Quarter-Pound Single Cheeseburger, Medium Fries, Medium Coke	
TOTAL CALORIES	1110
CALORIES FROM FAT	410
TOTAL FAT (G)	46
SATURATED FAT (G)	13
TRANS FAT (G)	2
SODIUM (MG)	1650

REGULAR MEAL

Big Mac, Medium Fries, Medium Coke, Oreo McFlurry	
TOTAL CALORIES	1690
CALORIES FROM FAT	590
TOTAL FAT (G)	66
SATURATED FAT (G)	23
TRANS FAT (G)	9
SODIUM (MG)	1520

CLEAN MEAL

Mandarin Chicken Salad (without almonds, noodles or dressing), Plain Baked Potato, Water	
TOTAL CALORIES	280
CALORIES FROM FAT	20
TOTAL FAT (G)	2
SATURATED FAT (G)	0.5
TRANS FAT (G)	0
SODIUM (MG)	630
Without Baked Potato	
TOTAL CALORIES	180
CALORIES FROM FAT	20
TOTAL FAT (G)	2
SATURATED FAT (G)	0.5
TRANS FAT (G)	0
SODIUM (MG)	630

CLEAN MEAL

Southwest Salad with Grilled Chicken (without cilantro lime glaze, cheese, and tortilla strips), Water, Fruit and Yogurt Parfait (without granola)	
TOTAL CALORIES	450
CALORIES FROM FAT	100
TOTAL FAT (G)	11
SATURATED FAT (G)	3.5
TRANS FAT (G)	0
SODIUM (MG)	1020

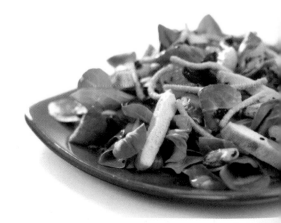

Websites for Wendy's, Chick-fil-A, McDonald's and Taco Bell offer nutritional information that can be personalized. The sites allow you to remove sauce, cheese and other ingredients from the food you wish to order and then recalculate nutritional numbers for that item. These food companies also post information encouraging a balanced diet in combination with exercise in addition to providing a nutrition guide for food sensitivities and food exchanges for people with diabetes. Most fast-food establishments offer suggestions to make meals healthier, including leaving cheese and mayo off of a sandwich and choosing salad instead of fries.

TIP Next time you and your kids are looking for a light meal or yummy treat, make some smoothies. Blend up some fruit, ice, yogurt and a touch of honey!

CHAPTER TEN

In the School Cafeteria

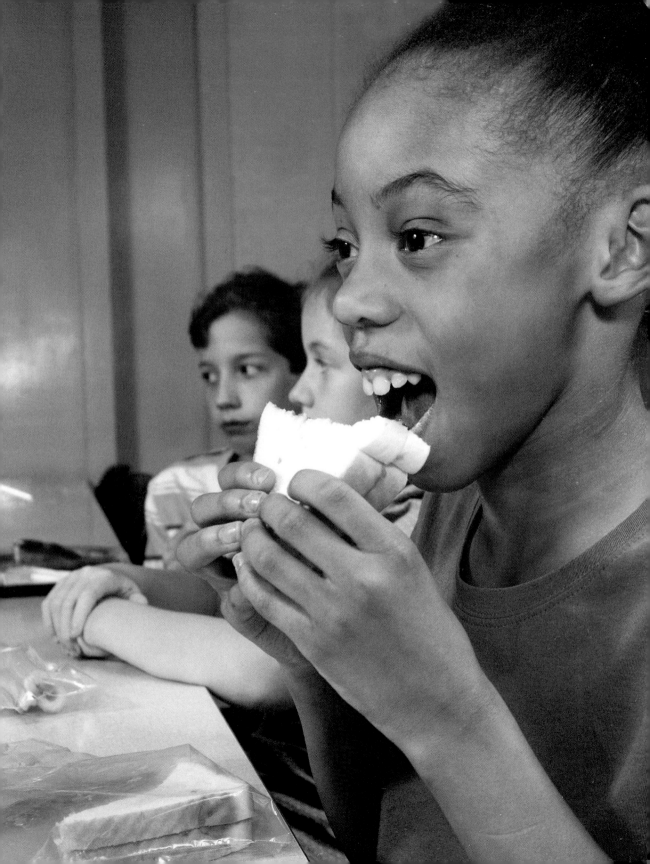

IN THE SCHOOL CAFETERIA

I remember being one of the few kids in high school who came with a packed lunch, and one that consisted of raw vegetables and fruit, at that. No ice-cream sandwiches or poutine for me!

Sadly, many school cafeterias lack a variety of healthy food options. You are more likely to come across a bank of vending machines spewing candy bars and carbonated beverages than find anything remotely resembling a salad. Even more disappointing is the fact that many schools depend on the deals they make with food companies to balance the fiscal budget, but that is another story. And of course what school is complete without its daily fare of burgers, pizza and fries?

Use the same eating-out strategies at school as you would when dining out. Stick to fresh fruit and vegetable options and other lighter foods. If you can get a sandwich made with whole-grain bread, then do so. Look for grilled chicken rather than greasy burgers. If you can find a salad, eat it without the dressing.

Of course there is always the option of packing your own lunch, which pretty much ensures you will be able to Eat Clean at home as well as at school. There are wonderful lunch selections in the recipe chapter of this book, but you can use the following handy guide to help you create a quick, healthy portable lunch.

PUT IT IN YOUR LUNCH PAIL!

* Whole-grain wraps with lean grilled chicken or turkey.
* Try alternative protein sources including natural nut butters (if allowed at your school), hummus or other bean spreads and legume-based dishes.
* Pack leftovers – I depend on these for lunch and always make too much of everything on purpose!
* Put plenty of in-season fruits and vegetables in your lunch.
* Small containers of low-fat yogurt are good lunch options too – don't forget the spoon!
* Homemade Clean protein bars, granola bars or muffins help kids avoid candy.

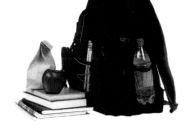

WRAP IT UP

In short, as long as you understand what good food is compared to bad you will do yourself a big favor by sticking to Clean-Eating foods and principles. Eat more good food, not less. Don't skip meals, and make sure to partner lean protein with complex carbohydrates at every meal. Drink it down with water and you are good to go. The result will be a leaner, happier and healthier family.

EXAMPLES OF CLEAN AND NOT-SO-CLEAN
INCENTIVES IN SCHOOLS

The movement toward eating better is starting to trickle into schools as administrators and concerned parents recognize the growing problem with overweight here in North America. Some schools are making positive changes, overhauling cafeteria menus and vending machines and offering healthier, less-processed foods. Other schools are still serving up fast food in all its greasy glory. I am certain the day will come when all schools will be forced to clean up their menus. The growing epidemic of overweight and sick children will be the motivating factor.

APTOS MIDDLE SCHOOL – SAN FRANCISCO, CALIFORNIA

This Californian school has 900 students spanning ages from 12 to 14. The San Francisco Unified School District selected Aptos Middle School as a pilot project in its attempt to make major changes to food options available to its middle-school students. Milk, water and juice have replaced all soft drinks in vending machines and in the cafeteria. Healthy options including turkey sandwiches, sushi, homemade soup, salads, and baked chicken with rice have replaced their high-fat, high-calorie counterparts.

Aptos Middle School has had great success with this program. The net revenue of the cafeteria has increased, resulting in a $6,000 surplus despite the fact that the healthy food options cost somewhat more. Student behavior has improved, especially after lunch, when sugar-highs used to fuel hyperactivity. More students sit down to eat and there is less litter. The school has been recognized by the State of California for their stellar advancements with the "Healthy Food, Healthy Kids" award. In the future, Aptos Middle School hopes to include more fruits and vegetables in their menu plans and eliminate all empty-calorie options.

"It's not enough to have foods that aren't bad for kids; we want foods and beverages to actually be good for them. Our motto is: No empty calories!"
~Dana Woldow, Parent and Chair, Aptos Student Nutrition Committee

At Byfield Elementary small steps are the key to success: *"Take baby steps rather than trying to change everything at once. Start by adding one nutrient-rich snack at every event, like a fresh fruit tray at every meeting,"* says Stewart Armstrong, the school's principle. Even with small steps, Byfield Elementary School, with a student population of 186, has made a significant difference with the implementation of a nutrition program for their students, aged four to nine.

Aside from their decision to sell juice, water and milk instead of soft drinks at the school, school officials have also developed several innovative solutions. Birthday parties are no longer supplied with sugary cupcakes, chips and treats. Rather, the school has made it policy for parents to bring cheese and crackers, fruit trays, and/or vegetables and dip to celebrate these occasions. Throughout the year "sample" days are held for students to try healthy items from a number of food companies who also have health on their minds.

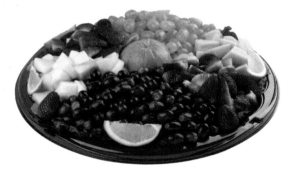

Parental knowledge of the nutrition plan is integral to the school's success and is increased by participation in meetings featuring chefs, and by offering suggestions for wholesome snacks. Students receive stickers and non-food rewards when they bring a healthy snack to school. Animal crackers and pretzels are available for students who do not bring food to school.

Like other schools making nutritional changes, Byfield has experienced an increase in food-service revenue for each year following the implementation of the program. In the future, Byfield Elementary would like to expand their program by adding "Dairy Dollars" coupons, "Caught Eating Healthy" awards, grab-and-go breakfast, soup-and-salad lunches, and morning milk service. With their marked success, Byfield is a shining example that a little goes a long way.

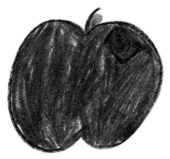

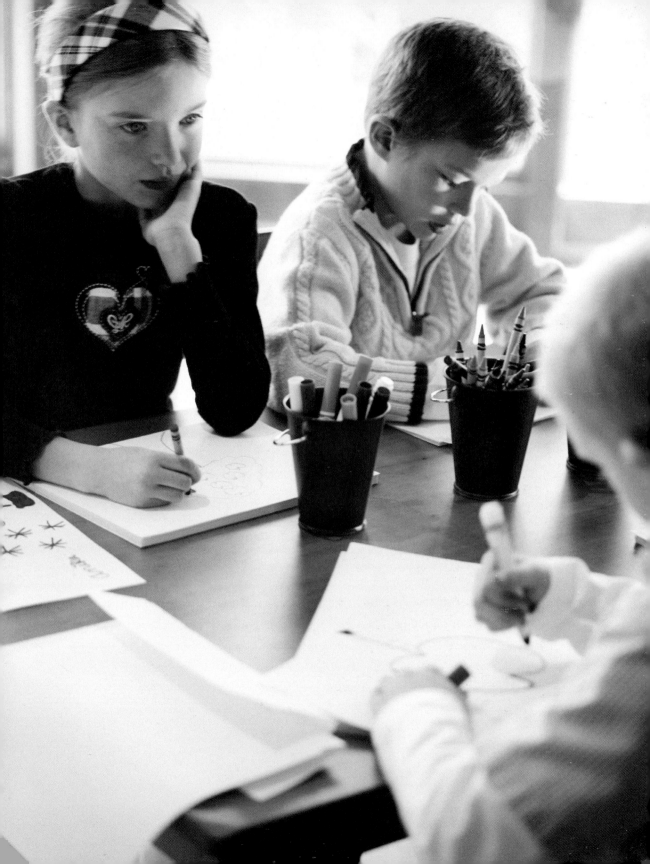

GREEN BAY AREA PUBLIC SCHOOL DISTRICT – GREEN BAY, WISCONSIN

The Green Bay public school district, which includes 20,000 students, is a prime example of how nutritional programs can be successful on a larger scale. The changes made in this school district were not drastic, but rather included a number of small alterations. Whole-wheat flour is now included in baked products, and deep fryers in all middle schools have been removed to encourage baked rather than fried foods.

A common solution for schools making nutritional changes is replacing low-nutrient items with fresh fruit and vegetables. However, the Green Bay school district has taken this idea one step further by providing nutritional fact cards for all food sold, and the school teaches the students how to understand these labels through nutritional lessons. This district also stands out from other school nutrition programs by producing active, healthy role models. Fifty percent of employees participate in staff wellness challenges that include eating at least five fruits and vegetables a day, eating breakfast, and walking more than 10,000 steps daily.

The Green Bay public school district has achieved success with this program by limiting the amount of items on the á là carte menu, which ultimately led to a 15 percent increase in school meal participation and an overall increase in revenue. In the future, this district would like to promote positive lunch experiences by ensuring enough time for students to eat, noise control in lunch areas and by having recess before the lunch period. Public schools in Green Bay have shown that small innovative changes impact the lives of countless others.

ST. LOUIS PUBLIC SCHOOLS – ST. LOUIS, MISSOURI

Menus saturated with high-fat foods such as pizza and corn dogs prompted the Physician Committee for Responsible Medicine (PCRM) to rank the public school district of St. Louis as the worst in its school lunch report card. The 95th school district received only 53 points out of a possible 100. A grade of "F" was based on menus that often lacked fresh fruit, vegetable sides, and vegetarian options. Insufficient nutritional education provided by the food-service department contributed to the failing grade.

Despite the failure of many school districts to offer healthy lunch options, the PCRM has observed an increase to 64 percent in the number of school districts that regularly offer vegetarian meals and 73 percent now offer alternatives to dairy milk.

CORTLAND ENLARGED CITY SCHOOL DISTRICT – CORTLAND, NEW YORK

The Cortland school district has not only made steps toward healthy food options, it has also placed an emphasis on physical activity and nutritional education. High-fat vending machine items were replaced with healthier options, and they took it one step further by eliminating these machines from all elementary schools. Fruit and vegetable sampling days are available to students and a healthy service bar was created in the high-school cafeteria to provide more nutritious options.

Phys. Ed. programs such as a walking club, jazzercise and yoga classes are encouraged in the school as well as the community. Experienced staff has been brought in to help with nutrition education and help with food-related disorders. Students have created a color-coded system for identifying whether a food is healthy or non-nutritious, and nutrition-related projects are displayed outside the cafeteria. Nutritional education is also extended to parents by providing lists of healthy snack foods.

Specific schools in the district have implemented their own innovative ideas, such as a grade-three field trip to a culinary arts school, where the students observe the planning and preparation of meals. In addition, another elementary school created a student hydration program that provided water bottles for all students.

The Cortland school district is a positive model to represent the direction schools should be headed. The focus on a healthy lifestyle through a combination of healthy eating, exercise and nutritional education is a product for success.

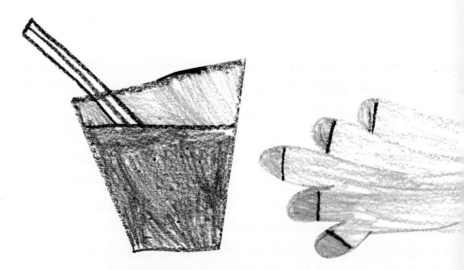

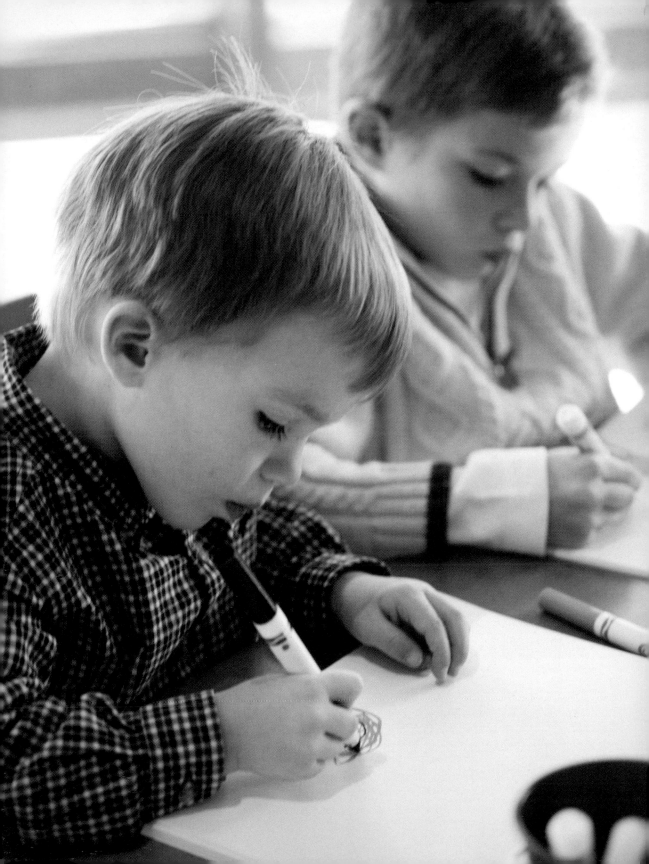

PINELLAS COUNTY SCHOOLS – FLORIDA

According to the Physicians' Committee for Responsible Medicine, Pinellas County is the top-rated school board of 2007. The school received 94 points out of a possible 100 based on three criteria: obesity and chronic disease prevention, health promotion and nutrition adequacy, and nutritional initiatives. Points were awarded for the daily availability of vegan options, vegetable sides, free juice, and available soymilk.

However, it was not just healthy food options that garnered the award for the school. Pinellas County encourages nutritional education through a program called "Teen Cuisine." Older students pair up with local chefs to create healthy recipes that are displayed in cooking shows for younger children. In addition, nutritional education specialists provided lessons on the benefits of fruits, vegetables, and whole grains for half of all elementary students.

The "A" grade received by Pinellas County schools is a testament to the importance of nutritional education beginning at an early age.

JORDAN COUNTY SCHOOL DISTRICT – UTAH

The Jordan County School District is the largest in Utah and also the worst in the state for providing unhealthy school lunches. According to the Physician Committee for Responsible Medicine School Lunch Report, Jordan County only scored 56 points out of a possible 100 based on three criteria: obesity and chronic disease prevention, health promotion and nutrition adequacy, and nutritional initiatives.

While fruits and vegetable are available at a side bar, menus include only one entrée, often a high-fat meal unnecessarily large in portion size such as a foot-long hot dog or a colossal burger. In this county a student must put in a special request for a vegan or vegetarian meal and a note is required to receive an alternative drink to dairy milk. Also, no nutritional education is offered.

A menu dominated by fatty food, failure to provide healthy alternatives and a lack of nutritional education for students and parents all contribute to a failing grade.

References:
www.healthyschoollunches.org/reports/pdfs/schoollunch_report2007.pdf • cdc.gov/HealthyYouth/nutrition/.../pdf/approach3-success.pdf

KAITLYN'S STORY
A reader's testimonial

"

Hello Tosca,

I know you probably receive hundreds if not thousands of e-mails from people everywhere thanking you for your Eat-Clean Diet, from the countless people who you have helped to lose weight or even those who you have just helped to enhance their lives. I just want to thank you personally for not only improving my life but for most likely saving it. I have battled an eating disorder for almost 10 years (I am only 24) and some days I thought anorexia would take my life in my sleep, as I could feel my heart struggling to beat. It was how I defined myself. It consumed my every waking moment.

While scouring the endless shelves of cookbooks one day, dreaming of the food I would never let cross my lips, I came across your book. I read it a matter of hours and then the next day I read it again. I loved the concept of eating clean from the moment I began the book. Everyone was always criticizing me for not wanting to eat things like ice cream and cookies, and time and time again eating-disorder specialists told me I must eat all of these things in order to consider myself even on the road to recovery. Cakes, chocolate, white bread, hamburgers, French fries – the list of things I was told to consume by nutritionists went on and on. I knew I could never eat such horrible things that made me feel ill and so I never committed to getting better and decided to continue my unhealthy habits of self-starvation.

The thing is, your book has given me new life. It has given me "the okay" to decide what I put in my body, to eat healthy and exclude those things that I know are not healthy. I no longer feel that if I don't eat garbage it means I can't conquer my disease. I don't feel ashamed or like a failure to say "no, I am eating clean" when a friend or relative puts in front of me a cheese-laden dish and then proceeds to make a concerned comment that I am starving myself again.

I have finally found a healthy way of life, even though most were skeptical at first. It is now clear that I am not on any diet, nor am I starving myself. I am giving my body what it needs. I now weigh almost 100 pounds. I am getting used to the idea of looking healthy, but more than anything I love the feeling of health.

Thank you for liberating me, for letting me know it is okay to say no to all that junk and just eat plain old healthy food and still be considered normal, and even healthy! I give myself permission to eat every day because most importantly I believe in the foods you promote and the values of eating clean.

I can't thank you enough for possibly saving my life.
Kaitlyn

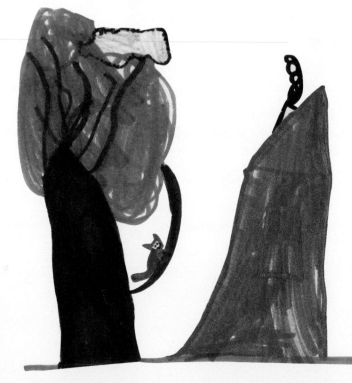

CHAPTER ELEVEN

Clean Eating on a Budget?

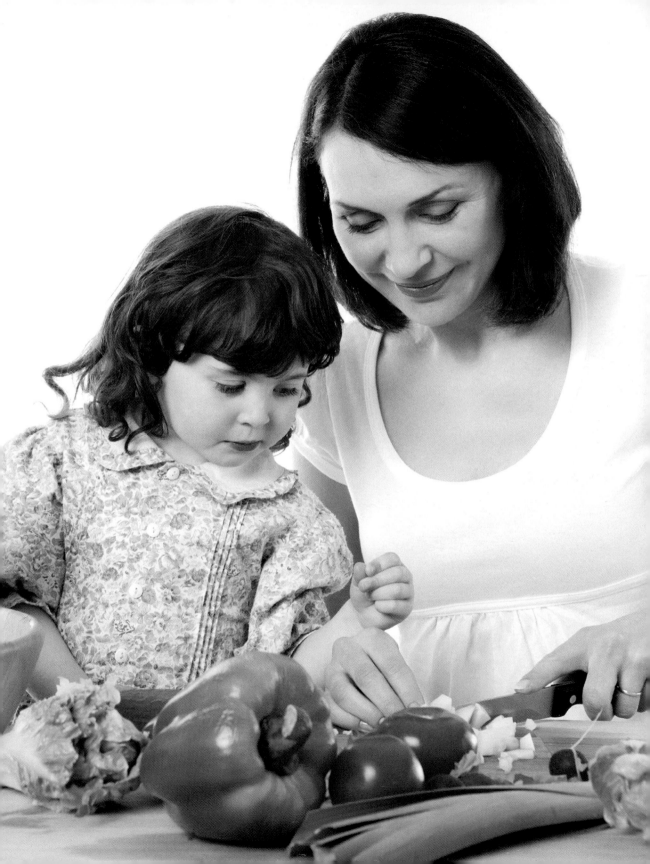

A COMMON QUESTION

One of the questions I field most often is: "Isn't Clean Eating expensive?" Many of you think that eating fresh, wholesome foods will cost more, and you worry the added expense will interfere with your weekly budget. Family income is under enough strain lately, so you should sigh with relief when I tell you Clean Eating will not break the bank. In fact, with a bit of planning Clean Eating is more economical than the way you've likely been eating, because you will not be relying on convenience foods and processed foods that usually carry a hefty price tag – both financially and on your health. Nor will you be driving a gas guzzler to get to a restaurant if you eat at home more frequently.

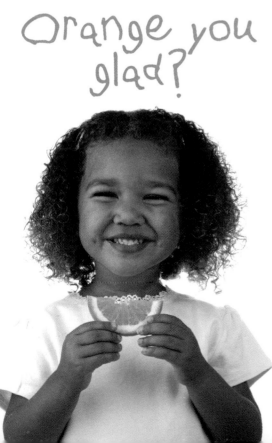

Remember that it took Someone or a lot of Someones a great deal of time and money to create a Twinkie. Another Someone had to come up with and create the packaging to store that Twinkie. The Twinkie then had to be shipped all across the country so that every North American had an opportunity to eat one. Then a load of expensive advertising was created to get that Twinkie out in the public eye. Someone has to pay for all this effort and that Someone, my friend, is YOU, if you buy a Twinkie. Far too many of us depend on convenience and processed foods such as the Twinkie, and that is one reason we are in the mess we find ourselves today. Clean Eating is efficient, inexpensive eating.

A POSITIVE ATTITUDE

Switch your dependence from processed to natural foods and you are immediately saving money. No one paid a food scientist to create the apple, no one designs a pretty plastic package for it, and you don't see all kinds of TV commercials trying to convince you to buy one. A diet based on whole foods in their unprocessed, natural state allows you to control what goes into the meals you are preparing for your loved ones and ultimately what goes into their tummies. Whole foods such as fresh fruit and vegetables, dried whole grains, legumes, nuts and seeds, fish and meats are far more nutritious than anything processed could ever be. Whole foods such as these also allow you to have more control over the food budget.

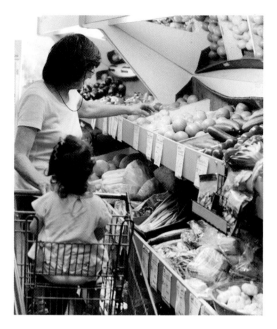

Give yourself a gentle reminder that Clean Eating is not hard. Eating on a budget is simple to do once you get the hang of it, and you will end up healthier and leaner in the long run. There is no need to worry that you can't manage to guide your family's nutrition into healthy waters. These pages are loaded with helpful ideas to keep your head above water and your pennies in your pocket.

Having a wide variety of natural foods in your pantry is the key to Clean Eating. Shopping for that variety of natural foods is easy and inexpensive if you follow my sage advice. Choose fresh fruit, vegetables, lean protein and whole grains and you will have the basics from which to create delicious meals.

COMPLEX CARBOHYDRATES FROM WHOLE GRAINS

Whole grains are the least expensive part of your food budget. Grains such as brown rice, quinoa, barley, oats, buckwheat and spelt are tiny nuggets of inexpensive food, densely packed with nutrition. Whole grains provide much-needed fiber and minerals and can easily be the focus of a perfect Clean-Eating meal.

➡ Skip rice and pastas drowning in sauce or flavorings. These are always more expensive (and not as healthy). Purchase whole grains on their own and add your own seasonings or sauce at home.

➡ Whole-grain cereals such as Cream of Wheat or oatmeal are more nutritious and far more economical than cereals with added sugar that come in cute little shapes and packages. Plus you can buy these cereals in bulk to save even more.

➡ Shop a local bakery for end-of-day sales on whole-grain breads, or purchase bread on sale and freeze.

➡ Stock up on whole-grain pastas when on sale. Pasta keeps unopened in your cupboard for years.

→ Always buy natural, long-grain rice rather than boxed "minute" or "converted" rice. The long-grain contains more nutrition and takes only a bit longer to cook. It's a snap if you bake rice in the oven!

→ If you buy a large loaf of bread, remove a few slices for the day and freeze the rest so the loaf won't go bad. Each day you can take a few slices out of the freezer for that day's use.

→ Better yet, bake your own bread. Once you get the hang of it you won't even need to look at the recipe book, and you'll know all the ingredients.

→ Make muffins and cookies from scratch rather than purchase store-bought goods or mixes.

→ Store whole-grain products in the refrigerator to extend their life span.

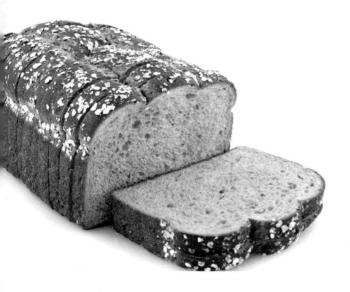

COMPLEX CARBOHYDRATES FROM FRESH FRUIT AND VEGETABLES

Fruit and veggies are essential to your family's nutrition since they are packed with phytochemicals, vitamins, minerals, fiber and enzymes that supercharge health. Be sure to select a wide variety of produce colors to get adequate amounts of every plant nutrient. Since I suggest eating fruit or vegetables at every meal when Eating Clean it is a good idea to stock up on the low-cost options such as apples, bananas, oranges, celery, carrots, beets, and cabbage.

→ Berries are wonderful for their antioxidant power but can be pricey. Purchase them in season and use immediately or freeze extras for those months when berries are ridiculously expensive.

→ Visit a pick-your-own farm for a real bargain – and a fun time with kids. Freeze extras for off season goodness and savings.

→ If you buy frozen fruits or vegetables, always purchase those that are not already doused in dressing, sauce or seasoning.

→ Cabbage is one of the cheapest vegetables no matter what time of year you buy it. I like to use nappa cabbage, which is softer, for salads, soups and stir-fries. Cabbage packs an enormous nutritional punch.

My brothers still like to push me around! It's all for fun, of course. They know I can lift more than they can in the gym!

→ Sprouts are power-packed foods that add nutritional power to sandwiches and salads. Buy these (or grow them yourself) instead of buying expensive lettuces.

→ Buy fresh fruit and vegetables in season. In winter buy oranges, grapefruit, bananas, turnips, onions, carrots, parsnips and potatoes. In spring buy berries, rhubarb, lettuce, spinach and root vegetable greens. In summer buy cherries, melons, berries, peaches, salad vegetables, tomatoes, corn, peas and beans. In fall buy apples, pears, plums, grapes, cauliflower and squash.

→ Try to buy from a local farm or co-op, again in season. If you have a chest freezer, you can blanch veggies quickly and then store them in Ziploc bags (suck as much air out as possible before freezing).

PROTEIN FROM DAIRY

Low-fat dairy products are an important source of lean protein and a great source of calcium. Skim milk, plain nonfat cottage cheese and yogurt, and kefir are ideal choices.

→ String cheese is a processed convenience-food item. Serve good-quality low-fat cheese, low-fat cottage cheese or plain yogurt instead.

→ Skim milk is cheaper than fuller fat milks.

→ Skim milk powder is useful as a milk substitute for cooking or baking.

→ Kefir is delicious and an excellent alternative to milk if your child or loved one is lactose intolerant.

→ Try milk alternatives such as rice milk, almond milk, soy milk or goat's milk for difficult tummies.

LEAN PROTEIN AND PROTEIN ALTERNATIVES

Protein is a must for building a strong healthy body, but it can also be the most expensive part of your food budget. There are numerous ways to get plenty of protein in your diet, not all of them animal based.

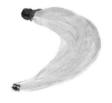

→ Less-costly protein sources include soy and other beans, tofu, nut butters, nuts, seeds, eggs, many frozen fish, water-packed canned tuna, sardines, rump roast and seaweed.

→ Meats are costly. Purchase chicken breasts or turkey breasts in bulk and when on sale to help bring cost down. Freeze extras.

→ Cheaper cuts of meats can always be improved by marinating and then cooking them in a slow cooker or via some other slow-cooking method with plenty of liquid.

→ Look for "utility" grade poultry, which simply means a leg or wing may be missing. The bird will be cheaper but provides the same meat as a fully limbed individual – often at a quarter of the cost.

⇢ Dried beans, legumes and lentils are excellent sources of protein and fiber that don't break the bank.

⇢ Look for plain, unbreaded cuts of white fish, even frozen varieties. Pollock and tilapia are excellent inexpensive choices.

⇢ Serve meat dishes made with less meat and more legumes, lentils or beans combined with whole grains such as brown rice, to cut down on meat cost.

⇢ Have eggs for dinner. We have "Breakfast for Dinner" at least once a week in our house.

GENERAL SHOPPING
STRATEGIES

✪ Buy in bulk.

✪ Plan meals ahead of time.

✪ Don't shop when hungry.

✪ Eat at home as much as possible.

✪ Pack your own lunch (that would be a Clean-Eating cooler) to take to work.

✪ Limit the amount of eating out you do.

TIP
• • • • • •

Have your kids make up a cooler's worth of food the night before. This way everyone will be out the door on time with healthy food to munch on throughout the day.

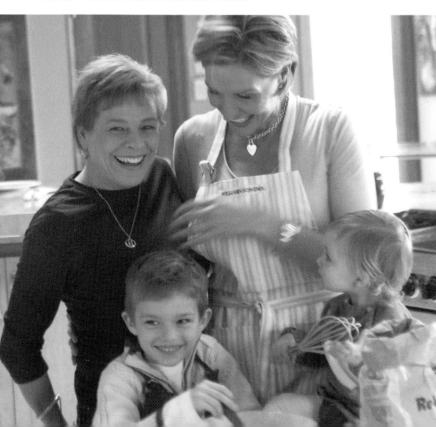

SMARTER SHOPPING

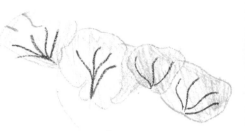

- ❖ Use coupons when possible.
- ❖ Buy what you can use, no more (unless freezing).
- ❖ Shop after you have eaten to reduce impulse purchases.
- ❖ Buy in bulk when possible.
- ❖ Buy locally if you can.
- ❖ Avoid convenience foods.
- ❖ Compare prices.
- ❖ Shop at farmers' markets for in-season foods.
- ❖ Join a food co-op where members receive a discount of 5% to 10%.
- ❖ Grow your own foods – why not? It's fun and healthy and keeps you lean.

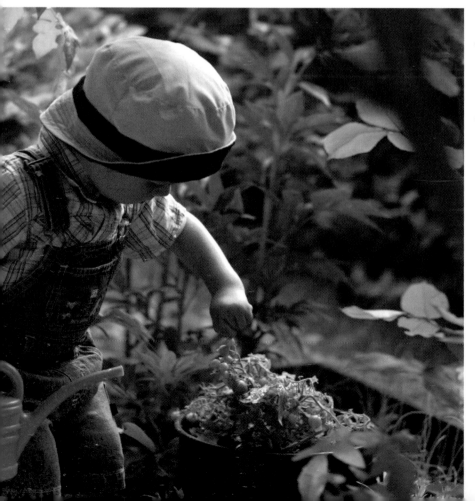

TIP
......

Invite your children to help you plant your garden. Kids love to play in the dirt and watch things grow.

I CAN'T AFFORD TO EAT CLEAN!

The initial stocking up of your kitchen may well cost you, depending how many of these items you have on hand to begin with. You may need to invest in spices, herbs and other foods that have not previously visited the interior of your home. However, once you get that part over with you will be pleasantly surprised to discover Clean Eating can be very cost effective.

TUSCAN SPICE

Thinking about preparing a fancy, flavorful meal, but don't know where to begin? Keep this spice mix in a glass Mason jar and throw it into soups, sauces, stock and meats. It's just the thing you've been looking for. Best of all, you won't have to buy those fancy high-sodium mixes in the store, which will save your pennies and your health! Fantastico!

INGREDIENTS

¼ cup / 60 ml dried rosemary, leaves only
2 Tbsp / 30 ml dried oregano leaves, crumbled
1 Tbsp / 15 ml dried sage
2 Tbsp / 30 ml dried garlic flakes
1 tsp / 15 ml celery seeds
Pinch chili flakes
¼ cup / 60 ml sea salt – not too coarse and not too fine
2 Tbsp / 30 ml black pepper, coarsely ground
Optional: dried orange peel

PREPARATION

In medium bowl, mix all ingredients until well blended. Pour mixture into a glass Mason jar with a tight-fitting lid. Label and store in a cool dark place.

Remember that convenience foods seduce you into buying them because there is little or no preparation time, especially if you are getting these foods at a fast-food place. But not one of these companies is giving you a discount on food and they certainly aren't making food for free. Their bottom line is always profit, and they are looking to get *your* dollars into *their* pockets. That means you are paying more for your food than you otherwise would be – period. You will also be doing a good thing for the environment by reducing the amount of time you spend in a car and reducing the amount of garbage you generate from all the packaging that comes with convenience and processes foods.

Be skeptical of convenience foods. If you stick to smart shopping and look for foods in season and in bulk you will probably spend less than you are presently spending on unhealthy foods. Remember to take not just your grocery bill into consideration, but also all the food bought at school cafeterias, off the lunch truck, at fast-food restaurants and anywhere else you or your family members buy food, snacks, coffee and other drinks each week. Once you tally it all up you'll probably be amazed at how much you have actually been spending on "food" each week.

TIP If there are no nut allergies at your kids' school, throw a bag of nuts and an apple in their backpack — there is no excuse for going hungry.

CHAPTER TWELVE

Kids Need to Go and So Do You

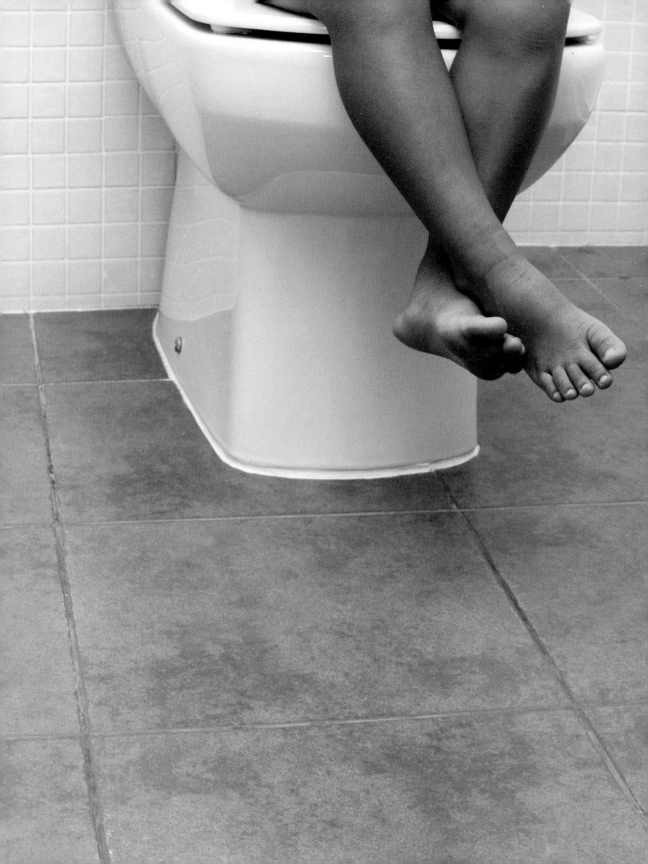

THE BENEFITS OF POOPING

> **Let food be your medicine and your medicine be your food.**
> **Hippocrates (460-377 BC)**

Sticky subject here folks, but everyone has got to do it, so let's talk. Elimination on a daily, regular basis is a must for optimal health. If you are one of those people who cannot eliminate frequently or readily it makes for a great deal of discomfort and a very cranky person. Folks like Dr. Mehmet Oz and Oprah Winfrey have been making the subject of "poop" less uncomfortable. It is a common denominator of all human beings after all, isn't it? I want to help clean out your pipes with some effective advice.

Optimal elimination should occur every day, and ideally more than once a day is healthy as long as the stool is soft and formed. As Dr. Oz likes to say: "Your feces should be S-shaped (the shape of your rectum as it nears your anus), as opposed to gumball-size pellets." (pg. 191, *You, The Owners' Manual*). So soft is best! No blood or mucus should appear in your stool – nor any other foreign objects either: think un-chewed food, pinworms and so on. If your deposit looks different then it is a sign that something is not quite right with your inner plumbing system. Most often the problems relate to insufficient fiber.

Far too many North Americans do not eliminate regularly. I have lead countless seminars where I discuss this stinky but quite normal subject openly. There hasn't been one instance when I haven't had several people approach me quietly on the side and tell me how difficult and painful it is to poop. One of my best friends (no names here) had issues similar to this. She had spent all her life not going to the bathroom more than once a week ... for 35 years! When I overhauled my diet to Clean Eating and included flaxseed every day I told her about the amazing benefits I had experienced. Elimination was tough for me too until flaxseed came along. Soon my friend was going every day and had lost 30 pounds (you can imagine what kind of weight she lost. The bowels and intestines can back up with pounds of un-eliminated waste). This was good news since she had just lost her father to colon cancer and she too was at risk. My friend is forever grateful that I introduced her to flax seed. She is also now 35 pounds lighter, and a regular eliminator.

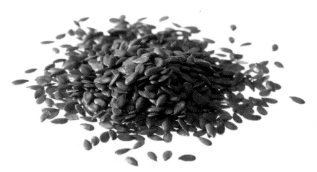

TOP-10 BODY ISSUES
AND THEIR SOLUTIONS

BODY ISSUE	SOLUTION
CONSTIPATED	FLAX SEED, OATMEAL
DEHYDRATED	WATER MIXED WITH PINCH OF SEA SALT
INSOMNIA	KEFIR
ACIDIC	BLUE-GREEN ALGAE, SAUERKRAUT, LEAFY GREENS
DIGESTIVE ISSUES	KEFIR, PLAIN YOGURT, FLAX SEED
ITCHY, DRY SKIN	ESSENTIAL FATTY ACIDS, WATER, SEEDS AND NUTS, HEART-HEALTHY OILS
CRAVINGS	75% OR DARKER CHOCOLATE AND SEA SALT
CRAMPS	ESSENTIAL FATTY ACIDS, MAGNESIUM-RICH FOODS (DARK CHOCOLATE IS RICH IN MAGNESIUM, WHICH MAY EXPLAIN THE PENCHANT FOR WOMEN TO EAT CHOCOLATE DURING THE EARLY PHASE OF THEIR CYCLE.) YOU CAN ALSO EAT WHOLE GRAINS, LEAFY GREENS, NUTS, SEEDS, VEGETABLES
BLEMISHED SKIN	OMEGA-2 FATTY ACIDS AND GLA-RICH FOODS, INCLUDING SEED OILS, LEAFY GREENS, COLD-RESISTANT CROPS (CARROT, BROCCOLI, BRUSSELS SPROUTS, KALE, ONONS AND SO ON)
MIGRAINE	SEED OILS, LEAFY GREENS, COLD-RESISTANT CROPS

FLAX SEED TO THE RESCUE!

Anybody who has been following the Clean-Eating movement (no pun intended) already knows that flax seed is my favorite Power Food. For a little guy this seed packs a mighty punch. Flax is an ancient superfood capable of healing anything from constipation, intestinal discomforts, high cholesterol and blood pressure to cardiovascular troubles and degenerative diseases. In studies performed in Toronto, Canada, doctors have found that consuming flax seed can reduce tumor size, prevent the growth of cancer cells and can lower cholesterol. This little power seed is not to be overlooked. The best part is that flax seed is an inexpensive source of health. You can buy it for pennies!

WHY DOES FLAX SEED HELP YOU GO?

The hard flax seed is loaded with healthy fats called essential fatty acids – EFAs. Essential fats like these don't make you fat. Instead they help keep you lean and build healthy muscle. And they help with a particular problem North Americans are having, and that is the constipation problem.

Flax seed works as a laxative because it contains fiber and has an enormous capacity to soak up water. Try this experiment at home. Place a few flax seeds in a small bowl and add water to cover. Now watch what happens. The outer coating of the flax seed absorbs water on contact. Soon you will notice

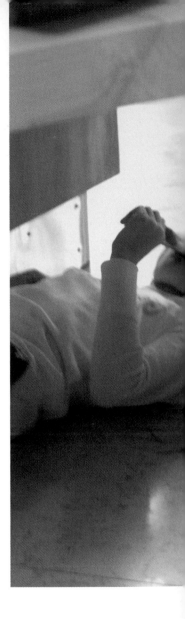

TIP Involve your friends, neighbors and their children in Clean Eating. If everyone is doing it your children will not feel left out and will be more excited about healthier foods.

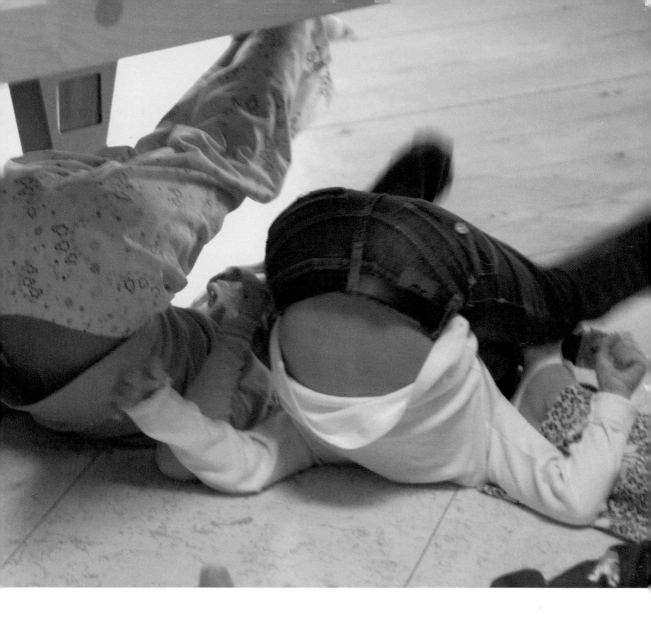

a gluey substance forming. Don't worry, this is not a sign that something is wrong. It is good. That gluey substance is healthy and is called a "mucilage." This same "glue" is formed inside you when you eat flax seed. You want this absorption to happen in your intestines rather than in the glass, to help you elmininate. If you have trouble with constipation, drink a glass of water containing a couple of tablespoons of flax seeds once or twice a day. Pretty soon you will notice the results.

Think also of the seeds as little scrub brushes that will pass through you and your inner pipes. These bits help scrub your inside pipes clean and move debris, waste and toxins away from the delicate tissues of your intestines and eventually out of the body.

Flax seed also contains fiber, another wonderful ingredient for helping you eliminate. Flax seed has two kinds of fiber – soluble and insoluble. Most of the fiber is insoluble – it cannot be digested by the body. This is part of the reason flax seed helps you have a bowel movement. The fiber sweeps the intestines clean. Soluble fiber has more benefit in the blood since it helps keep blood in good shape. Lately flax seed has been recommended for diabetics, since blood-glucose levels are significantly reduced if flax seed is ingested on a regular basis.

A LITTLE TIP: the seeds need to be broken down slightly in order to be useful. Otherwise they can pass right through your system before the outer casing opens. I use a coffee grinder to coarsely chop the seeds and then store them in a glass Mason jar in the fridge. Remember to drink plenty of water as well.

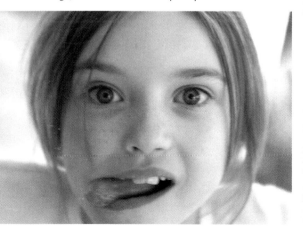

GINA'S STORY
A reader's testimonial

"

Hi Tosca,

I could write for days on why I love The Eat-Clean Diet Cookbook. *I've attempted to sum it all up in just a few sentences.*

I recommend The Eat-Clean Diet Cookbook *to all my clients. As a dietician I find it can be a challenge to teach and convince clients that the foods they love can be modified into a healthier and cleaner version. Many of my clients are used to trying every diet out there and "clean eating" is a new concept to most, if not all, of my clients. Your cookbook helps me teach them to continue eating some of the foods they love, but just cleaner, modified versions of the foods. Once my clients start experimenting with a few recipes in* The Eat-Clean Diet Cookbook, *they are hooked on the concept of clean eating. The rewarding part of my job is seeing the changes in clients' energy levels from eating clean, and then following them as they achieve their fitness and lifestyle goals.*

"

Thanks Tosca!

Gina Juenger, RD, CSDS
The HIT Center – St. Peters
Lighten-Up/HIT FIT Director

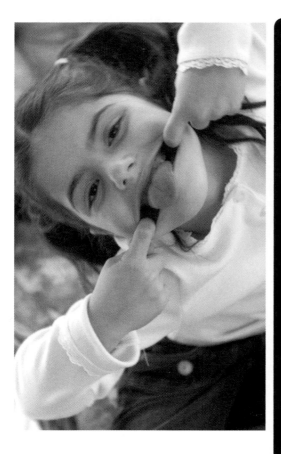

WHAT CAN FLAX SEED DO FOR YOU?

- ✪ **Help build lean muscle tissue**
- ✪ **Promote regular, healthy elimination**
- ✪ **Stimulate lazy bowels**
- ✪ **Prevent blood platelets from sticking**
- ✪ **Prevent blood clots from forming**
- ✪ **Reduce high blood pressure**
- ✪ **Promote weight loss**
- ✪ **Increase energy levels**
- ✪ **Increase metabolism**
- ✪ **Promote optimal organ function – brain, nervous system, skin, sexual organs**
- ✪ **Provide energy**

TIP Take Sundays to prepare healthy ingredients for lunches and snacks. If your kids make their own lunches, make sure to have pre-made Clean foods such as brown rice, grilled chicken, and pre-cut and cooked vegetables. This way your kids can grab and go without feeling the need to resort to not-so-clean choices — especially if they are pressed for time in the morning.

CHAPTER THIRTEEN

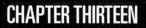

Ready! Set! Action!

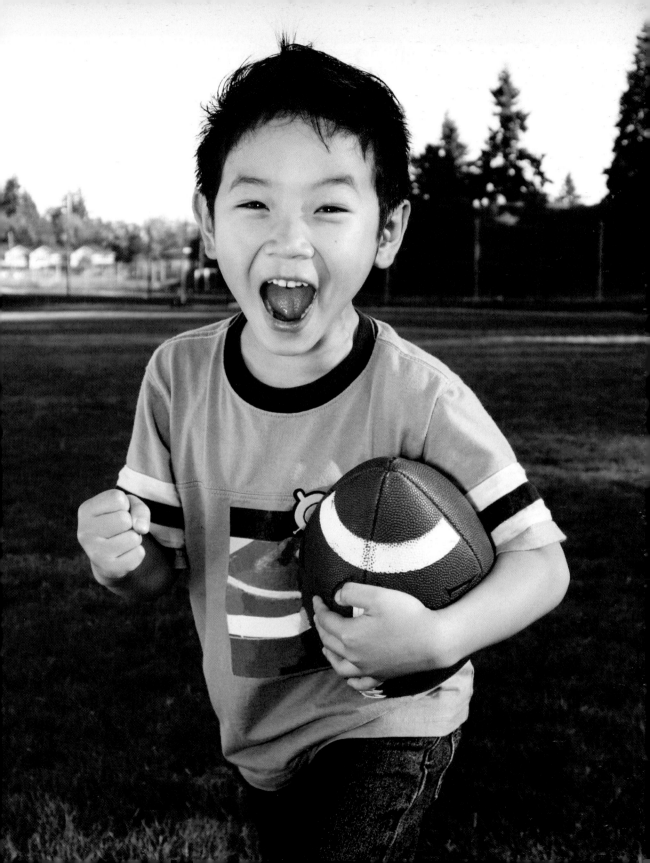

READY! SET! ACTION!

No, we are not on the set of a new TV show or movie. These next pages can be considered a call to action for you and your family. It is not enough to simply eat well, although I will remind you that excellent nutrition choices account for 80 percent of your physical appearance and health. But to maximize the potential of these things we too often take for granted – our health, fitness and well-being – we must hit the problem from all angles. Eating Clean will solve many health issues, as we have already seen, and 10 percent of your health and fitness comes thanks to your genes, which you can do nothing about. But that final 10 percent needs attention, too. Today 28 percent of American adults get zero physical activity each day, and roughly 42 percent get less than the suggested 30 minutes each day as recommended by the US Department of Health and Human Services. If you add those numbers you get about 70 percent, which looks remarkably like the number of overweight or obese people in this country – children and older folks alike. This is not a coincidence.

HOW IT WAS

It was a rare day when my siblings and I as kids were indoors parked in front of the television. My brothers Rene and Ron and my sister Martina and I were always busy doing something, and that something was always physical. Those were the days before computers, video games and iPods. With less entertainment coming at us, we had to make our own fun. That meant getting outdoors at every opportunity, even when the weather turned frigid. Our activities ran the gamut: ice-skating, swimming, gymnastics,

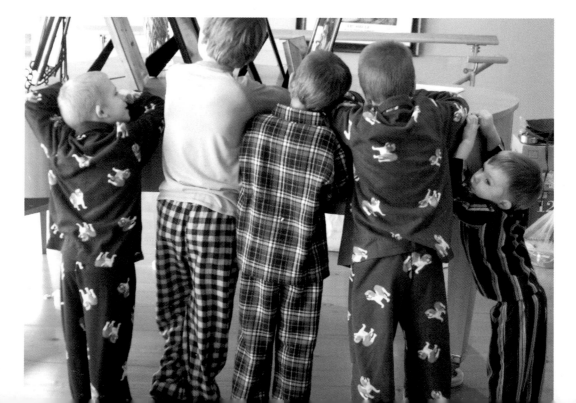

soccer and wrestling. My dad was a swim instructor at the local YMCA and he was adamant that we all learned how to swim, which we did of course. We also got around using our own two feet either walking or cycling. Needless to say there wasn't much sitting around time and none of us were overweight.

My parents were healthy role models who led by example. Each night after supper, no matter what the weather, they went for a long walk together. The five-mile loop from Sunset Boulevard in Kingston, Ontario to the lakeshore and back again took them an hour to complete and they looked forward to those walks. My mom would also jump on her bike with us kids and go to the farmers' market in the center of town every Saturday to pick up fresh fruit and vegetables. Let me just add that the bike ride was 10 miles one way and that there were significant hills on the way. The ride back home was always harder — must have been the weight of all those vegetables!

Every summer we would cottage at a beautiful lake where the daily activities would include swimming, rowing, hiking, diving and fishing all day long. We would also do a family swim where we would all get in the water and swim from the beach in front of our little cottage to the island in the distance, which was about one kilometer. Someone always had to take a turn rowing while the rest of us swam. It was a long distance for any of us to swim, especially as children, but we did it with a proud sense of accomplishment.

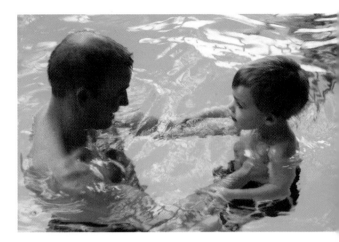

HOW IT IS

If this sounds like an idyllic backwoods kind of lifestyle, it probably was. It even sounds that way to me now as I write it. I know life has changed a lot, and is certainly lived at a much quicker pace in the past few decades, but the point I am trying to make is that my parents were exceptional role models for us, and role models are exactly what is needed today if we are going to keep our kids out of the kind of trouble they are currently finding themselves in. Children must be able to depend on their parents as a guide for living this wonderful life in a healthy way. I took the lessons my parents taught me and shared them with my own children. All three of my daughters were required to learn how to swim. They danced competitively for years, and my youngest daughter Kelsey Lynn is now receiving dance training at the Quinte Ballet School of Canada. She wants to be a professional ballet dancer, and to that end she trains

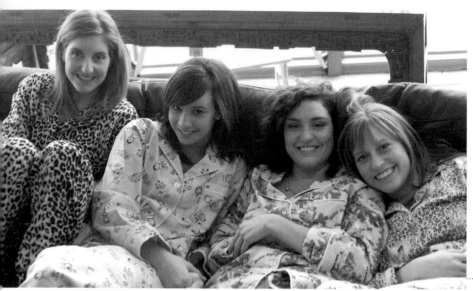

My girls are as different as night and day, but they are united by their love for being in the kitchen making good food. We spend more time in the kitchen than anywhere else in the house.

ABOVE IMAGE (left to right): Rachel, Chelsea, Kiersten, Kelsey

five hours every day, six days a week. Kiersten and Rachel train with weights and run practically every day. Chelsea is my volleyball fanatic. It seems like the good lessons are really paying off. My brothers' and sister's children are also involved in all sorts of sports, and that is what it takes. My parents lived an active and healthy lifestyle, particularly after my father suffered a heart attack at the age of 34. Role models are of the utmost importance – necessary to set the path upon which your children will tread.

HOW IT CAN BE

Your child will pick up whatever attitudes you have about exercise, or even the simple act of moving about. If you are loafing about on the couch enjoying Seinfeld reruns and munching incessantly, odds are your kids are going to end up the same way. On the other hand, when you go to the gym for your workout do you do it with a round of complaints or do you go willingly? If you are one of those who gives the impression training is a punishment or a Must Do, remember your kids are watching and drinking in that negativity. Try to change that way of thinking. Aren't you lucky to be able to get outdoors and enjoy the weather, the fresh air and the positively energizing feelings you get from being able to do so? I never look at training as a punishment. When it is time to train I can't wait. It is something I want to do in order to achieve my best health, and even after all this time I get excited about it. I don't do it for my appearance as much as I do it for the positive way it makes me feel. If you take the outward appearance factor out of the equation, the chance is much greater that your child will pick up this positive attitude towards exercise.

SHERRY'S STORY

A reader's testimonial

"

Tosca,

I run a personal-training studio that also offers open fitness and group classes. Our main focus is training. We train young and mature clients who have a wide variety of goals and issues. Our clients may have high or low BMIs, they may be athletes post-rehab, or they may be experiencing MS, Parkinson's, or other neuromuscular or autoimmune dysfunctions. A large proportion of those we work with are women reaching their pre-menopausal, menopausal or post-menopausal years. We have recently become part of a team working with individuals receiving the lap-band procedure. I even recommend your books to them!

Here is our story! Our facility is in Vienna, WV, a community bordering Ohio. All of my staff members have promoted your books. We love them! Finally we can suggest a book that is easy to read and follows what we believe. Every client, including fitness and group fitness clients, are directed to the books that sit on our bookshelf at the entrance to the studio. We have sent many individuals to Borders to buy your books. They can't keep them in stock. Recently a client came back to her second training session, reporting that the bookstore was out of stock again. Borders informed her they cannot keep up with the demand because a personal trainer in the community is sending everyone to buy it! That would be me … we love your books and Oxygen magazine.

"

You have changed so many lives!

Sherry McCay,
Personal Trainer & RN

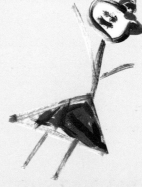

Involve your child in team sports or other physical activities. If you have a shy child who does not want to take the risk of playing in front of others, find something you can do with him or her, such as playing golf or Frisbee, or even running around the playground. Be sure to plan for these activities in your schedule in ink, otherwise you won't get to them. Sometimes in this busy life you have to schedule free time with as much importance and regularity as work time. And it's amazing how often we will take the time for work activities and not for family activities.

ANYTHING IS BETTER THAN NOTHING

I suspect some of you will already have your children involved in activities that keep them physically active, but there is a greater segment of the population that is quite content to sit on their collective butts and be entertained by video games, movies, cellular phones, computers and more. So in love are we with technological toys such as these, and with being entertained, there remains very little time for moving about. Fortunately, we can change all that as easily as making a decision to move around. Stop everything you are doing and open your front door. Get outside. Walk, run, ride, jump or move in some way that gets your heart pumping. Do it now! Then come back and finish this book.

The only way to get your children and the rest of your family in better shape and health is to pay attention to the food they are eating and the amount of physical activity they are getting. So there it is again – it's a combination of diet and exercise that will clinch the deal of wellness. The longer a person stays overweight and inactive, the less they believe they have a chance of turning the situation around. The sense of powerlessness paralyzes them and they feel committed to an unhealthy life forever. That is why parents must step in early and make changes if they recognize their child is at risk of becoming one of these sedentary kids. Think of it this way: if you or your child is currently doing nothing, a big fat ZERO, nada, zip, then any amount of exercise is better than nothing. That means simply getting up off the couch, away from the TV or the computer, walking past the refrigerator, down the hall and out the front door, right down the driveway and around the block. This is a very good thing indeed! You have just increased your physical activity level by 100 percent. Now all you have to do is repeat that tomorrow. If you made it without too much trouble and your heart is still in your chest, walk a little further. Each day of walking that little bit further becomes a victorious day, a day worth living and a day worth repeating. If you can manage this 10 times in a row, you have now made walking a healthy habit. The same way you got yourself into this messy lifestyle of poor eating and no exercise also took 10 times to make it a bad habit. It only takes 10 times to make doing something a habit. So come on! Just undo it! Don't wait one more minute! Start your healthy habits going today.

"It only takes 10 times to make doing something a habit."

THE BENEFITS OF EXERCISE

It can't be stressed enough. Exercise is necessary for optimum health. Hundreds of thousands of reports substantiate these claims. But since neither you nor I want to read them all, here are some of the best reasons to include exercise in your daily routine:

Getting enough exercise – that means a minimum of three 30-minute sessions per week – will help you and your child strengthen your cardiovascular systems, or your heart and lungs. In doing so you will place less strain on your heart and lungs and you will lower your cholesterol.

Exercise helps you lower your blood pressure. A healthy blood-pressure reading (taken at the doctor's office with a blood-pressure cuff) means your heart does not have to work hard to push your blood through your blood vessels. During a physical exam your doctor will let you know if your blood pressure is too high. Increasingly, overweight and obese children are suffering from the (unhealthy) grown-up condition of high blood pressure. Strive for a number close to 120 / 60.

Exercise encourages the proper development of bones and muscles in children. If you doubt the value of exercise in fostering good health, have a look at anyone who is wheelchair bound or unable to support his or her bodyweight. The lower limbs will be underdeveloped and prone to breakage. There is no reason for

TIP Ask your kids to help you wash the car on Saturday morning. Washing the car burns lots of calories and it's fun, too!

the body to strengthen its bones and muscles if they are not being used. The upper body may be affected as well, depending on the type of injury or illness. It is critical to challenge the body daily by "stressing" it during exercise.

Type II diabetes is a rapidly spreading epidemic that is taking the entire world by storm. It's having devastating affects on today's youth, too. Exercise decreases the risk of developing Type II diabetes by lowering blood-sugar levels, and it does this in many ways, including creating an increased need and processing time for glucose, especially in muscle cells. According to the Diabetes Prevention Program study by the National Institute for Health (NIH), a healthy diet and moderate exercise resulting in weight loss will delay and prevent the prevalence of Type II diabetes.

Does Grandpa stoop over? Did Grandma break her hip? Both of these result from osteoporosis. There is no time like the present to offset the chance of developing osteoporosis, and that doesn't mean just drinking a glass of milk a day. Exercise encourages bone growth, and the best time to maximize this development is at a young age when bones are maturing. Children who develop good exercise habits now are more likely to keep them up, which will offset bone loss as they age. If Grandma had exercised she may not have broken her hip, since regular exercise decreases falls by 25 percent (Bulletin of the World Health Organization). P.S. Quinoa is a super grain that contains more calcium ounce for ounce than milk.

MORE BENEFITS FROM EXERCISE

BETTER SLEEP

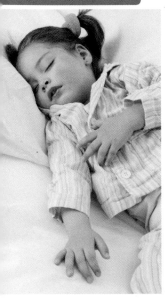

Rest easy, exercise will have you sleeping well in no time. It helps us transition between each phase of sleep until we hit that perfect REM stage. Working hard during the day will have you physically "stressed"... in a good way! Your brain recognizes this and keeps you in a deep sleep longer. This means more time to repair and rebuild your body tissues for the next day.

IMMUNITY BOOSTER

With all of the germs that are spread in the classroom and on the playground, kids are literally playing in a bacteria soup. A strong immune system acts as a superpower shield against illness. You'll notice with increased activity your kids won't get sick as often.

Why is this? According to Dr. David Neiman, immune cells travel through the body fighting bacteria and viruses better and faster in exercisers than in non-exercisers. There's no better way to get yours kids outside and active than to tell them they'll develop superhero, bacteria-fighting powers doing it!

SKIN HEALTH

Preteens, teens and even adults are affected by acne. Having dealt with it in one of my children, I know how frustrating and damaging it can be to one's self-esteem. Regular exercise can help. It stimulates detoxification by enhancing circulation, nutrient delivery and waste removal for the skin. When oxygen is delivered by increased circulation it produces collagen, which gives you that nice, plump look. Don't believe me? Get up and do five minutes of stair climbing. Is your face red? That's due to increased blood flow to your skin! Who knew it was so easy?

MOOD LIFTER

If you are having a down day, exercise is one of the surest ways to improve your mood. It can also decrease anxiety and stress. During and after exercise, endorphins — the body's own mood elevators — are released into the bloodstream. You then feel a "rush" or a "high" that many people equate with euphoria. I look forward to that feeling every time I train — and I get it, drug free! Consider exercise as your Prozac without the pill. In fact, studies have shown exercise to be as effective as antidepressants at relieving clinical depression. The body soon becomes accustomed to this wonderful feeling. If you happen to miss a few days of training your body will let you know. I become cranky and irritable when I miss my training sessions. Try it! You will soon see what I mean.

Making time for exercise every day, or as often as possible, starts the positive cycle of "looking after oneself." You would not hesitate to teach your child how to brush his or her teeth and you would not skip brushing yours. You taught your youngsters how to do it and it is now a healthy habit. The same applies to exercise. Introducing your family to physical activity helps the gang feel like they are doing something good for themselves. In the beginning you may get groans, but stay the course and know things will turn around as soon as everyone starts feeling good. After all, the family who plays together stays together. And you know something? Most kids would choose playing sports, running, biking, walking, playing at the park or even simply shooting hoops in the driveway with their parents over playing a video game. You may be shocked at how happy your kids become by you simply playing with them.

And let's not forget the fat-burning potential! From the moment your family begins to move more frequently, run, play, jump and swim, fuel – stored as fat in our bodies – will begin to burn up, away and out.

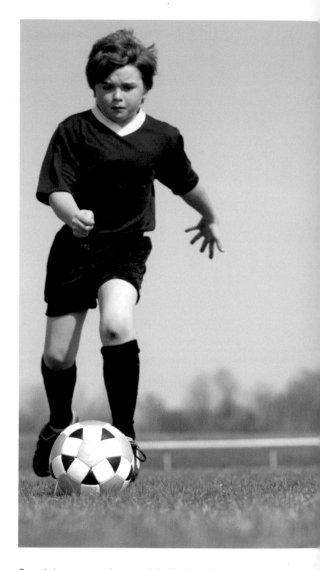

Certainly you can lose weight/fat by other means, such as counting and reducing your caloric intake. However, this method has not proven to be universally successful and certainly not long lasting. Look around you – at any given moment 52 percent of us are on such a diet, and the results are poor. We are still overweight and unhealthy. It is far better to adopt a healthy lifestyle that includes Clean Eating and exercise as its backbone.

Finally, your child (or even you) may discover, through exercise, his or her passion or particular skill at sport. This is what happened to me. I went from being horizontal on a couch for most of my adult life to this RENO-vated life I live now. Through the disciplines of training I discovered the potential that lay hidden underneath pounds of unwanted weight and years of damaged self-esteem. I could not envision my life otherwise today. If nothing else, let exercise help you discover the potential hidden within you. I can't wait to hear your success story. Remember I am always listening.

ARE YOU ACTIVE, SEDENTARY OR SOMEWHERE IN BETWEEN?

Most often your child's family physician is the one who notices weight gain, particularly if the child is becoming excessively heavy for his or her height. Some weight gain is normal, of course, during active growing years. But too much is too much and that is why doctors take the time to measure height and weight and plot these measurements against a standard stature-for-age and weight-for-age charts, also known as growth charts. Doctors will also ask a child how active he or she is during a typical day.

See if you can assess how active you or your children are based on these descriptions:

- ☸ **ACTIVE:** Intense play for prolonged periods of time.
- ☸ **MODERATELY ACTIVE:** An additional 30 minutes of physical activity on top of a day's regular activities.
- ☸ **SEDENTARY:** You guessed it! Sitting on your sitter doing not much at all.

Consider this and any information you get from your doctor as a baseline indicator of where you or your child fit on the "Am I overweight and not active enough?" scale. Once you face the truth it is easier to accept that changes must be made.

HOW TO MAKE CHANGE

I am not talking about making change from a dollar here, folks. Now that you know it is time to do something about your inactivity, you have to consider your options. Parents, don't throw the household into an uproar by forcing all concerned to join you on the Back Nine for a 10-mile run. That's like going from zero to 60 in three seconds. You will get a lot of complaining and not much participation. It is best to introduce small changes to your family's lifestyle. Remember, this is not a punishment. In the end increased activity levels for the whole family translates into FUN and improved health – don't tell your kids the last part, they probably won't buy it, but they do like fun.

⭐ Walk your dog(s).

⭐ When it snows get outside with the kids and clear snow (and throw it, too!).

⭐ When you have built a pile of snow, go tobogganing.

⭐ Have the children help you with house-cleaning jobs, both inside and outside.

⭐ Use the stairs at any public venues.

⭐ Park your car as far away as possible from the place you need to be to encourage walking.

⭐ Plan a hike or walk in a nearby park.

⭐ Play with your kids on the swings, slides and monkey bars!

⭐ Make sure each of your family members has a bike and a helmet and go for a group ride.

⭐ Install a trampoline in your backyard complete with safety nets and join the fun.

⭐ Find a beautiful walking path or nature trail and explore what it has to offer.

⭐ Most local pools offer a Family Swim session. Make good use of these.

⭐ Put on some music and dance around the kitchen or living room with your kids.

⭐ Install sports equipment at your home. Consider a basketball hoop, a ping pong table, a skateboard ramp or even the new Nintendo Wii – yes it is a video game but you have to move around to play it.

These are some basic activities you can introduce your family to, but keep your eye on the prize. Once you get them active they can participate in any sport or activity they like. It is just a matter of getting started.

My best friend, Franca, and I battle it out on the Wii! →

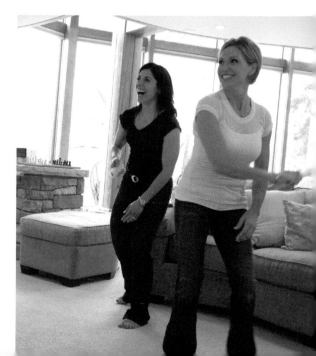

HIDDEN BENEFIT

All three of my daughters competed in dance. They danced six days a week and competed several times a year. There are many benefits to having your children involved in organized sports, but perhaps one of the best is that it keeps kids off the street. Whenever their friends called and asked if they could "hang out at the mall" I was relieved to hear them say: "No, I can't. I have dance class." Being involved in team sports gives kids a reason to say NO to some of the unsavory things they could otherwise involve themselves in. My girls developed a strong sense of team commitment and confidence through dance.

STEP IT UP

You and your child may soon find yourselves ready to participate in organized sports. When your child develops an interest in a sport, run with the idea. My philosophy when raising my own daughters was to introduce them to a variety of sports and through that process discover which ones they ultimately loved. Interestingly, none of them loved sports in the strict sense of the word, but they did discover dance, and

to my mind that is a sport too. Dance is incredibly physically demanding, especially if it is taken to the competitive or professional level. Currently dance is experiencing something of a comeback, thanks to the popularity of such shows as *So You Think You Can Dance, Dancing With the Stars* and *America's Best Dance Crew*. And any noteworthy dancer has an amazing physique.

Whatever your son or daughter loves to do, let them experience the sport to its fullness. You will find the results as satisfying as they will.

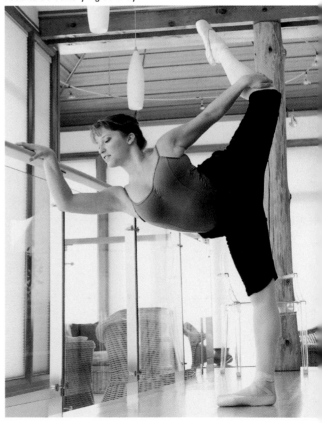

TIP Get involved in your children's extra-curricular activities. Sign up for an adult lesson in whatever activity he or she participates in. Lots of sports have non-competitive adult leagues, and kids love cheering on their parents!

CHAPTER FOURTEEN

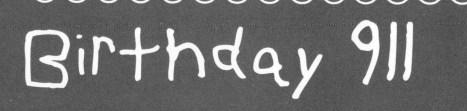

Birthday 911

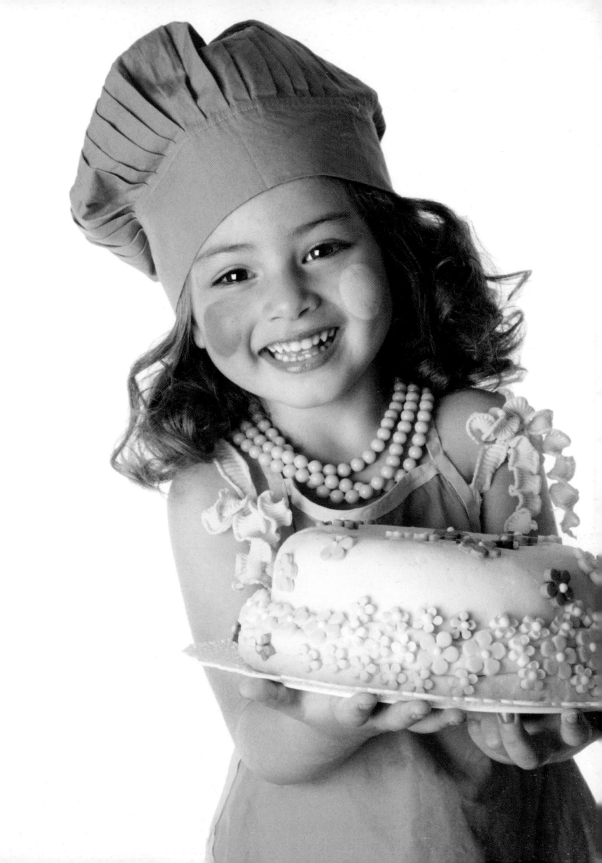

I KNOW THEY ARE COMING BUT I'M STILL CAUGHT OFF GUARD!

Although I do know the dates (of the birthdays) of those close to me, somehow when the actual moment draws near I find myself scrambling to pull something amazing out of the hat. To be completely honest, the same happens to me at Christmas. It's not that I don't care; there are just so many demands on my time that I am left scrambling. Many of you feel the same way, judging by the e-mails I receive. To add salt to the wound there is pressure to give green, Eat Clean and to impress with gifts that will awe. Wow! I am freaked out thinking about it and I just got through birthday season in my house.

Let's take a step backwards here. Remember birthdays are just that, a day to celebrate the birth of you or your loved ones, not tea with the Queen. Have you ever noticed the simpler you keep things the better they turn out? I have made the mistake of attempting to perfect every aspect of a celebration down to the minutest detail – even the toilet paper had to be folded just so and it had to be the right kind. Did anyone notice? Did anyone care? Hardly! And it had little effect on the party-goers. They simply ran amok! Now I keep things reasonable. For goodness sake, let's be reasonable!

These days I like to catch my breath and enjoy the celebrant's big day without emerging hours later in a shambles of emotion and a raft of "If onlies!" and "Why didn't I's?" Memorable parties at my home recently have included nothing more than simple fare such as Crispy Chicken Bites (page 282), Crudités the Clean Eating Way (page 255), Protein Smoothie Popsicles (page 310) and fresh fruit. The Birthday Cupcakes on page 193 are delicious and can be made in advance. I depend heavily on fresh flowers and greens for natural decorations, particularly those that herald whatever season you happen to be in – daffodils and tulips for spring, plenty of greenery and poinsettias for the festive season and so on. Fresh plants and flowers breathe life into the space and are readily available at most supermarkets – where you have to be anyway to pick up the foods you need for the party.

Toscareno.com forum member, Barb, shares: "For food ideas you could always "health up" spaghetti or sloppy joes or use Clean-Eating pizza ideas." (See my Whole-Grain Pasta with Turkey Meatballs recipe on page 293, Sloppy Joe recipe on page 243, and my Homemade Pizza recipe on page 247).

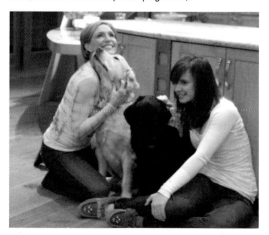

GRANDMA TINA TURNS 70

GUEST LIST:

- ❀ Martina, Warren & children Tayler and Alissa
- ❀ Ron, Tammy & children Ryan and Reid
- ❀ Rene, Jody & children Anika, William and Ethan
- ❀ Tosca, Robert & children Braden, Chelsea, Rachel, Kiersten and Kelsey-Lynn
- ❀ Tina Van Diepen (my feisty Mom) as the guest of honor

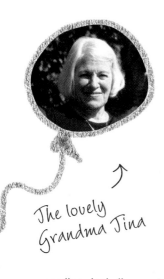

The lovely Grandma Tina

THE PARTY

At my mother's 70th birthday party held recently, my entire family gathered for a pool party. Her greatest desire was not to be wowed with fancy dining. She wanted everyone to be part of the celebration. She wanted an intimate family affair. We bought loads of pool toys and noodles, including water pistols, and partied all day long. We lit a wood fire in the outdoor grill and cooked up platters of marinated grilled chicken breasts, roasted vegetables of all descriptions and then tossed up a crisp summer salad loaded with the freshest ingredients. Grilled peaches and apricots were a huge hit. Birthday cake was served poolside under the twinkling lights of a brilliant summer evening. It was joyful and simple. Even the adults behaved like kids. More importantly, it was memorable and that is what a celebration should be about.

As the host of that party I was happy to have accomplished what seemed on first glance to be a daunting task – feeding 21 people. All food served was Clean food and as fresh and in season as possible.

GREAT EXPECTATIONS

The point here is not to be too clever. A party is enjoyable for everyone if the details are kept simple and of excellent quality. This way you don't have big expectations of yourself and the pressure that goes alongside. It isn't necessary to prepare batches of gourmet foods. They won't be appreciated nearly as much as you might think.

I recall my attempt to celebrate Chelsea's 13th birthday. She requested pizza. I wanted to shine and give her the best party I could. Off I went in search of gourmet pizza. I had heard that a local caterer was "to die for" and thought I would have him do up the pizza. "She is going to love this wood-oven thin-crust pizza," I thought. The pizza arrived on cue and each one looked, in my mind anyway, scrumptious. There was one with goat cheese and arugula and another with mushrooms and a load of vegetables. Too bad no one liked the pizza. I was trying to be clever and it backfired. Those kids wanted cheesy, pepperoni-encrusted, good-old pizza. They did not want to be impressed. I learned my lesson. Now I ask what each of the children would like in the way of food to celebrate their birthday and work along those lines. Today I will make a "good-old pizza" – cleaned up of course – and stick to simple, well-accepted foods that my kids already know and love. A birthday is not the time to try out new recipes.

ANOTHER MOTHER SHARES HER WISDOM

As a mother of six children ages 15 to 28 I have put on quite a few parties. I cannot say all of them were Clean Eating but here are a few things I have tried through the years: Keep it active. Have a swim party with a beach theme including fruit kabobs, grilled lean meats and veggies. In your back yard or park have a picnic with outdoor games including sports or relay races, balloon toss, egg- or marshmallow-on-a-spoon run and other fun games. Make a piñata filled with birdseed and take turns breaking it just for fun. It's good for the environment too! For food ideas why not a breakfast or brunch celebration? We did that one year for my daughter and her friends and they loved the pancakes, eggs, fruit and muffins. In this day and age I think there is pressure on parents to put on an elaborate birthday party with constant entertainment. I prefer to keep it simple and the kids seem to enjoy their special day. Especially when the kids are young; too much sugar and stimulation are a bad combination.

— *Carol Cuomo, Rochester, New York*

ACTIVE BIRTHDAY CELEBRATIONS

Don't forget to spice up your child's birthday party with activities. Partygoers will want a memorable experience and one that they have shared with their friends. Recently I attended a birthday party where I was certain I had arrived at the wrong house. The party was for my friend's 11-year-old son and there was not a sound to be heard anywhere except for the occasional "ping." As I entered I saw 10 little boys sitting beside each other each playing with their own Nintendo DS handheld units. Not one child was interacting with another. They were all simply involved in their own games. It saddened me. Where was the activity and the excitement, the interaction, that normally accompanies a child's birthday? As an aside (or perhaps not), most of the kids at the party were also carrying excess weight.

A birthday party can be active if that is what you enjoy, and the kids will love it. When my daughter turned sixteen in the middle of February we had a skating party. The real fun lay in the fact that our pond had iced 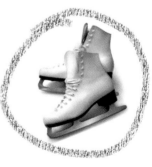 over thanks to a brutally cold Canadian winter and that the skating happened outdoors on that little pond. We set up a bonfire to keep the skaters warm and had plenty of hot chocolate (see my Happy Hot Chocolate recipe on page 306) for warming up off the ice. This was a memorable party because everyone had a chance to skate and be active, be silly and just be kids. Afterwards we enjoyed zippy Friday Night Chili (page 290) served with hearty bread and plenty of crudités and hummus (page 255) served at our dining table, where everyone piled in for a wonderful feast. I made a decadent carrot cake with Yogurt Cheese Icing (page 118) and had fruit to go with it. The party was a success even by my daughter's admission.

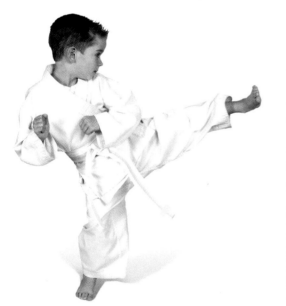

TIP Make birthday parties active! Rent the town pool, skating rink or gymnasium, or make your own outdoor party outside. You can have sledding parties, or set up an obstacle course and other games in your back yard.

TWO MOMS SAY:

For my son's 5th birthday we took it to the gym! We had a party at the local gymnastics center where the kids had two instructors guide them through trampoline activities and floor exercises. There was a huge pit filled with foam to jump in ... the the kids were aged 4 through 13 and they had an awesome time! I served water, apple juice boxes (100 % juice), pasta salad and healthy pizzas.
— Jean Pereda, South Elgin, Illinois

....

We own a karate school and we host at least one birthday party every weekend. The kids have a great time! Sometimes the kids are our students, so they enjoy showing their friends what they can do. Sometimes the kids have no experience. One of the most popular events is the obstacle course we set up. Some parents bring the typical food but other parents take the opportunity to introduce Japanese or other Asian foods to the children. Most parents bring water bottles for the kids. I have seen some pretty healthy pizzas. Peanut butter in celery with raisins (Ants on a Log), apple and orange slices and other healthy foods are also common. Hummus with veggies and healthy cookies are good too. They have also made some fun, kid-friendly sushi. Coconut balls are a hit. And of course the ever popular "power balls" made with nut butter, protein powder and honey and rolled in anything from granola to coconut to mini chocolate chips ... kids love them.
— Victoria Larioza, Fowlerville, Michigan

YOUR ACTIVE BIRTHDAY

⭐ Skiing, skating, tobogganing, tubing – any winter activities are great fun for an active party.

⭐ Swimming – check out your local YMCA or community pool for public swim times. Some have private swim times and party rooms available.

⭐ Ping pong, air hockey, billiards or Wii – if you happen to have the equipment.

⭐ Bowling – you can contact a local bowling alley and reserve it for your child's celebration.

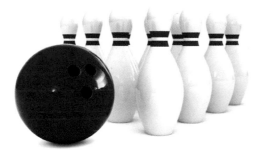

⭐ Bocce ball, horseshoes, baseball, soccer … even cricket can be fun for all ages.

⭐ Scavenger hunt around your home – searching for the items can be quite physical depending on the age of your child.

⭐ Surfing lessons – when I was on the beach in Santa Monica recently I noticed you could drop your child off for surfing lessons. Gather a group of friends and sign them up for a day in the waves.

⭐ Dance lessons – have a dance instructor come to the house to teach kids how to do a certain dance. This is all the more popular with such shows as *So You Think You Can Dance* climbing the charts.

⭐ Set up an obstacle course in your backyard and have guests run it until they are pooped.

⭐ Contact a local gym and have guests do a fitness class tailored for the specific age group. They can learn some basic gymnastics tricks and possibly do a trampoline work too.

BARB SAYS:

When my son had his first birthday I made him a small carrot cake sweetened with applesauce. I didn't want to just hand over a piece of regulation chocolate cake. We also played "active" games at the party that even adults could enjoy – 3-legged races, wheelbarrow races, relay races – and for summer birthdays we went to a local park, used the pavilion and the kids used the equipment while we played softball or volleyball. It's both cheap and healthy!
— *Barb Stegenga, Dyer, Indiana*

There are thousands of engaging ideas for activities to help your child celebrate his or her big day. Use your imagination or follow up on the kinds of physical activities your child likes to participate in, and then use those ideas as the basis for the event.

ERIN SAYS:

"Something I do at every birthday and it has evolved as my kids have been getting bigger is a treasure hunt/scavenger hunt. The kids have such a great time and it not only gets their bodies active but their minds as well. When the kids are really young I use pictures and as they got older, pictures with words. Another game the kids love when they are young is charades. Again using pictures of animals. They get to pick a picture, act it out, and then the other kids guess which animal they are.

— *Erin Di Loreto, Sherwood Park, Alberta*

ELIZABETH SAYS:

I fill the treat bags for our little guests with inexpensive toys, pencils and stickers. NO candy! Toys are better than candy any day. I also rent a jumper. The kids are outside burning energy! Perfect!

— *Elizabeth Shepherd, French Valley, California*

RECIPE FOR BIRTHDAY SLIME

Somehow things that are gross and disgusting always capture the attention of even the most adult birthday celebrant. Here is a recipe for homemade slime that will be the center of attention at your next big party.

INGREDIENTS

1 tsp Borax (found in laundry soap aisle)
1 ½ cups water, separated
½ cup Elmer's glue
Food coloring

PREPARATION

In large metal or plastic bowl pour Borax into 1 cup of water. Mix well. Add Elmer's glue and ½ cup water to Borax mixture. Mix well. Add food coloring of choice and mix well.

Get ready to be slimed!

BIRTHDAY MENU

The recipes in this book will help you prepare a Clean-Eating spread for your partygoers that will keep them fed and happy not wired, hyper and emotional. Use any combination of recipes, depending on the kind of party you are throwing and the age of the guests. The following is an ideal menu.

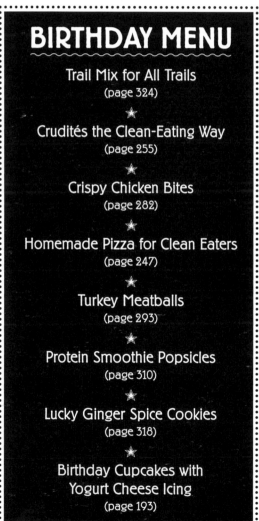

BIRTHDAY MENU

Trail Mix for All Trails
(page 324)

★

Crudités the Clean-Eating Way
(page 255)

★

Crispy Chicken Bites
(page 282)

★

Homemade Pizza for Clean Eaters
(page 247)

★

Turkey Meatballs
(page 293)

★

Protein Smoothie Popsicles
(page 310)

★

Lucky Ginger Spice Cookies
(page 318)

★

Birthday Cupcakes with Yogurt Cheese Icing
(page 193)

POWER FLOUR

Although wheat-based flours are the standard in the baking world, many other flours can be used. Some flours work better than others in baking. Power Flour is made of a combination of flours, to optimize nutrition and effectiveness.

INGREDIENTS

¼ cup/ 60 ml **brown rice flour**

¼ cup/ 60 ml **amaranth flour**

¼ cup/ 60 ml **spelt flour** (if not gluten intolerant)

¼ cup/ 60 ml **kamut flour** (if not gluten intolerant)

¼ cup/ 60 ml **barley flour** (if not gluten intolerant)

¼ cup/ 60 ml **unbleached wheat flour**
   (if not gluten intolerant)

PREPARATION

Mix all ingredients together in an airtight container and store in the refrigerator.

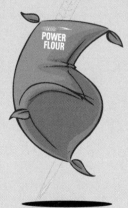

TIP Freeze Protein Smoothie mixture in decorative ice-cube trays for a perfect bite-sized serving.

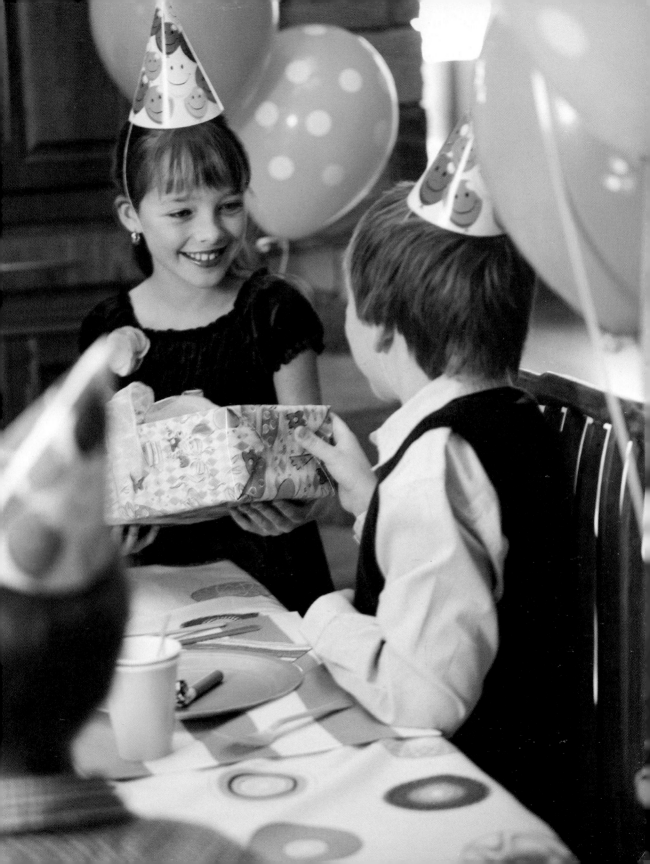

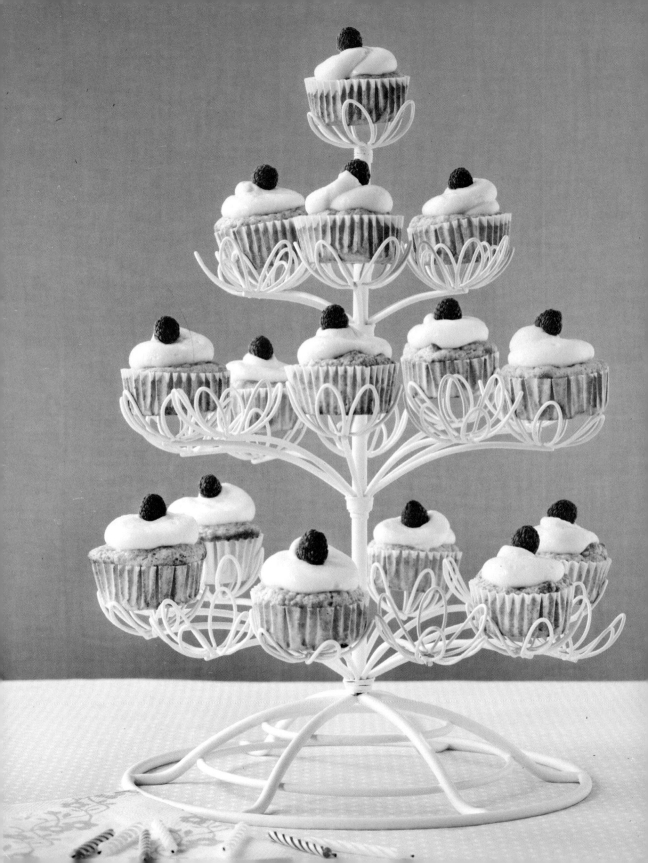

BIRTHDAY CUPCAKES AND A BAKING LESSON TOO

Makes 12 cupcakes • Prep Time: 10 min. • Cook Time: 15-20 min.

How many times have you bought a huge birthday cake slathered in frosting? You may notice a strange thing once the kids have finished eating and gone back to their play. Plates are strewn about with the cake eaten and the frosting still sitting there. Admit it! You've seen it a hundred times. Here's my version of this childhood treat (remember it is a treat) complete with a frosting that will get eaten.

INGREDIENTS FOR CAKE

½ cup / 120 ml egg whites or 5 large egg whites*

2 ¼ tsp / 11.25 ml lemon juice OR white vinegar**

¼ tsp / 1.25 ml sea salt

½ cup / 120 ml unbleached all purpose flour OR
   gluten-free flour OR Power Flour (see page 190)

¼ cup / 60 ml agave nectar***

1 tsp / 5 ml best-quality vanilla

¼ cup / 60 ml cooked, puréed sweet carrots

1 tsp / 5 ml finely grated lemon rind

1 ½ tsp / 7.5 ml baking powder

INGREDIENTS FOR FROSTING

2 cups / 480 ml yogurt cheese (recipe page 255)

½ tsp / 2.5 ml vanilla

½ to 1 cup / 120 – 240 ml sifted confectioners' sugar

NUTRITIONAL INFORMATION FOR ONE TBSP OF FROSTING:
Calories: 23 | Calories from Fat: 0.5 | Fat: 0g | Saturated Fat: 0g | Trans Fat: 0g | Protein: 1g | Carbs: 4g | Dietary Fiber: 0g | Sodium: 20mg | Cholesterol: 0mg

NUTRITIONAL INFORMATION FOR ONE CUPCAKE WITH ONE TBSP OF FROSTING:
Calories: 39 | Calories from Fat: 1 | Eat: 0g | Saturated Fat: 0g | Trans Fat: 0g | Protein: 1g | Carbs: 8g | Dietary Fiber: 0.5g | Sodium: 60mg | Cholesterol: 0mg

PREPARATION FOR CAKE

1. Preheat oven to 350˚F/ 171˚C. Line a muffin tin with Silpat reusable muffin liners or unbleached paper liners. In a large bowl combine egg whites, lemon juice or vinegar, and sea salt.

2. Beat whites at high speed until stiff peaks form. This will take a few minutes – about 4 or 5 – so be patient. When you are finished you should have doubled the volume.

3. Fold the egg whites and the rest of the ingredients together so everything is just combined. Don't over mix or you will lose the volume in your egg whites. Fill muffin cups with batter.

4. Bake in preheated oven for about 20 minutes. Check about 15 minutes into baking to check their progress. The muffins should be golden brown, not dark. You can do the bounce test, too. Place your finger gently on top of one muffin and press down. If the muffin springs back, it's done. Remove from heat and let cool on wire rack.

METHOD FOR FROSTING

1. Mix all ingredients together until smooth and creamy. Frost cupcakes and refrigerate.

Recipe continued on next page…

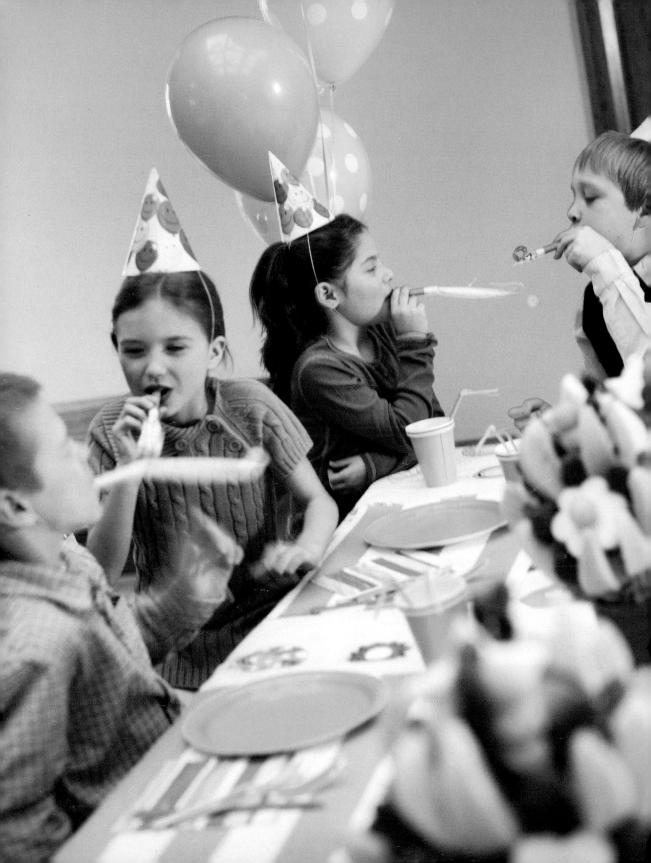

TIP For Frosting: start with ½ cup / 120ml of confectioners' sugar but you may need to add a bit more — this will depend on how much water has drained from your yogurt and how stiff it is. You can adjust accordingly. This will not be the sickeningly sweet frosting you normally expect from a conventional birthday cake or cupcake.

* **Egg whites**: Liquid egg whites can be purchased in cartons and are a convenient and neat way of working with them.

½ cup / 120 ml liquid egg whites = 4 to 5 egg whites
2 Tbsp / 30 ml liquid egg whites = 1 egg white

** **Cream of tartar:** Normally called for in a fluffy cake and muffin recipe such as this, cream of tartar is the lay term for potassium acid tartrate, or potassium bi-tartrate. This sounds like a dangerous chemical, but it is actually a by-product of making wine. This acid forms on the inside of the barrels where wine is aged and then scraped away and processed to make the end product.

Cream of tartar is used to stabilize egg whites. When egg whites are beaten they incorporate air and become fluffy. Cream of tartar helps keep them that way. In this recipe we use a substitute.

Cream of tartar substitutes: Lemon juice or vinegar – use 3 times the amount of cream of tartar called for.

***Agave Nectar:** This light-colored liquid comes from the agave plant and has a glycemic index much lower than that of table sugar. Use it in this or other recipes to keep the sugar content low.

TIP I remember being fascinated by the way my mother could turn egg whites into gorgeous piles of fluffy white air. She had a few tricks up her sleeve to recreate this magic time and time again. She would put the mixing bowl and beaters into the refrigerator for an hour before she was going to use them. Of course the egg whites would stay in the refrigerator too. Then she would mix everything together and hold the beater at an angle in the bowl so she could incorporate more air into her creation. As far as I recall these tips never failed her.

Happy Birthday!
I will be thinking of you!
Best Wishes,
Josca

Clean-Eating Recipes

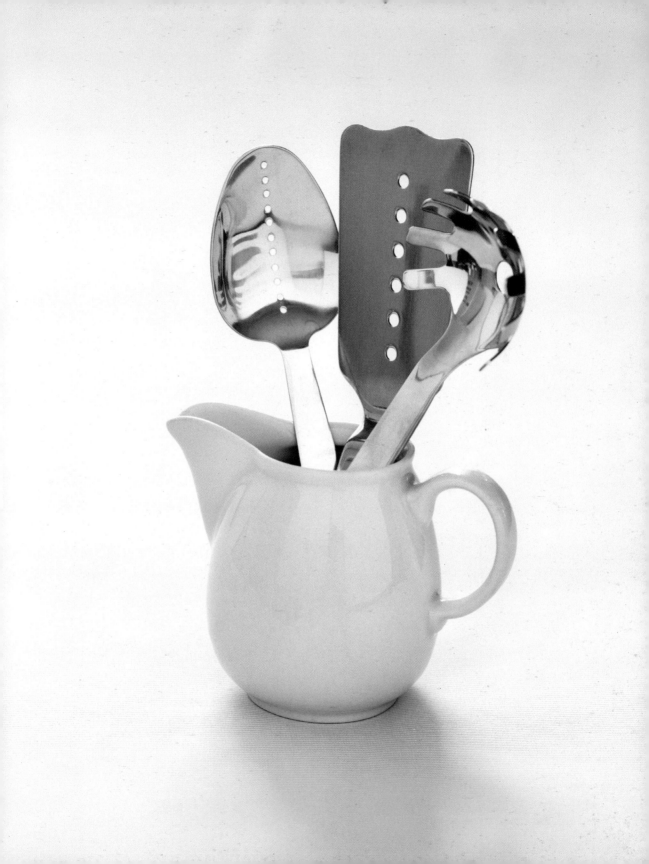

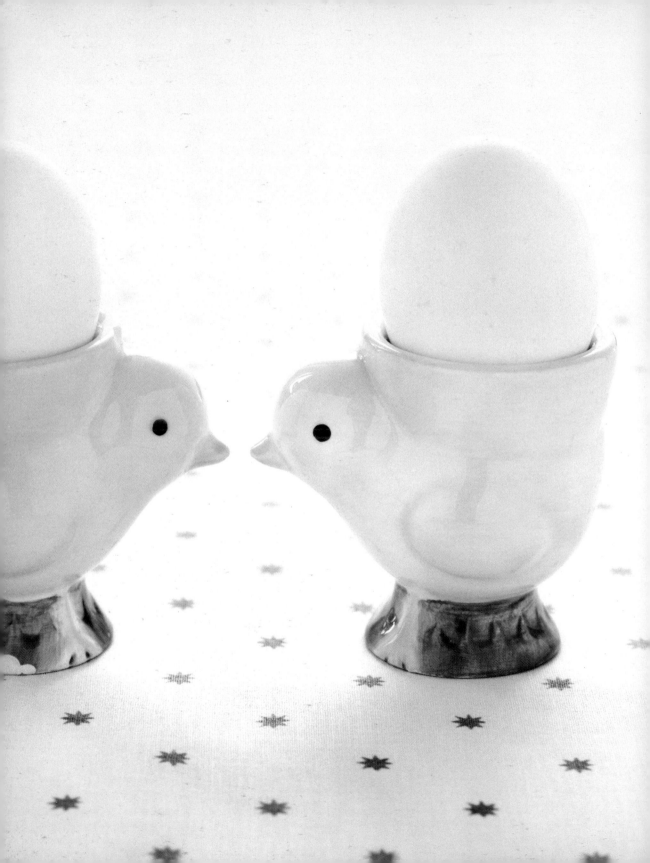

Breakfast

· ·

BREAKFAST HERMITS

Yield: 5 dozen cookies • Prep Time: 20 min. • Chill Time: 2 hrs. • Cooking Time: 10 min.

Eating a cookie is just plain fun. Eating a cookie for breakfast feels a bit naughty but it sure helps nutrients go down. This cleaned-up version of hermit cookies chases fat and sugar with a helping of delicious dried fruits and spices.

INGREDIENTS

2 ½ cups / 600 ml whole wheat flour

½ cup / 120 ml protein powder

2 tsp / 10 ml baking powder (look for a brand that contains no alum)

¼ tsp / 1.25 ml ground cloves

¼ tsp / 1.25 ml ground cinnamon

½ tsp/ 2.5 ml ground nutmeg

⅛ tsp / 0.6 ml ground mace

⅛ tsp / 0.6 ml ground cardamom

¼ tsp / 1.25 ml sea salt

½ cup / 120 ml agave nectar

½ cup / 120 ml best-quality olive oil

4 egg whites

½ cup / 120 ml unsulfured blackstrap molasses

½ cup / 120 ml apple butter (see recipe page 302) or applesauce

1 Tbsp/ 15ml best-quality vanilla

2 Tbsp / 30 ml plain low-fat yogurt

1 cup / 240 ml organic sultana raisins

1 cup / 240 ml unsalted, raw, slivered almonds

½ cup / 120 ml dried unsweetened cranberries

PREPARATION

1. Preheat oven to 350°F / 171°C. Prepare cookie sheets by lining with Silpat or parchment paper.

2. Sift all dry ingredients and spices together in a large mixing bowl. Cream olive oil and agave nectar together until smooth.

3. In separate bowl beat eggs together and then add to olive oil mixture. Mix well. Add molasses, applesauce, vanilla and yogurt and mix well again.

4. Add raisins, cranberries and almonds. Mix well. You may have to use your own clean hands coated lightly with olive oil to mix this properly. The dough should form a ball.

5. Wrap with plastic and refrigerate for an hour or two. Remove from refrigerator.

6. Using a soup spoon, make small balls with the batter. Place on cookie sheet and press down lightly with a fork. Bake 10 minutes or until lightly browned.

NUTRITIONAL VALUE FOR ONE COOKIE:
Calories: 87 | Calories from Fat: 43 | Fat: 5g | Saturated Fat: 0.5g | Trans Fat: 0g | Protein: 3g | Carbs: 11g | Dietary Fiber: 1.5g | Sodium: 10mg | Cholesterol: 0mg

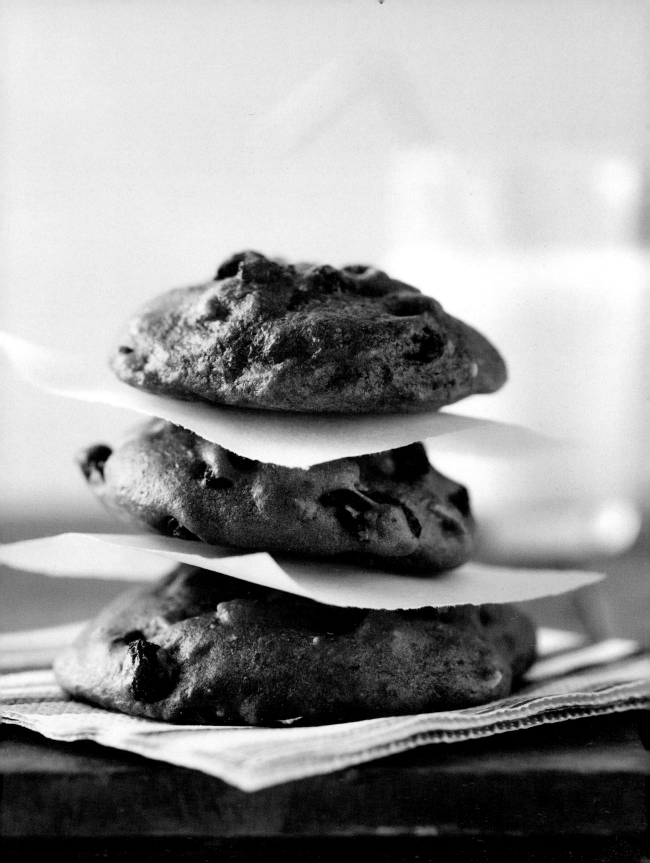

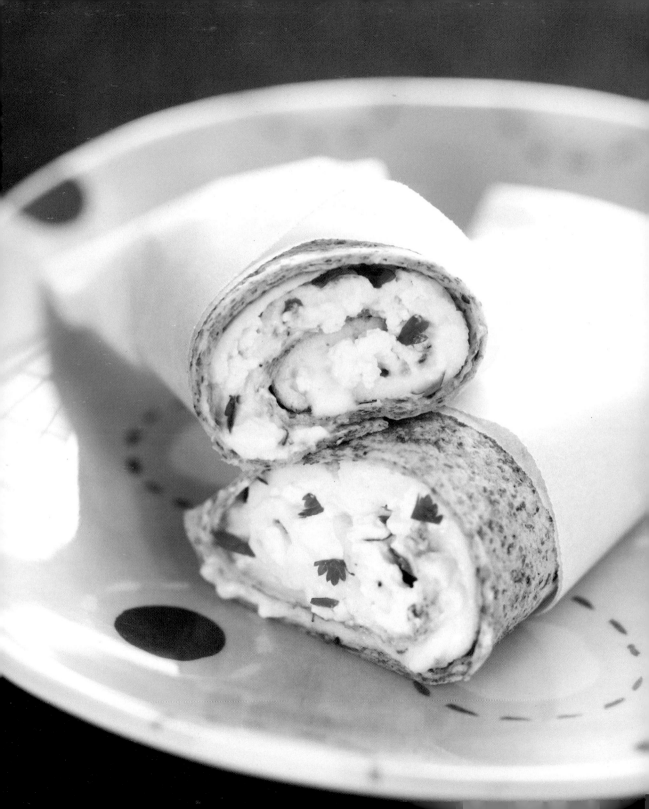

OMELET ROLL UPS

Yield: One roll up • Prep Time: 5 min. • Cook Time: 1 min.

Too many of us spend less than 10 minutes preparing breakfast, and that means you probably pop something unhealthy into your mouth. This egg-based roll-up takes only a couple of minutes to prepare, a minute to cook and it's loaded with nutrients, but the best part is that it's fun – to make and to eat. Make extra to pack into lunches. Your kids will love it.

INGREDIENTS

3 egg whites

1 whole egg

1 Tbsp / 15 ml skim milk

Sea salt and pepper

1 Tbsp / 15 ml low-fat yogurt cheese (see recipe page 255)

1 tsp / 5 ml chopped fresh cilantro or other fresh herb

1 seven-inch / 18 cm brown rice wrap

Eat-Clean cooking spray (see page 23)

PREPARATION

1. Whisk together egg, milk, salt and pepper.

2. Heat skillet over medium-high heat. Coat with cooking spray. Pour in egg mixture, tilting to spread evenly. Cook, piercing any bubbles, for about one minute or until set.

3. Spread the omelet with yogurt cheese and sprinkle with cilantro or other herbs. Slide the omelet onto the brown-rice wrap. Roll up!

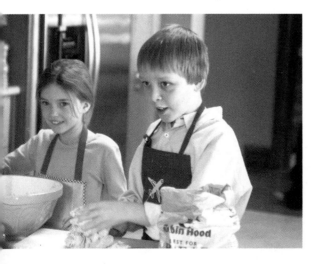

NUTRITIONAL VALUE FOR ONE ROLLUP:
Calories: 328 | Calories from Fat: 111 | Fat: 12.3g | Saturated Fat: 2.5g| Trans Fat: 0g | Protein: 24.5g | Carbs: 31g | Dietary Fiber: 5g | Sodium: 775mg | Cholesterol: 213mg

DUTCH MUESLI

Yield: 12 cups • Prep Time: 15 min. • Soak Time: overnight • Cooking Time: 0

The real name for this whole grain and fruit mix is Birchermuesli, so named for the person who invented it at the turn of the 19th Century. A German doctor, Dr. Bircher-Brenner, popularized muesli (the German word for mixture) throughout Europe and Britain as the ideal breakfast cereal. It's not hard to see why, since a traditional muesli recipe contains rolled oats, wheat germ, nuts and dried fruit – the perfect Clean-Eating breakfast! Recipes vary greatly, since you can add virtually anything to the mix. My preference is the wet version of muesli, which is made with yogurt. The mixture is soaked overnight, allowing the whole grains and dried fruits to plump up nicely by morning. The dry version of muesli is called granola.

INGREDIENTS

½ cup / 120 ml barley flakes

2 cups / 480 ml large-flake rolled oats, not quick or instant

¼ cup / 60 ml flax seed, coarsely ground

¼ cup / 60 ml wheat germ

¼ cup / 60 ml oat bran

3 cups / 720 ml boiling water

¼ cup / 60 ml raw, unsalted almonds, coarsely chopped

¼ cup / 60 ml sultana raisins

½ cup / 120 ml chopped, pitted dates

Juice of one fresh orange (grate rind and reserve)

¼ cup / 60 ml agave nectar or honey

1 cup / 240 ml plain, nonfat yogurt

½ tsp / 2.5 ml ground cinnamon

1 large crisp apple, washed well, unpeeled, grated

PREPARATION

1. Place barley, oatmeal, flax seed, wheat germ and oat bran in a medium-sized glass bowl. Mix well to combine.

2. Pour boiling water over all and let sit overnight or until water is completely absorbed.

3. Meanwhile, in another glass bowl, measure remaining ingredients. Mix well to combine.

4. Add wet grains to fruit mixture and mix well. Serve immediately or refrigerate. Muesli keeps well for about four days … if it lasts that long!

NUTRITIONAL VALUE FOR ONE-CUP SERVING:
Calories: 253 | Calories from Fat: 30 | Fat: 3g | Saturated Fat: 0.6g |
Trans Fat: 0g | Protein: 9g | Carbs: 47g | Dietary Fiber: 7g |
Sodium: 22mg | Cholesterol: 0mg

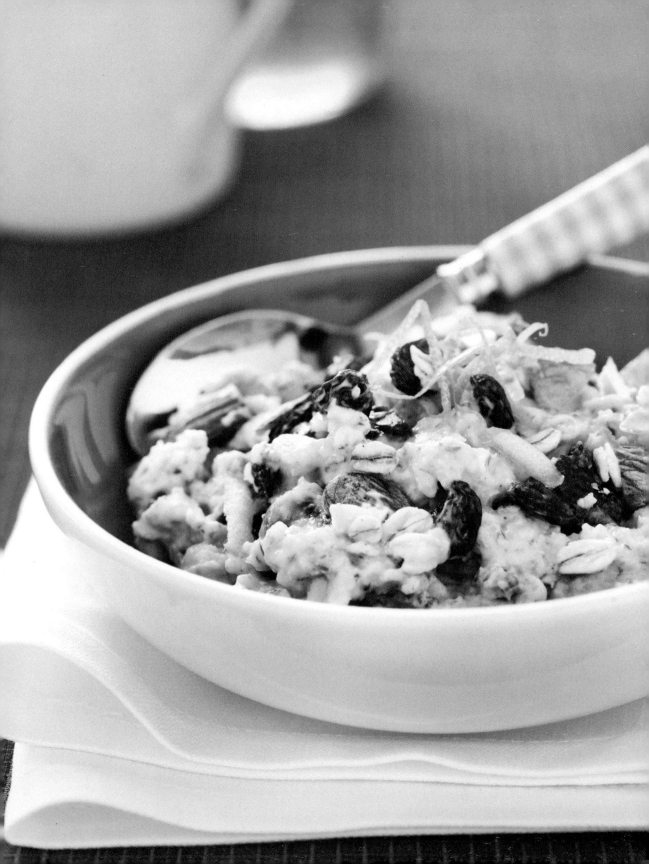

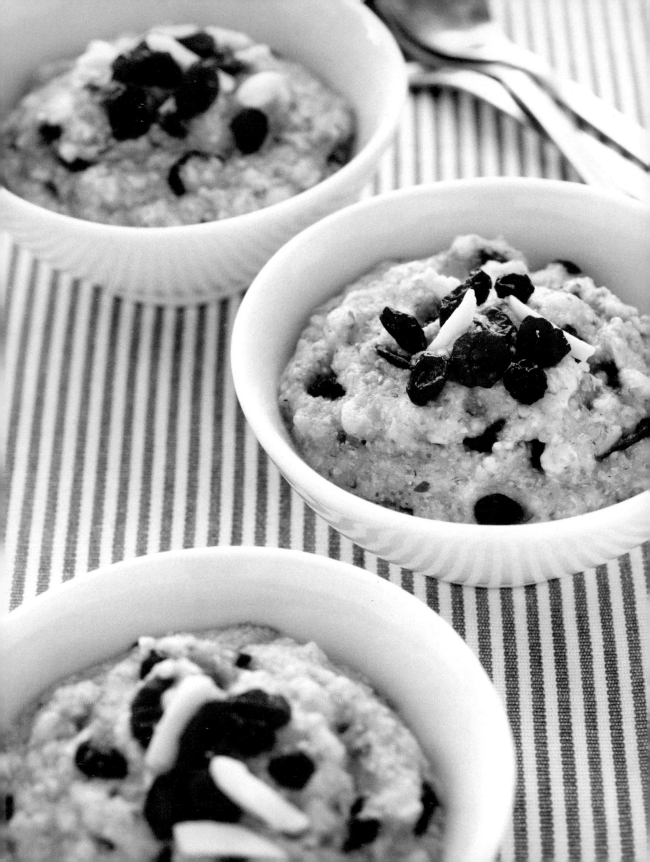

MORNING HOT CEREAL MIX

Yield 8 cups cooked cereal • Prep Time: 5 min. • Cook Time: 8 min.

This recipe comes from a firecracker of a gal called Izzie. She created this no-nonsense hot cereal mix for a nutritionally loaded breakfast sure to keep you fired up all morning as it does for Izzie and her family!

INGREDIENTS

½ cup / 120 ml oatmeal

½ cup / 120 ml Cream of Wheat cereal

½ cup / 120 ml Red River or other multigrain hot cereal mix

½ cup / 120 ml wheat germ

½ cup / 120 ml oat bran

½ cup / 120 ml raisins

½ cup / 120 ml mixed dried fruit: cranberries, cherries and blueberries

½ cup / 120 ml slivered almonds

¼ cup / 60 ml protein powder *(optional)*

PREPARATION

1. Mix all ingredients together in a large airtight container to keep for weeks.

PREPARATION FOR COOKING:

1. To make breakfast use ½ cup / 120 ml dried mixture and from 1 to 1 ½ cups / 240 – 360 ml water to make 1 cup / 240 ml of cooked cereal.

2. Mix and heat on medium-high until boiling. Continue cooking on low heat until mixture thickens to a porridge-like consistency.

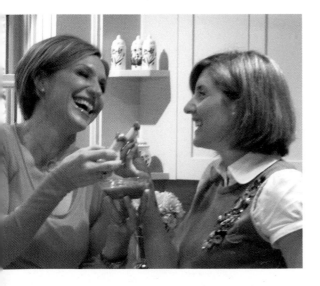

NUTRITIONAL VALUE FOR ONE CUP OF COOKED CEREAL WITHOUT PROTEIN POWDER:
Calories: 305 | Calories from Fat: 90 | Fat: 10g | Saturated Fat: 1g | Trans Fat: 0g | Protein: 10g | Carbs: 49g | Dietary Fiber: 8g | Sodium: 87mg | Cholesterol: 0mg

SWEET WHOLE-GRAIN BREAKFAST PANCAKES

Yield: 9 x 4" / 10 cm pancakes • Prep Time: 6 min. • Soak Time: 30 min. • Cook Time: 15-20 min. (cooking 3 at a time)

It is important to eat several servings of whole grains every day. They help offset the many hormone-related imbalances we see today, particularly diabetes. I like to serve these oatmeal-based pancakes because it is just one more way I can get whole grains into my kids. If we have leftovers, all the better. I just warm them up and serve them next day.

INGREDIENTS

1 ½ cups / 360 ml rolled oats

¾ cup / 180 ml whole-wheat flour

1 cup / 240 ml buckwheat flour

1 ¼ Tbsp / 19 ml baking powder

⅛ tsp / 0.6 ml sea salt

4 egg whites

2 ½ cups / 600 ml buttermilk or plain kefir

2 Tbsp / 30 ml avocado, sunflower or safflower oil

1 Tbsp / 15 ml best-quality vanilla

1 ½ Tbsp / 22 ml organic honey

Eat-Clean cooking spray (see page 23)

PREPARATION

1. Place all dry ingredients in a medium-sized mixing bowl. In another medium mixing bowl place all wet ingredients. Add wet ingredients to dry and mix until just blended. The mixture could still be lumpy. Let sit on the counter for half an hour so the oats can soften.

2. Spray a skillet or griddle with cooking spray. Set over medium heat. Using a ladle, measure ½ cup / 120 ml of batter onto hot skillet. Let cook until edges are lightly browned and bubbles start to appear on top of the pancake surface. Flip and continue cooking until both sides are golden brown.

TIP Use cookie cutters to make fun shapes. Spray the interior of the cookie cutter with cooking spray to keep the batter from sticking. Pour the batter into the cookie cutter. Let cook until bubbles form. Remove cookie cutter and flip the pancake. Make sure to use metal cookie cutters — plastic will melt.

NUTRITIONAL VALUE PER PANCAKE:
Calories: 210 | Calories from Fat: 46.5 | Fat: 5g | Saturated Fat: 1g | Trans Fat: 0g | Protein: 11g | Carbs: 30g | Dietary Fiber: 5g | Sodium: 80mg | Cholesterol: 0mg

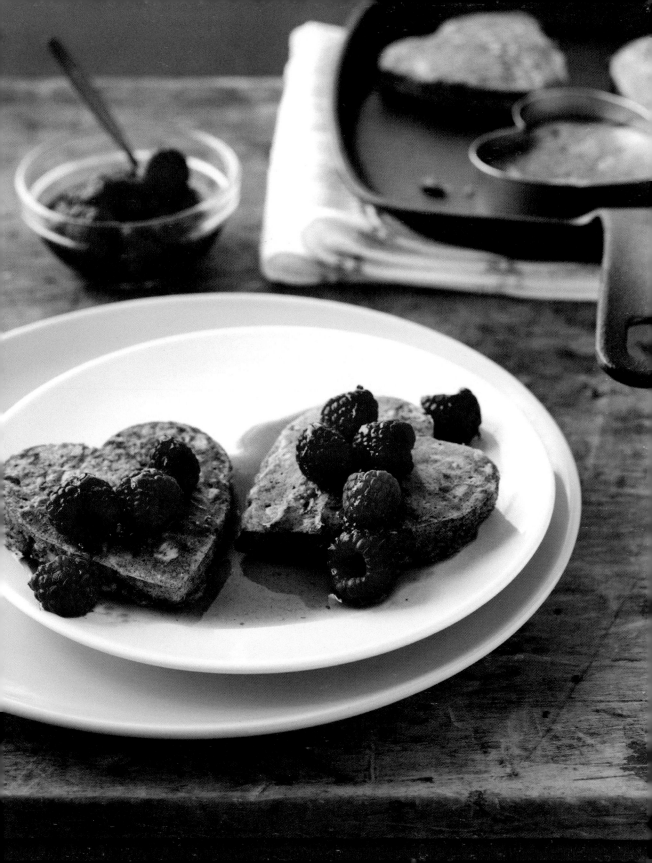

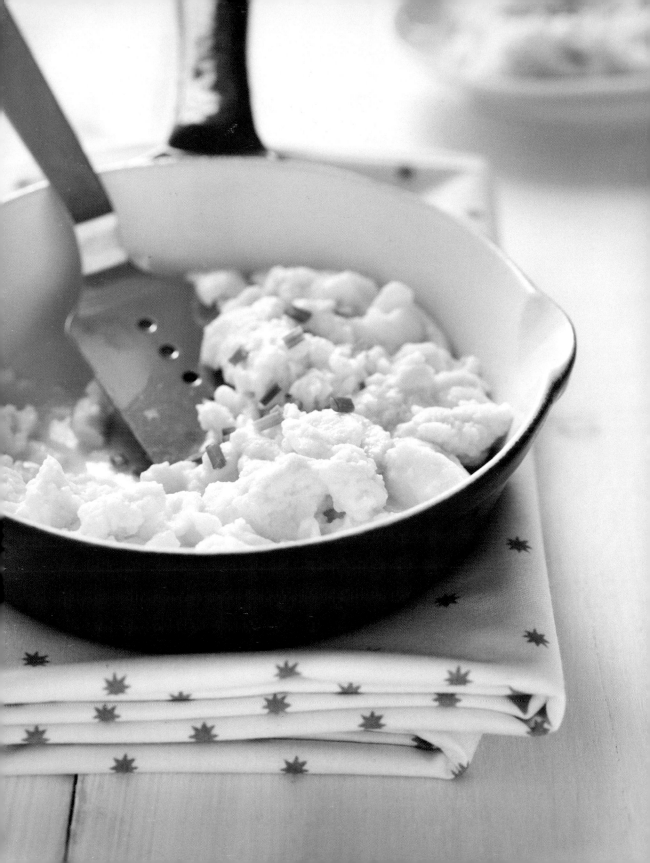

SCRAMBLED EGG WHITES – A BREAKFAST STAPLE

Yield: 1 serving • Prep Time: 5 min. • Cook Time: 2-3 min.

The last thing you want for breakfast is rubbery scrambled eggs. Fluffy, piping-hot clouds of scrambled eggs are a delicious, nearly perfect food. Have them for breakfast, lunch or dinner. Opt for the freshest eggs possible. I often seek out farm-fresh eggs close to where I live, or buy from a farmer's market. The less they have to travel, the fresher they are.

INGREDIENTS

3 egg whites

1 whole egg

¼ cup / 60 ml yogurt cheese (see page 255)

¼ tsp / 1.25 ml sea salt

Freshly ground white pepper

Eat-Clean cooking spray (see page 23)

TIP Multiply the recipe to serve more.

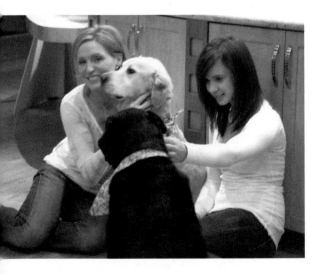

PREPARATION

1. Crack three eggs over a medium bowl, separating whites into the bowl and discarding the yolks.

2. Crack one whole egg into the bowl. Add remaining ingredients.

3. Coat a skillet with cooking spray. Heat on medium.

4. Pour egg mixture into skillet and reduce heat to low. Cook eggs, stirring constantly with a spatula. This will take 2 or 3 minutes. Don't let eggs overcook. When the eggs are just dry they are ready to serve.

NUTRITIONAL VALUE FOR ONE SERVING:
Calories: 194 | Calories from Fat: 49 | Fat: 5g | Saturated Fat: 1.6g | Trans Fat: 0g | Protein: 24g | Carbs: 10.5g | Dietary Fiber: 0g | Sodium: 720mg | Cholesterol: 214mg

 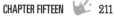

EGGS WITH BLACK BEAN SALSA

Yield: 2 servings • Prep Time: 5 min. • Cook Time: 12 min.

Kids love spicy food as long as it's not too hot. Salsa and jalapeno pepper spice up scrambled egg whites, while black beans add a healthy and much-needed dose of fiber, protein and flavor.

INGREDIENTS

1 Tbsp / 30 ml best-quality olive oil

1 small onion, chopped

1 clove garlic, passed through a garlic press

1 tsp / 5 ml minced fresh jalapeno pepper

1 19 oz. / 540ml can of black beans, drained and rinsed

2 plum tomatoes, chopped

1 cup / 235 ml salsa

2 Tbsp / 30 ml chopped fresh cilantro

Dash Worcestershire sauce

5 egg whites

1 whole egg

Eat-Clean cooking spray (see page 23)

PREPARATION

1. In saucepan, heat oil over medium heat; cook onion, garlic and jalapeno for 3 to 5 minutes or until softened.

2. Stir in beans, tomatoes and salsa. Cook for several minutes or until thickened. Stir in cilantro and Worcestershire sauce.

3. Meanwhile, whip egg whites and whole egg together in bowl. Spray large skillet and heat over medium. Pour eggs into hot skillet and cook till just done.

4. Spoon salsa onto heated plates. Settle eggs on top of the salsa.

NUTRITIONAL VALUE FOR HALF RECIPE:
Calories: 372 | Calories from Fat: 54 | Fat: 6g | Saturated Fat: 1g | Trans Fat: 0g | Protein: 28g | Carbs: 51g | Dietary Fiber: 14g | Sodium: 2mg | Cholesterol: 105mg

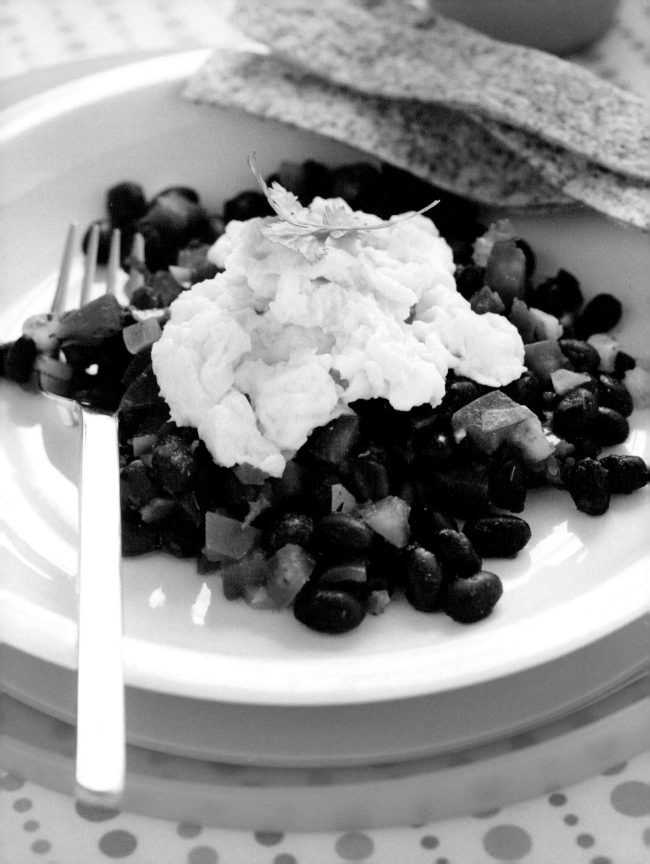

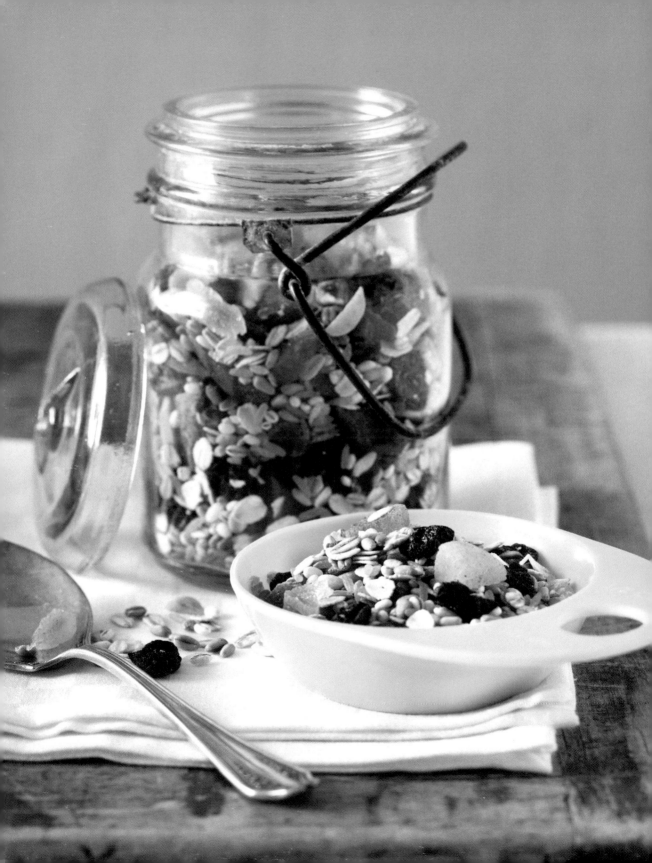

WHOLE LOTTA GRAINS CEREAL

Yeild: 13 cups of cooked cereal • Prep Time: 5 min. • Cook Time: 15 min.

Hot cereal is perfect for those chilly mornings when you need something substantial to fuel your furnace. Don't compromise on nutrition by serving commercial cereals. Try this breakfast cereal that is chock full of delicious goodness but not drowning in sugar. Make sure the dried fruit is unsulfured and without added sugar.

INGREDIENTS

1 ½ cups/ 360 ml old-fashioned rolled oats (large
   flake and not quick cooking is best)

1 cup / 240 ml quick-cooking barley

1 cup / 240 ml quick-cooking brown rice

1 cup / 240 ml triticale flakes

½ cup / 120 ml chopped pitted dates

½ cup / 120 ml dried unsweetened cranberries

½ cup / 120 ml chopped dried apricots

½ cup / 120 ml slivered almonds, toasted

1 Tbsp / 15 ml ground cinnamon

Pinch nutmeg

PREPARATION

Combine all ingredients and place in an airtight container. This mix can be stored for several weeks.

PREPARATION FOR COOKING

1. Cook ½ cup / 120 ml cereal with 1 cup / 240 ml of water. You may have to add a bit more water if your porridge is too stiff.

2. Once the whole grains are soft, remove the porridge from the heat source and serve.

3. Top with fresh berries or unsweetened applesauce.

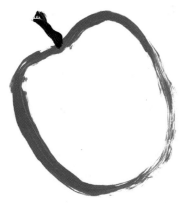

NUTRITIONAL VALUE FOR ONE CUP COOKED CEREAL:
Calories: 242 | Calories from Fat: 25 | Fat: 3g | Saturated Fat: 0.3g | Trans Fat: 0g | Protein: 7g | Carbs: 49g | Dietary Fiber: 7.5g | Sodium: 10mg | Cholesterol: 0mg

BEANS ON TOAST

Yield: 10 servings • Prep Time: 15 min. • Cook Time: 10 min.

This is a Clean-Eating version of a long-favored comfort food originating from Britain. Beans on toast can be much better than it sounds, especially if you get creative with the ingredients. Using kidney beans instead of canned baked beans ups the nutrition content significantly. Serve it on multigrain toast and you've upped it again.

INGREDIENTS

2 Tbsp / 30 ml best-quality olive oil

½ cup / 120 ml finely chopped sweet onion

2 cloves garlic, passed through a garlic press

½ cup / 120 ml tomato paste

1 Tbsp / 15 ml amber agave nectar

1 – 2 Tbsp / 15 – 30 ml unsulfured blackstrap
   molasses

1 Tbsp / 15 ml Dijon mustard

½ cup / 120 ml water

2 x 19 oz. / 540 g cans white kidney beans, rinsed
   and drained

1 multigrain baguette cut on the diagonal in ¼-inch/
   0.5 cm slices

2 cups / 480 ml fresh salad greens – mesclun mix,
   baby spring mix, baby spinach, arugula, or your
   choice

2 Tbsp / 30 ml chopped cilantro *(optional)*

PREPARATION

1. In medium skillet heat olive oil over medium heat. Sautée chopped onion and garlic until soft, about 4 minutes.

2. Add tomato paste, agave nectar, molasses, Dijon mustard, water and kidney beans. Heat through. Turn off heat and let sit.

3. Meanwhile, toast baguette until crispy. Set aside.

4. Prepare plates for two. Place a cup of salad greens on each plate. Arrange toast at the side.

5. Spoon bean mixture over each piece of toast. Garnish with chopped cilantro. Serve.

NOTE: Beans on toast can be made into a full Clean-Eating meal by adding scrambled egg whites.

**NUTRITIONAL INFORMATION PER HALF-CUP BEANS,
TWO SLICES OF BAGUETTE AND GREENS:**
Calories: 197 | Calories from Fat: 25 | Fat: 3g | Saturated Fat: 0.4g | Trans Fat: 0g | Protein: 8g | Carbs: 33g | Dietary Fiber: 8g | Sodium: 395mg | Cholesterol: 0mg

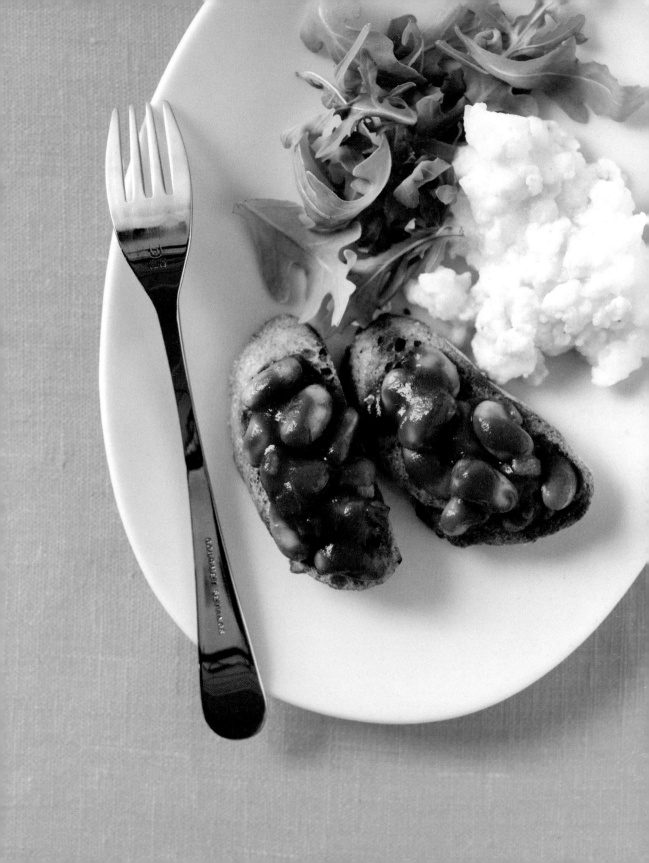

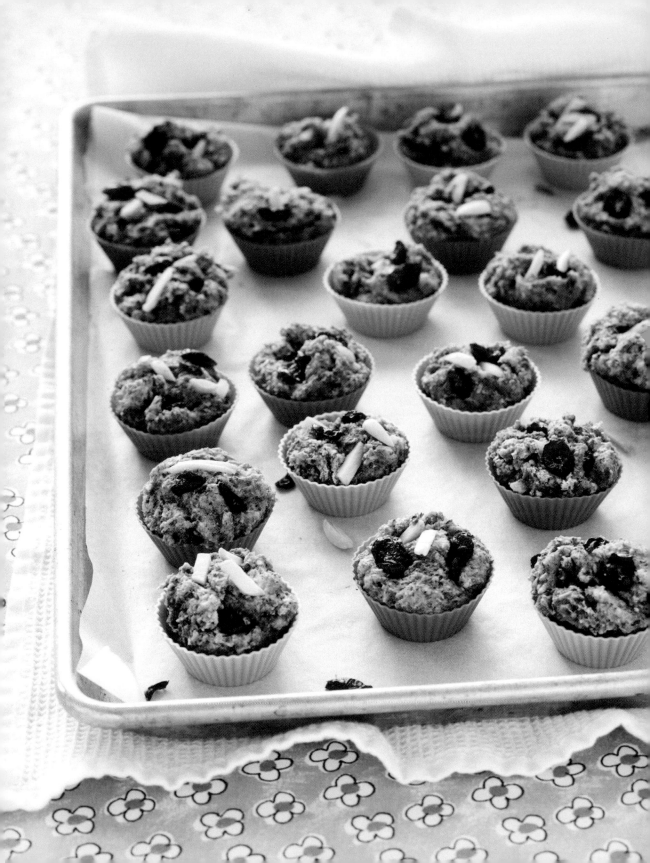

CRANBERRY FLAX SEED BREAKFAST MUFFINS

Makes 12 muffins or 24-36 mini muffins • Prep Time: 15 min. • Cook Time: 15 min. (for mini) & 25 min. (for full)

You know how I feel about flax seed. If your family is balking at eating this tiny powerhouse food, don't worry. You can hide them in these delicious muffins and no one but you will be the wiser … unless you had a little help making them!

INGREDIENTS

1 cup / 240 ml flax seeds

1 cup / 240 ml oat bran

1 cup / 240 ml whole grain flour

1 cup / 240 ml Power Flour (see recipe pg 190)

1 Tbsp / 15 ml baking powder

1 tsp / 5 ml ground cinnamon

Pinch ginger

1 tsp / 5 ml baking soda

½ tsp / 2.5 ml sea salt

2 egg whites

1 cup / 240 ml unsweetened applesauce

1 ½ cups / 360 ml plain kefir

⅓ cup / 80 ml best-quality olive oil or safflower oil

1 ½ cups / 360 ml dried unsweetened cranberries (unsulfured if possible)

½ cup / 120 ml slivered almonds

NOTE: These muffins are high in healthy, unsaturated fats with lots of Omega 3's. If you are going to enjoy these, balance the rest of your meals for the day by limiting nuts, nut butters and other healthy oils.

PREPARATION

1. Preheat oven to 375˚F / 191˚C. Prepare muffin tins with unbleached paper liners, Silpat reusable cups or a light coating of cooking spray.

2. Grind flax seeds to a meal in a coffee grinder or food processor. Place in large mixing bowl. Add flours, bran, baking powder, baking soda, cinnamon, ginger and salt. Use a fork or whisk to mix dry ingredients until well blended.

3. In another bowl mix egg whites, applesauce, kefir and oil. Pour wet ingredients into dry. Add almonds and cranberries and mix until just combined. Do not over mix or your batter will make rubbery muffins.

4. Fill muffin cups with batter about ¾ full. Bake in preheated oven for about 20 to 25 minutes. Check the top of your muffins. If they are firm and bounce back when touched, they are done. Remove from oven and let cool on a wire cooling rack.

NUTRITIONAL VALUE FOR ONE FULL-SIZE MUFFIN:
Calories: 363 | Calories from Fat: 177 | Fat: 19g | Saturated Fat: 2g | Trans Fat: 0g | Protein: 11.5g | Carbs: 43g | Dietary Fiber: 11g | Sodium: 200mg | Cholesterol: 0mg

THE YES BREAKFAST SANDWICH (YOGURT CHEESE, EGG AND SPINACH)

Yield: 4 sandwiches • Prep Time: 5 min. • Cook Time: 15 min.

Everyone loves the breakfast sandwich, but I sure don't love the high fat and nitrates that normally go along with it. The YES breakfast sandwich gives you a crunchy toasted English muffin spread with creamy yogurt cheese, loaded with nutritious spinach and protein-packed egg whites, and topped with a juicy tomato. The perfect on-the-go breakfast!

INGREDIENTS

4 whole-grain English muffins, split

4 whole eggs

8 egg whites

½ cup / 120 ml yogurt cheese (see page 255)

1 large ripe tomato, sliced thickly

2 - 3 cups / 480-720 ml spinach, cleaned

Fresh cilantro, optional

Sea salt and black pepper

Eat-Clean cooking spray (see page 23)

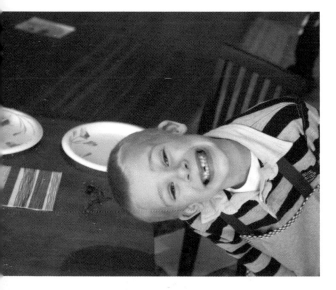

PREPARATION

1. Preheat oven or toaster oven to 350°F / 177°C.

2. Toast English muffins in heated oven for about 4 minutes or until golden brown and crispy. Remove from oven and set aside on wire cooling rack.

3. Meanwhile, steam the spinach: Bring about ½ cup / 120 ml of water to a boil in a large skillet with a tight-fitting lid. Add spinach. Place lid on top and reduce heat. Cook for about 5 minutes. Remove from heat and set in a colander to drain all excess liquid.

4. Separate the eggs in a medium bowl. Keep the whites of all 12 eggs and the yolks of four. Mix well. Spray a medium-sized skillet with cooking spray and make four small egg-white omelets to fit on the English muffin. Set aside.

5. Spread both sides of the toasted English muffin with yogurt cheese. Place one omelet on the bottom half, divide the spinach between them, then top with a large slice of tomato and chopped fresh cilantro. Sprinkle with salt and pepper and serve immediately.

NUTRITIONAL VALUE FOR ONE SANDWICH:

Calories: 280 | Calories from Fat: 53 | Fat: 6g | Saturated Fat: 1.75g | Trans Fat: 0g | Protein: 19.5g | Carbs: 8g | Dietary Fiber: 3.6g | Sodium: 500mg | Cholesterol: 0mg

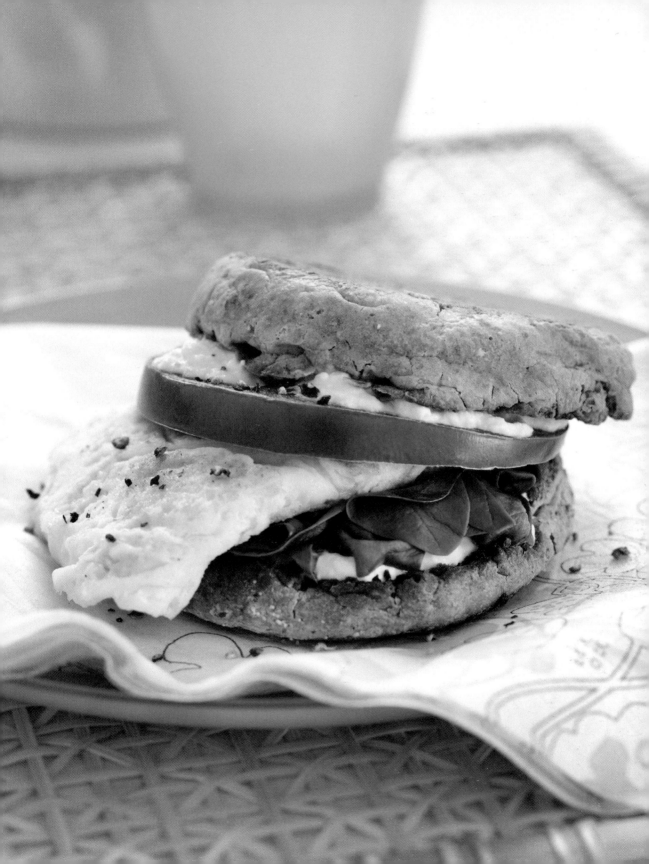

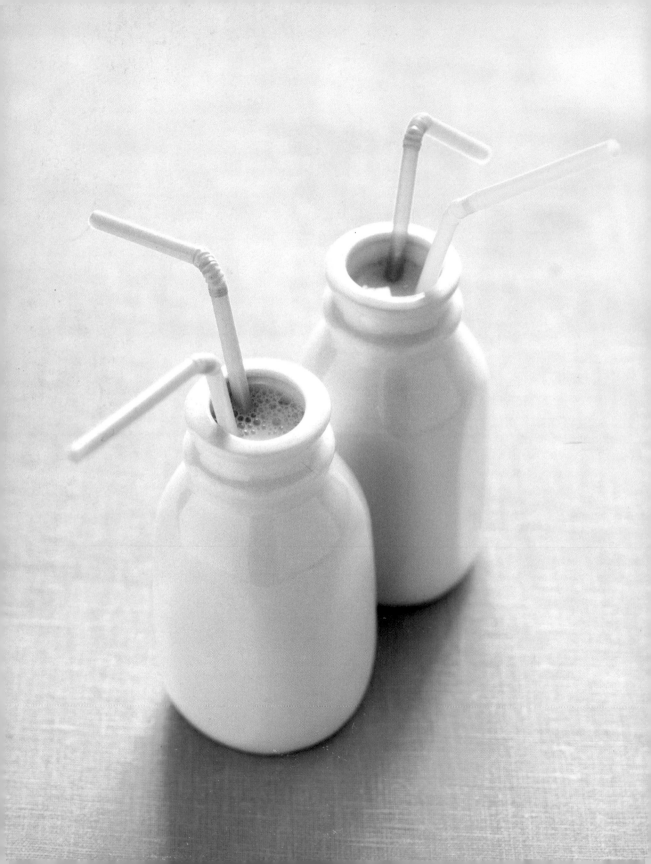

Lunch

CRISPY TUNA TRIANGLES

Yield: 8 triangles • Prep Time: 10 min. • Cook Time: 2-3 min.

This dish is low in fat and a good source of iron. Better than that, it is a delicious take on an old staple – the good old tuna sandwich. These "quesadillas" also offer a boost of fiber by incorporating whole-wheat or brown-rice wraps.

INGREDIENTS

2 cans (each 6 oz. / 170 g) water-packed tuna, drained

2 cloves garlic, minced

2 tsp / 10 ml lime juice

½ tsp / 2.5 ml each salt, pepper and ground cumin

¼ cup / 60 ml each chopped fresh cilantro and green onion

½ cup / 120 ml yogurt cheese (see page 255)

4 six-inch / 15 cm whole-grain wraps

Eat-Clean cooking spray (see page 23)

PREPARATION

1. In small bowl mix together tuna, garlic, lime juice, salt, pepper, cumin, cilantro and green onion.

2. Spread yogurt cheese on one side of each wrap.

3. Spoon one-quarter tuna mixture over half of each wrap. Sprinkle evenly with cilantro and green onion. Fold the uncovered half of wrap over filling and press together.

4. Heat skillet, spray with cooking spray, place quesadillas in skillet and cook over medium-high heat. Use spatula to press down, browning, and then flip. Cook until golden – 2 to 3 minutes per side. Cut each folded wrap in half.

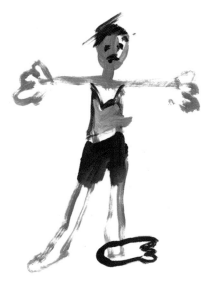

NUTRITIONAL VALUE FOR TWO TRIANGLES:
Calories: 223 | Calories from Fat: 40 | Fat: 4.5g | Saturated Fat: 1g | Trans Fat: 0g | Protein: 17g | Carbs: 30g | Dietary Fiber: 2g | Sodium: 378mg | Cholesterol: 26mg

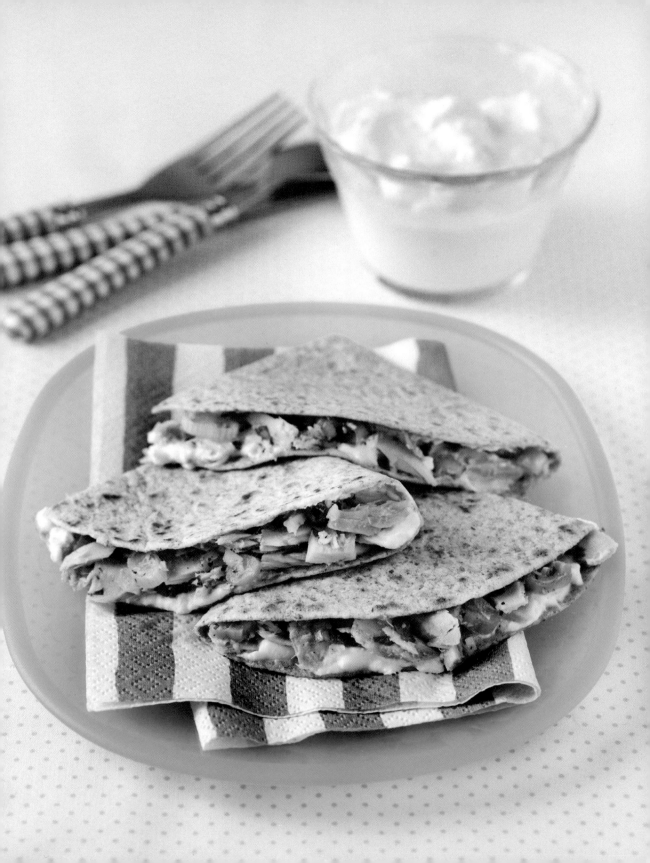

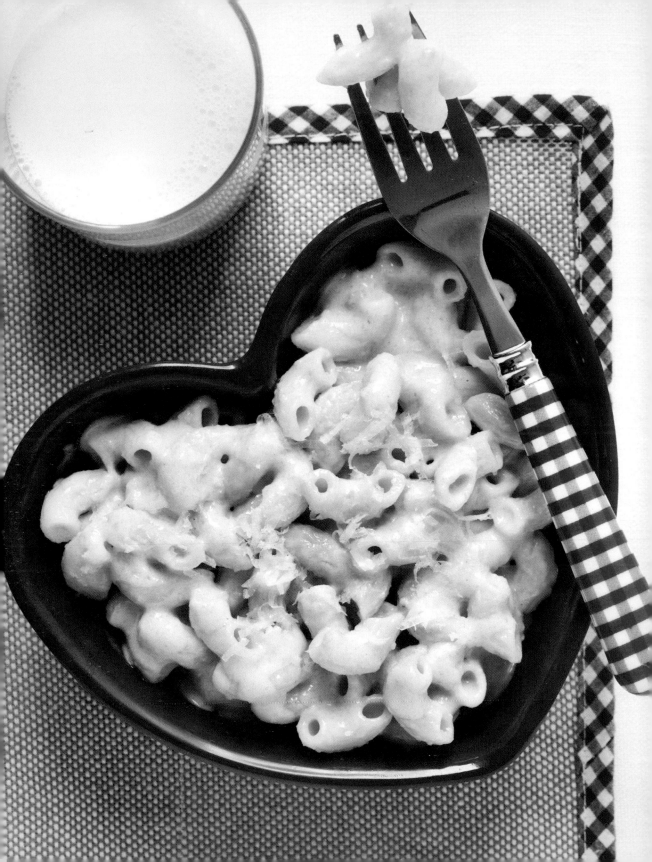

HEALTHY MAC AND CHEESE, BELIEVE IT!

Yield: 9 cups • Prep Time: 25 min. • Cook Time: 30 min.

Conventional macaroni and cheese contains sodium, fat, and questionable cheese. This Eat-Clean version replaces whole milk with skim or even chicken stock, "cheese product" with a hard parmesan cheese – the harder the cheese the less fat – and offers macaroni made from whole grains rather than refined white flour. Lunch is served!

INGREDIENTS

2 Tbsp / 30 ml best-quality olive oil

2 Tbsp / 30 ml flour: whole wheat, gluten free or Power Flour (see page 190)

¾ cup / 180 ml cooked, mashed sweet potato or regular potato

¾ cup / 180 ml low-fat milk (heated until just warm)

1 cup / 240 ml yogurt cheese (see page 255)

2 Tbsp / 30 ml grated parmesan cheese – look for a very old variety

Sea salt

Freshly ground black pepper

¾ pound / 345 g whole-grain noodles: use spiral, elbow or other

NOTE: You can also finish the cooking in the oven. Set your oven to 225°F/ 107°C. Coat a casserole dish lightly with olive oil and fill with macaroni mixture. Cover and bake for 10 to 15 minutes.

MAKE IT A MEAL: I like to steam some broccoli and snow peas and toss them into the dish along with cooked sliced chicken breast. You could also serve these alongside, of course.

TIP For a creamier sauce, purée the potatoes.

PREPARATION

1. Cook macaroni noodles according to instructions on package. Drain and set aside.

2. Meanwhile, heat olive oil over medium heat in a medium skillet. Add flour. Using a wire whisk, make a paste (called a roux). Don't let the roux burn. Add the warm milk gradually, whisking all the while, until you see the sauce begin to thicken. Add the mashed sweet or regular potato. Keep stirring.

3. Now add the grated parmesan cheese, yogurt cheese, sea salt and pepper. Your sauce should look smooth. When that mixture is nicely heated through, add the drained, cooked noodles. Stir to coat the noodles. Serve piping hot.

Jessica Seinfeld recommends adding puréed canned white beans of any variety to increase the protein and fiber content. I like that idea! Check out her book *Deceptively Delicious* (Collins, an imprint of HarperCollins Publishers) for more healthy-kid recipes.

NUTRITIONAL VALUE FOR HALF-CUP SERVING:
Calories: 91 | Calories from Fat: 22 | Fat: 2.5g | Saturated Fat: 0.5g | Trans Fat: 0g | Protein: 4.5g | Carbs: 14g | Dietary Fiber: 1.5g | Sodium: 40mg | Cholesterol: 10mg

TOMATO SOUP

Yield: 8 servings • Prep Time: 25 min. • Cook Time: 1 hr.

I call soup a "walk-away-from-the-kitchen dish," because once the chopping and sautéing are done, you can walk away and let it cook. I always plan leftovers so we can enjoy the soup another day.

INGREDIENTS

2 Tbsp / 15 ml best-quality olive oil

1 large sweet cooking onion, peeled and coarsely chopped

4 ribs celery, trimmed, tough strings removed, coarsely chopped

2 sweet carrots, peeled, coarsely chopped

3 – 4 cloves garlic, peeled

1 medium sweet potato, peeled, coarsely chopped

2 cups / 480 ml chopped fresh Roma tomatoes or one 28-ounce / 800 g can plum tomatoes

4 cups / 960 low-sodium chicken or vegetable stock or water

1 Tbsp / 15 ml crumbled dried basil

1 Tbsp / 15 ml crumbled dried oregano

1 tsp / 5 ml sea salt

Freshly ground black pepper

Pinch good-quality curry powder

2 low-sodium chicken or vegetable natural bouillon cubes

PREPARATION

1. In heavy stockpot or Dutch oven, heat olive oil over medium-high. Add all chopped vegetables and sauté until soft and onion is translucent.

2. Reduce heat to medium and add tomatoes, stock or water, basil, oregano, sea salt, black pepper, curry powder and boullion cubes. Bring to boil and reduce heat to low. Simmer for 30 minutes, stirring occasionally.

3. Using a hand-held blender, purée soup to uniform consistency.

4. Remove from heat and serve. Garnish with a dollop of low-fat plain yogurt or yogurt cheese.

OPTIONAL ADDITIONS:

PROTEIN:

Try cooked, diced chicken breast, canned beans of your choice, or small meatballs made from lean ground chicken, turkey or bison. Kids love meatballs!

COMPLEX CARBOHYDRATES:

Kids love fun small pasta shapes such as bow-tie or rotini. Rice works well, too.

POPEYE'S FAVORITE:

Place some baby spinach in the soup bowl and then ladle the soup on top.

SALBA CRACKERS?:

Crackers can be atrocious, but Salba crackers are made with chia seed, a superfood.

NUTRITIONAL VALUE FOR ONE-CUP SERVING:
Calories: 170 | Calories from Fat: 32 | Fat: 3.5g | Saturated Fat: 0.5g | Trans Fat: 0g | Protein: 1.5g | Carbs: 10.5g | Dietary Fiber: 2.5g | Sodium: 500mg | Cholesterol: 0mg

 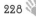

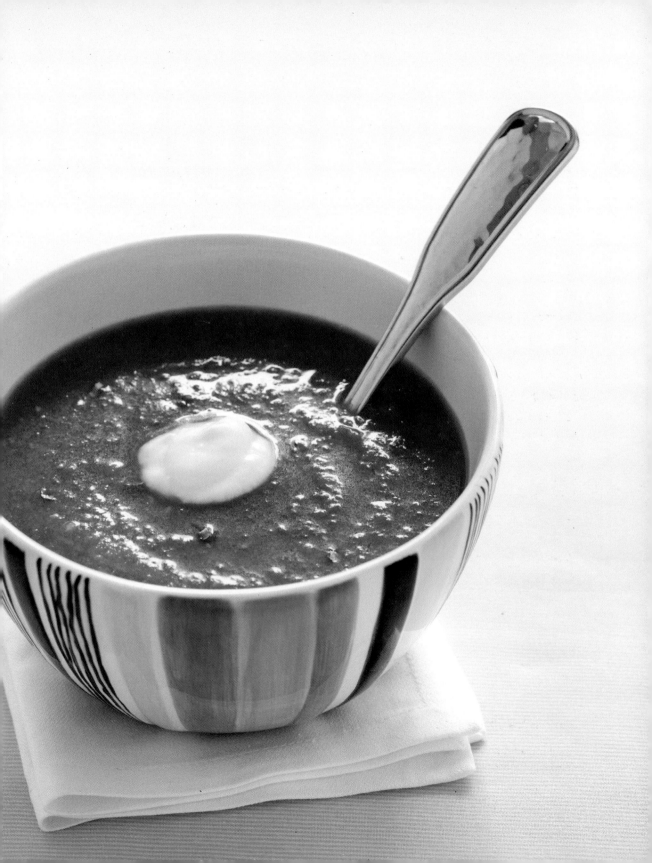

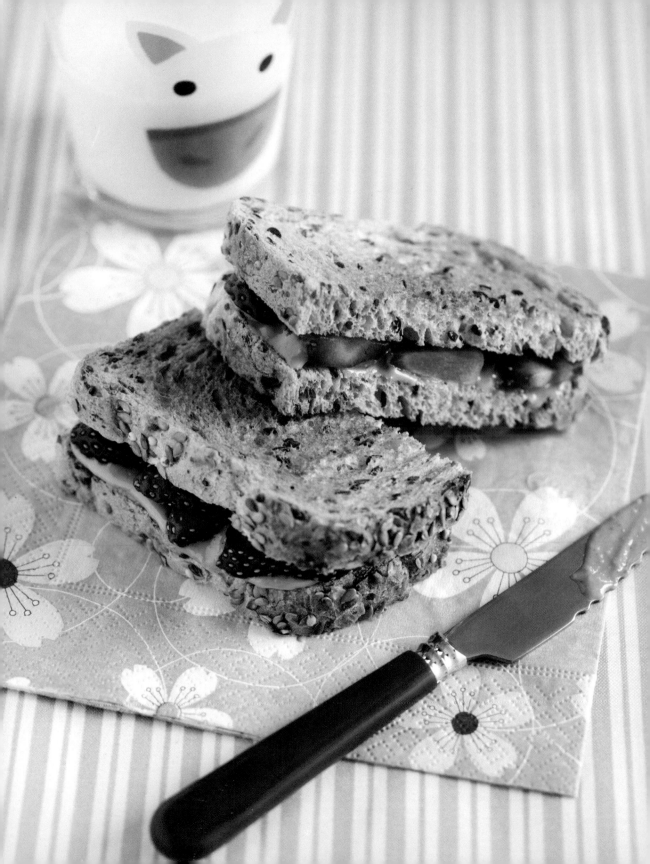

PB & J ALL CLEANED UP

Yield: 1 Sandwich • Prep Time: 2 min. • Cook Time: 0 min.

A delicious peanut butter and jelly sandwich is one of life's little pleasures. The wonderful blending of nutty sweet flavors is an unforgettable childhood favorite. But there are nasty surprises in most commercially made brands of peanut butter and jelly. Both contain high levels of sugar, and peanut butter is often charged with trans and saturated fats. Clean up your PB & J with these tips and you can once again love your childhood favorite.

INGREDIENTS

2 slices bread (Ezekiel bread, rye or any hearty whole-grain bread)

2 Tbsp / 30 ml natural nut butter (almond, peanut or cashew)

4 or 5 fresh strawberries, hulled and sliced

PREPARATION

1. Toast two slices of your selected bread. Spread the toasted bread with nut butter.

2. Place sliced strawberries on top of nut butter so the nut butter is completely covered with berries.

3. Place the second piece of toast on top of the first. Cut and serve.

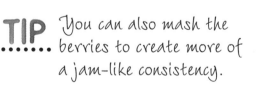

TIP You can also mash the berries to create more of a jam-like consistency.

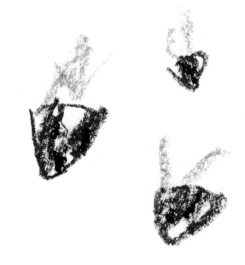

NUTRITIONAL INFORMATION FOR ONE SANDWICH:
Calories: 386 | Calories from Fat: 60 | Fat: 20g | Saturated Fat: 2g | Trans Fat: 0g | Protein: 13.5g | Carbs: 43g | Dietary Fiber: 9g | Sodium: 155mg | Cholesterol: 0mg

EAT-CLEAN EGG SALAD

Yield: 1 cup • Prep Time: 5 min. Cook Time: 20 min.

Egg salad is a long-time kid favorite. It gets a bad rap because of its high fat content and not-so-subtle smell. This recipe was provided by *Oxygen* fan Carolyn Kay. I have made a few minor changes but it is sure to please without the extra fat.

INGREDIENTS

¼ cup / 60 ml fat-free cottage cheese

1 Tbsp / 15 ml skim milk

1 tsp / 5 ml mustard

4 hardboiled egg whites, diced

1 hardboiled yolk

2 Tbsp / 30 ml chopped green onion

2 Tbsp / 30 ml chopped celery

Dash curry powder

¼ tsp / 1 ml sea salt

PREPARATION

1. Whip cottage cheese and milk until smooth in medium-sized mixing bowl.

2. Blend remaining ingredients except egg whites with cottage cheese mixture.

3. Add diced egg whites to cottage cheese mixture. Mix well.

TIP Serve in a bowl alongside crudités or as a sandwich on toasted Ezekiel bread.

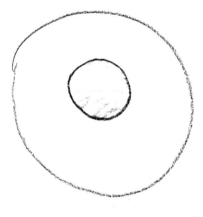

NUTRITIONAL INFORMATION FOR HALF-CUP SERVING:
Calories: 170 | Calories from Fat: 30 | Fat: 3.5g | Saturated Fat: 1g | Trans Fat: 0g | Protein: 17g | Carbs: 18g | Dietary Fiber: 3.5g | Sodium: 528mg | Cholesterol: 106mg

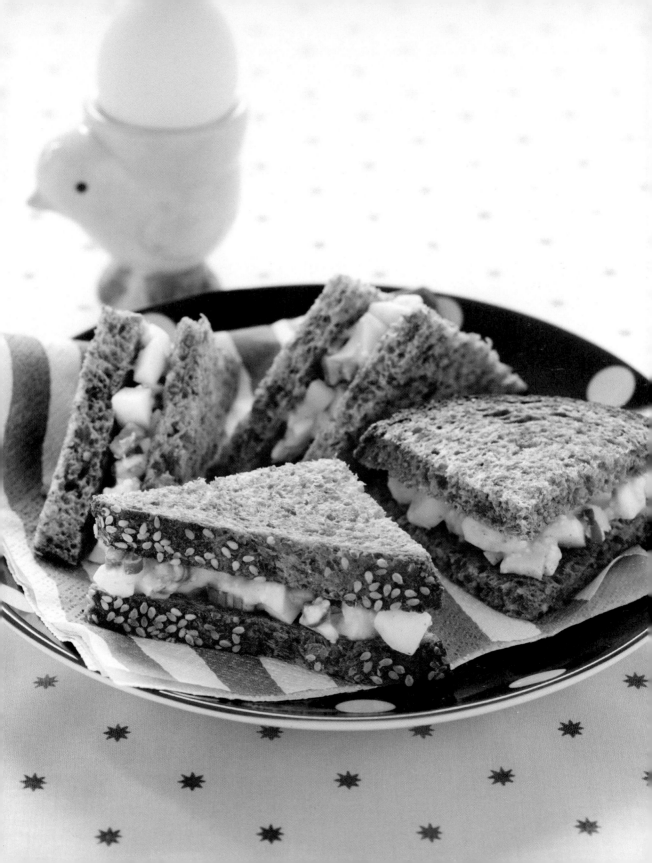

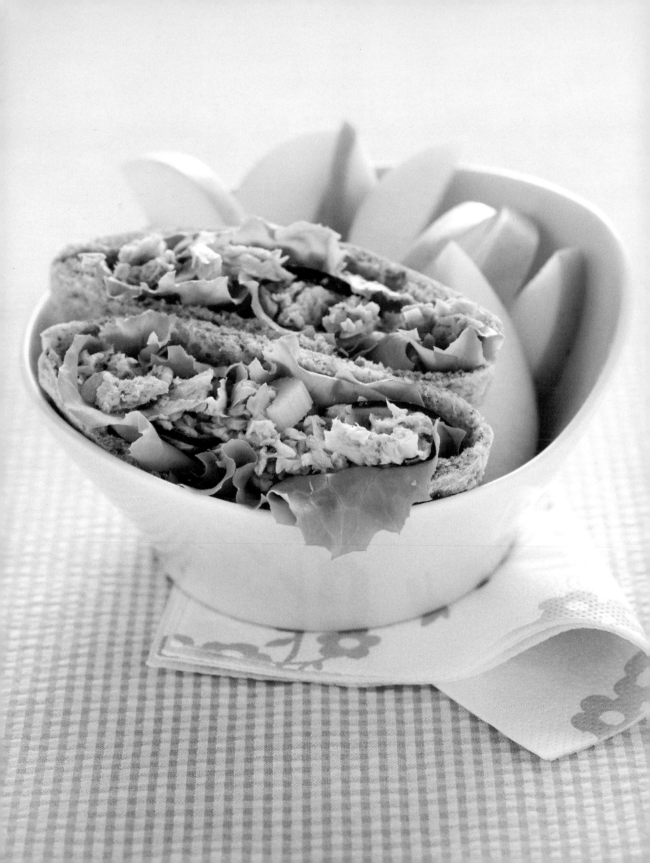

SALMON PITAS WITH CELERY HEART SALAD

Yield: 4 pitas • Prep Time: 10 min. • Cook Time: 0

Kids of all ages will love this salmon wrap charged with zippy vinegar and loaded with health. My mom always mashed the soft salmon bones for added calcium. The kids will never know! You and yours will love these for lunch.

INGREDIENTS

2 Tbsp / 30 ml chopped fresh dill

2 Tbsp / 30 ml fresh lemon juice

1 Tbsp / 15 ml best-quality olive oil

¼ tsp / 1.25 ml each sea salt and pepper

1 small celery heart

½ cup / 120 ml thinly sliced radishes

½ cup / 120 ml thinly sliced sweet onion

¼ cup / 60 ml plain low-fat yogurt

2 cans (each 7 ½ oz. / 213 g) wild salmon, drained

1 cup / 240 ml leafy salad greens

4 whole-grain pita pockets or brown-rice wraps

PREPARATION

1. Finely chop the tender celery heart along with the leaves.

2. Combine all ingredients but wraps and salad greens in a medium-sized bowl. Mix well to combine all ingredients.

3. Line pita pocket with salad greens, then spoon a quarter of the salmon mixture into each pita.

4. Cut in half and serve.

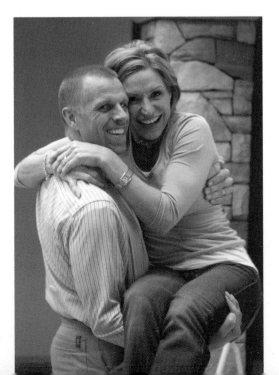

NUTRITIONAL INFORMATION FOR ONE PITA:
Calories: 400 | Calories from Fat: 141 | Fat: 15.5g | Saturated Fat: 26g | Trans Fat: 0g | Protein: 35g | Carbs: 29g | Dietary Fiber: 5.5g | Sodium: 320mg | Cholesterol: 75.5mg

 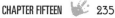

LOADED TURKEY BURRITO

Yield: 6 wraps • Prep Time: 10 min. • Cook Time: 7 min.

These wraps are bursting with flavor and can be made in advance, which is a great help to your morning lunch-making machine. Use any lean ground meat or even soy or tempeh in these wraps to get your family through the day.

INGREDIENTS

8 oz. / 225g lean ground turkey, cooked and drained

½ cup / 120 ml each: grated carrot, zucchini and apple

½ cup / 120 ml low-sodium, sugar-free salsa

6 six-inch / 15 cm whole-wheat or brown-rice wraps

¼ cup / 60 ml Yogurt Cheese (page 255) or Homemade Hummus (page 240)

Salad greens and/or sprouts

PREPARATION

1. Combine salsa with cooked ground turkey in a small bowl. Set aside.

2. Spread each wrap with two tablespoons yogurt cheese or hummus. Place a handful of sprouts and salad greens on top.

3. Divide the grated mixture among the wraps and top with ground turkey/salsa mixture. Fold the bottom of the wrap up and then roll tightly toward the center. Wrap each wrap in waxed or parchment paper. Pack into lunches or refrigerate for later use.

NUTRITIONAL INFORMATION FOR ONE WRAP:
Calories: 274 | Calories from Fat: 77 | Fat: 8.5g | Saturated Fat: 1.5g | Trans Fat: 0g | Protein: 17.5g | Carbs: 9g | Dietary Fiber: 7g | Sodium: 233mg | Cholesterol: 39mg

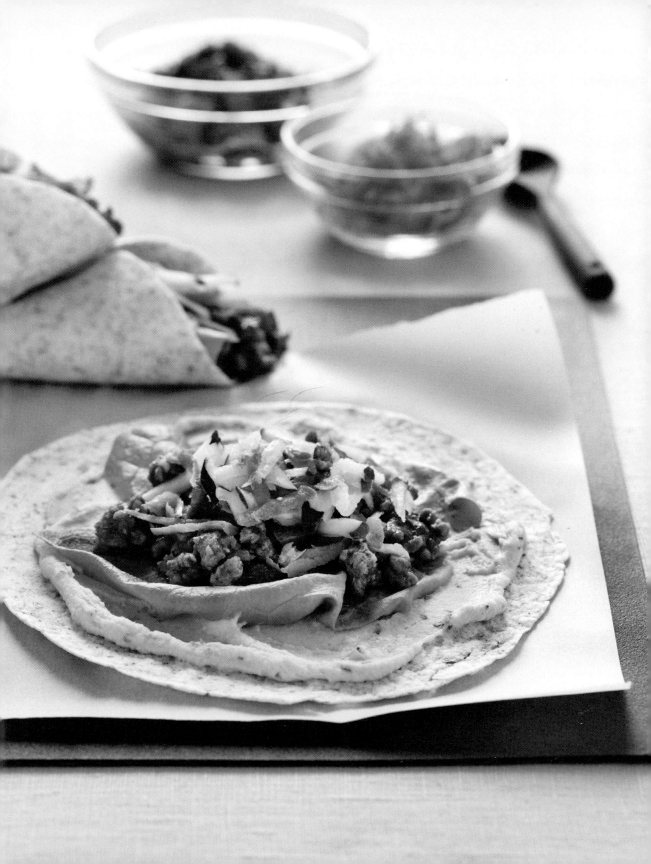

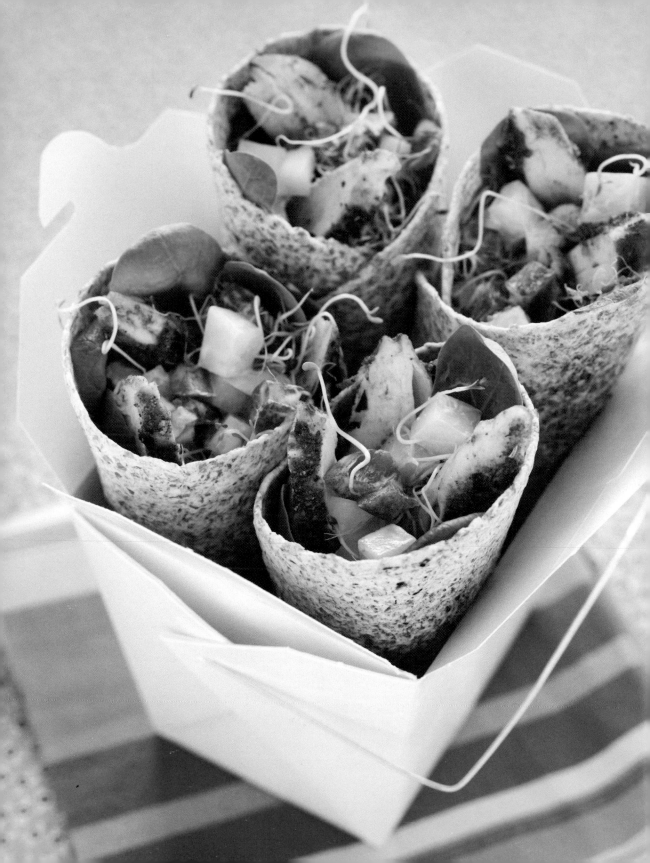

MANGO CHICKEN SALAD WRAP

Yield: 4 wraps • Prep Time: 10 min. • Cook Time: 12 min.

Mango can be sweet, sour or savory and is delicious served every way. Tossing it with chicken is even better – complex carbs and lean protein all at once.

INGREDIENTS

1 Tbsp / 15 ml jerk seasoning

1 Tbsp / 15 ml best-quality olive oil

2 boneless skinless chicken breasts

1 cup / 240 ml sprouts

1 cup / 240 ml baby spinach greens

1 mango, peeled, pitted and diced

½ sweet red pepper, diced

¼ cup / 60 ml low-fat plain yogurt

Juice and grated rind from ½ fresh lime

4 six-inch Ezekiel, multi-grain or brown-rice wraps

PREPARATION

1. In a bowl whisk jerk seasoning with oil. Add both chicken breasts and turn to coat.

2. Place chicken on parchment-lined baking sheet. Broil, turning once, for a total of 12 minutes or until no longer pink inside. This is easier to do when the chicken breast is of uniform thickness.

3. Let cool slightly; cut into thin strips. In a large bowl, toss together mango, red pepper, yogurt, lime rind and juice. Lay one-quarter of the spinach and chicken in each wrap.

4. Divide the mango mixture among wraps, placing in center of each. Place ¼ cup / 60 ml sprouts on each wrap. Fold both sides over filling. Roll up tightly from the end.

NUTRITIONAL INFORMATION FOR ONE WRAP:
Calories: 387 | Calories from Fat: 85 | Fat: 9.4g | Saturated Fat: 1g | Trans Fat: 0g | Protein: 16g | Carbs: 36g | Dietary Fiber: 7g | Sodium: 320mg | Cholesterol: 0mg

HUMMUS AND VEGGIE WRAP

Yield: 4 wraps • Prep Time: 10 min. • Cook Time: 0

Hummus is easy to make and a staple in my kitchen. You will often find me whizzing up a batch in my Clean Eating kitchen. I always keep a can or two of chickpeas in the cupboard so I can whip up a batch in a hurry.

INGREDIENTS

4 six-inch whole-grain or rice wraps

1 cup / 240 ml shredded romaine lettuce

½ cup / 120 ml each chopped tomato, cucumber, and green onion

½ cup / 120 ml each grated carrot and zucchini

1 cup / 240 ml Homemade Hummus

PREPARATION

1. Spread ¼ cup / 60 ml hummus over each wrap.

2. Sprinkle with lettuce, tomato, cucumber, carrot, zucchini and green onion.

3. Fold bottom of wrap up about 1 ½ inches / 4 cm. Roll sides tightly toward center.

4. Wrap each bundle in parchment or wax paper.

HOMEMADE HUMMUS
Yield 2 ½ cups/ 540 ml

INGREDIENTS

1 19 oz. / 540 g can **chickpeas, drained** and **rinsed**

¼ cup / 60 ml **fresh lemon juice**

⅓ cup / 80 ml **tahini**

2 Tbsp / 30 ml **fresh cilantro**

2 Tbsp / 30 ml **best-quality olive oil**

1 **clove garlic**

½ tsp / 2.5 ml **ground cumin**

¼ tsp / 1.25 ml each **sea salt** and **black pepper**

PREPARATION

1. Place chickpeas in food processor. Purée coarsely.

2. Add lemon juice, tahini, cilantro, olive oil, garlic, cumin, salt and pepper. Process. Add lemon juice to thin if necessary.

NUTRITIONAL INFORMATION FOR ONE TABLESPOON:
Calories: 38 | Calories from Fat: 17 | Fat: 2g | Saturated Fat: 0.2g | Trans Fat: 0g | Protein: 1g | Carbs: 4.5g | Dietary Fiber: 1g | Sodium: 60mg | Cholesterol: 0mg

NUTRITIONAL INFORMATION FOR ONE WRAP:
Calories: 282 | Calories from Fat: 36 | Fat: 4g | Saturated Fat: 1g | Trans Fat: 0g | Protein: 11g | Carbs: 45g | Dietary Fiber: 11g | Sodium: 350mg | Cholesterol: 0mg

 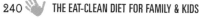

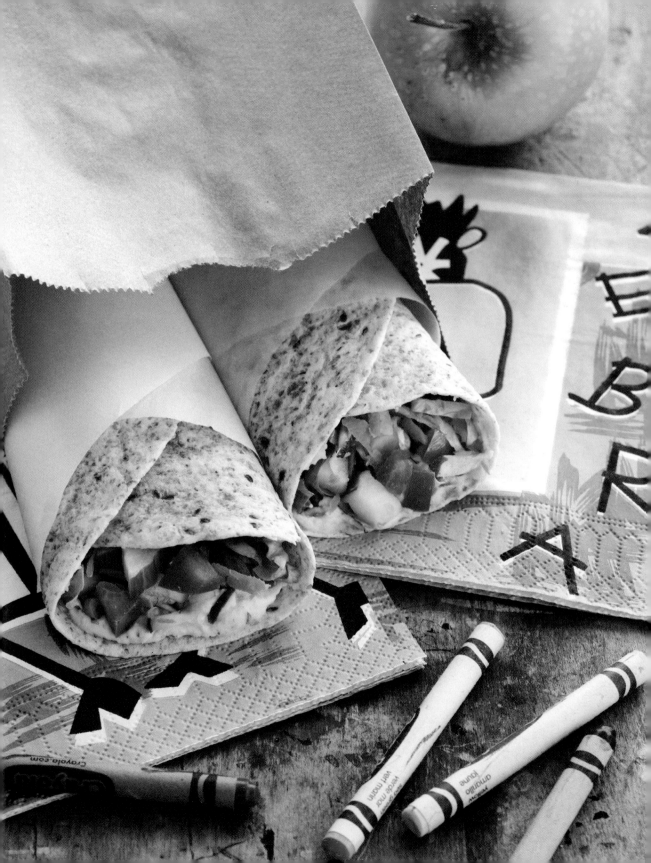

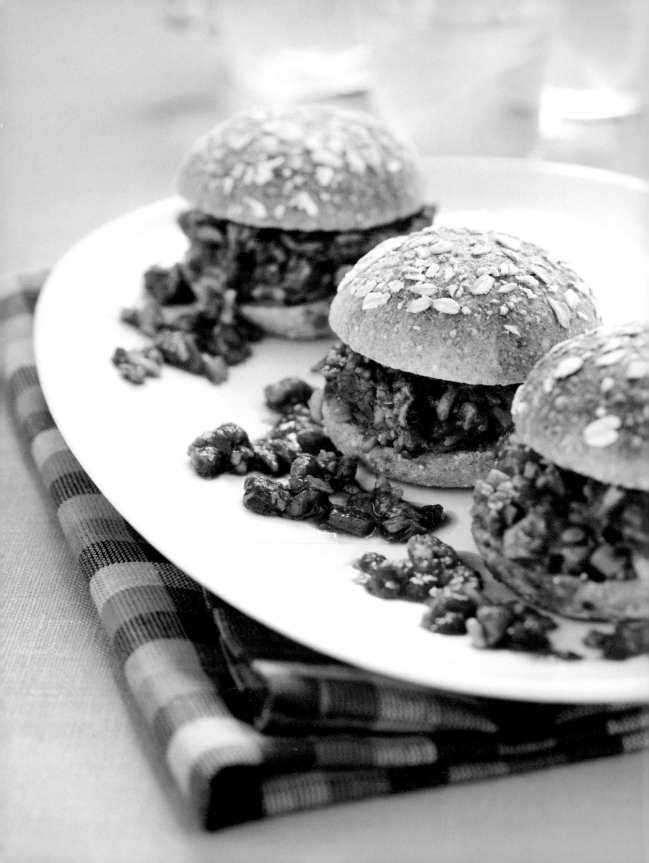

SLOPPY JOES

Yeild 4 sandwiches • Prep Time: 15 min. • Cook Time: 10 min.

Most kids have fond memories of oozy, yummy Sloppy Joe meals. There is something fun and slightly naughty about eating messy food with your hands! Sloppy Joes are sublime comfort food for kids. This recipe contains none of the unwanted ingredients that make most recipes decidedly un-Clean.

INGREDIENTS

½ cup / 120 ml low-sodium chili sauce

2 Tbsp / 30 ml tomato paste

1 Tbsp / 15 ml Worcestershire sauce

1 tsp / 5 ml each cumin, sea salt, black pepper and chili powder

1 Tbsp / 15 ml white wine vinegar

1 Tbsp / 15 ml dried, crumbled oregano

1 Tbsp / 15 ml best-quality olive oil

¼ cup / 60 ml finely chopped sweet onion

¼ cup / 60 ml finely chopped celery

1 clove garlic, passed through a garlic press

1 pound lean ground turkey or bison

¾ cup / 180 ml cooked brown rice

Handful chopped scallions

4 multi-grain buns, cut in half

¼ cup / 60 ml Homemade Hummus (see page 240)

PREPARATION

1. In a small bowl combine chili sauce, tomato paste, Worcestershire sauce, spices, vinegar and oregano. Mix well. Set aside.

2. Heat olive oil in a medium skillet. Sauté onion, celery and garlic for 5 minutes. Add ground meat, let brown for 5 minutes. Drain excess oil.

3. Combine browned meat with spice mixture, cooked brown rice and scallions and mix gently.

4. Spread each side of the bun with a tablespoon of hummus. Spoon about 1 cup / 240 ml of the meat mixture onto one side of the bun. Top with the other bun. Cut in half.

MAKE IT VEGETARIAN: substitute tofu or tempeh for the turkey or bison.

NOTE: This is a spicy dish; make less spicy by using ¼ cup / 60 ml of chili sauce and ¼ cup / 60 ml of Clean Ketchup (see page 286)

TIP You can also make this a to-go meal by securing the meat mixture in a wrap rather than a bun. Roll the wrap in parchment or wax paper and cut in half for a perfect, spill-free meal on the run.

NUTRITIONAL INFORMATION FOR HALF A SLOPPY JOE:
Calories: 235 | Calories from Fat: 85 | Fat: 9.5g | Saturated Fat: 2g | Trans Fat: 0g | Protein: 16g | Carbs: 16.5g | Dietary Fiber: 2.5g | Sodium: 630mg | Cholesterol: 40mg

CHICKEN SOUP – HUMBLE BUT DIVINE

Yield: 10 cups • Prep Time: stock – 15 min., soup – 20 min. • Chill Time: 4-6 hrs. •
Cook Time: stock – 2-3 hrs., soup – 20 min.

Everyone loves chicken soup. It's good-for-the-soul food. The best chicken soup is made with homemade stock. Making it takes some effort but it's worth it, and your efforts will be noted. Chicken soup says love!

INGREDIENTS FOR STOCK

1 x 5-pound / 2.25 kg chicken carcass, organic or
  naturally raised

Enough water to cover the chicken – about 10 to 12
  cups / 2.35 – 2.8 L

2 large onions, peeled and cut into large chunks

4 ribs celery, tough ends removed – keep the leaves
  on the stalks, they are loaded with flavor

2 thick sweet carrots, peeled and cut into large
  chunks

2 parsnips, peeled and cut into chunks

5 cloves garlic left whole

5 bay leaves

1 Tbsp / 15 ml sea salt

INGREDIENTS FOR SOUP

2 carrots, peeled and chopped

3 ribs celery, cleaned and chopped, include leaves

4 Brussels sprouts, chopped fine

1 cup / 240 ml orzo pasta

Handful fresh parsley, chopped fine

2 low-sodium, natural chicken bouillon cubes

PREPARATION FOR STOCK

1. Place all ingredients in large stockpot or Dutch oven. Bring to a boil. Reduce heat. Place lid on pot, allowing steam to escape. Let simmer over low heat for 2 to 3 hours. Let cool. Put pot in the fridge for a few hours to allow fat to congeal on top of the liquid.

2. Remove the congealed fat, return stock to stove and bring to a boil. This is now all protein, and is the makings of an excellent soup stock. Once the gelatin has liquefied, strain the liquid through a fine mesh sieve into another soup pot. Discard cooked vegetables. Remove meat from chicken bones for use in the soup.

METHOD FOR SOUP

1. Add chopped vegetables, orzo and bouillon cubes to soup stock and bring to a boil. Reduce heat and cook for 20 minutes or until vegetables and pasta are soft.

2. Correct soup flavor with sea salt and black pepper. Ladle into bowls and serve hot.

NUTRITIONAL VALUE FOR ONE CUP:
Calories: 119 | Calories from Fat: 7 | Fat: 1g | Saturated Fat: 0.1g | Trans Fat: 0g | Protein: 8.5g | Carbs: 20g | Dietary Fiber: 2g | Sodium: 550mg | Cholesterol: 10mg

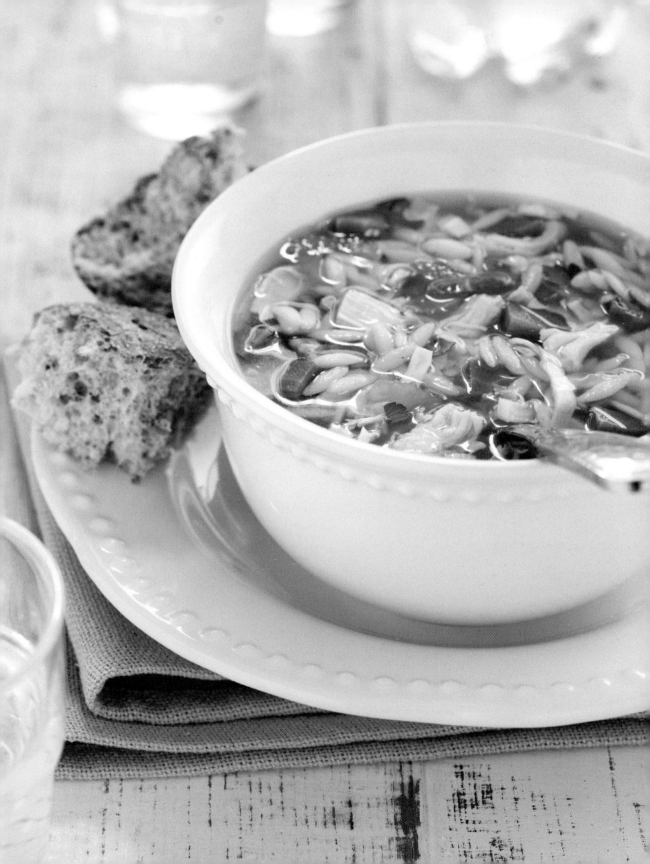

NOTE: Be sure to involve your family in the pizza-making activity. Each of you can choose a favorite topping. It's fun, and even better when you are all sitting down to a homemade slice.

HOMEMADE PIZZA FOR CLEAN EATERS

Yield: 1 large pizza (8-12 slices) • Prep Time: dough – 20 min., pizza – 20 min. • Rising Time: 1 hr. • Cook Time: 15 min.

Most pizzas are loaded with unhealthy fats and white-flour crust. Clean up your pizza with this version, sure to please your loved ones. Kids can help make the dough and load the pizza with chopped veggies. Double the recipe so you don't have to prepare lunch the next day.

INGREDIENTS FOR ONE PIZZA

1 cup / 240 ml whole-wheat flour (or use Power Flour (page 190) or gluten-free flour)

1 cup / 240 ml unbleached, unrefined all-purpose flour or gluten-free flour

1 package, or 2 ¼ tsp / 11.25 ml , fast-rising dry yeast

1 tsp / 5 ml sea salt

½ tsp / 2.5 ml Sucanat

¾ cup / 180 ml warm water

1 to 2 tsp/ 5 – 10 ml best-quality olive oil

Sauce*

Toppings (see page 127 for great topping ideas.)

MAKING THE PIZZA DOUGH

1. Place flours, salt and sugar in the bowl of a food processor. Use the pulse button to combine. Then change the blade to kneading. In a measuring cup combine hot water, oil, yeast and Sucanat. Let stand for five minutes until mixture becomes foamy.

2. Add this liquid to the flour in the food processor while it is running. Soon the dough will turn into a soft-looking ball. If it appears crumbly add more

NUTRITIONAL VALUE FOR ¹⁄₁₀ OF PIZZA WITH CHICKEN, TOMATO SAUCE, SPINACH AND GRATED MOZZARELLA (ONE CUP USED OVER ENTIRE PIZZA):
Calories: 171 | Calories from Fat: 50 | Fat: 5.5g | Saturated Fat: 2g | Trans Fat: 0g | Protein: 11.5g | Carbs: 21g | Dietary Fiber: 4g | Sodium: 420mg | Cholesterol: 20mg

water. Allow the food processor to knead the dough for about 5 minutes.

3. With lightly oiled hands remove the dough from the food processor. Place it in a large bowl. Rub a bit of olive oil on your hands and then rub the surface of the dough. Place a dampened kitchen towel over the dough and let rise for one hour.

4. Remove dough from bowl and place on a surface dusted with flour. Roll it out to fit your pizza stone or baking sheet.

METHOD FOR BAKING PIZZA

1. Make sure you have a rack on the lowest position in the oven. Preheat oven to 500°F / 260°C.

2. Bake pizzas until crust is golden brown, about 15 minutes.

METHOD FOR GRILLING PIZZA

1. Grill pizza dough before dressing with pizza ingredients. Grill until golden on both sides. This takes about 2 minutes.

2. Now dress pizza and then finish by placing on grill and cooking until toppings become warm and cheese melts. You may have to place a sheet of foil over the pizza to keep the heat from escaping.

* This can be a low-sodium sauce from a can or make your own using tomato paste diluted with a bit of rice wine vinegar. Add fresh or dried basil and oregano and a dash of fresh minced garlic. Yum!

HARVEST SOUP

Yield: 12-16 cups • Prep Time: 20 min. & 10 min. • Cook Time: 3.5 hrs. for stock, 1hr. for soup

When the holiday turkey meal is finished the best is yet to come: soup! I love everything about soup – making it, cooking it and eating it. Soup is the ultimate in convenience food because once you have made a batch it is ready to go for you no matter when you need it. Highly portable, loaded with nutrients and packed with lean protein and complex carbohydrates, soup is good food for you and yours.

INGREDIENTS FOR STOCK

2 large turkey legs or one carcass

Water to cover the meat

1 large onion, peeled and coarsely chopped

2 large carrots, peeled and coarsely chopped

1 parsnip, peeled and coarsely chopped

3 whole cloves garlic

5 bay leaves

1 tsp / 5 ml sea salt

INGREDIENTS FOR SOUP

Stock

1 large onion, peeled and chopped

2 large carrots, peeled and chopped

4 ribs celery, trimmed and chopped

2 tart green apples or hard red apples, cored and diced (leave skin on)

2 good-sized sweet potatoes, peeled and chopped

6 Brussels sprouts, trimmed, hard ends removed, shredded

2 Tbsp / 30 ml olive oil

1 tsp / 5 ml sea salt

Freshly ground black pepper

½ cup / 120 ml apple cider

1 tsp / 5 ml dried, crumbled basil

1 tsp / 5 ml dried, crumbled parsley

PREPARATION FOR STOCK

1. Place all ingredients in large soup kettle. Bring to a boil. Reduce heat and let simmer for 3 hours. Let sit until cool. Refrigerate overnight.

2. In the morning, remove fat that has congealed on top. Strain liquid into a clean soup kettle. Place on stove and bring to a simmer.

3. Remove leftover meat from bones, cut into pieces and add to strained liquid. Add any other chopped meat left over from turkey dinner. Discard the remaining bones and vegetables.

PREPARATION FOR SOUP

1. Put olive oil in a large sauté pan and place over medium heat. Add all chopped vegetables and cook briskly until soft. Add chopped apples and continue to cook, stirring frequently. When vegetables and apple are cooked al dente, add to soup.

2. Add remaining spices, salt and cider. Bring to a boil and reduce. Let simmer for 20 minutes. Ladle into bowls and serve hot.

NUTRITIONAL VALUE FOR ONE CUP OF SOUP:
Calories: 93 | Calories from Fat: 24 | Fat: 3g | Saturated Fat: 0.5g | Trans Fat: 0g | Protein: 5g | Carbs: 13g | Dietary Fiber: 2.5g | Sodium: 340mg | Cholesterol: 10mg

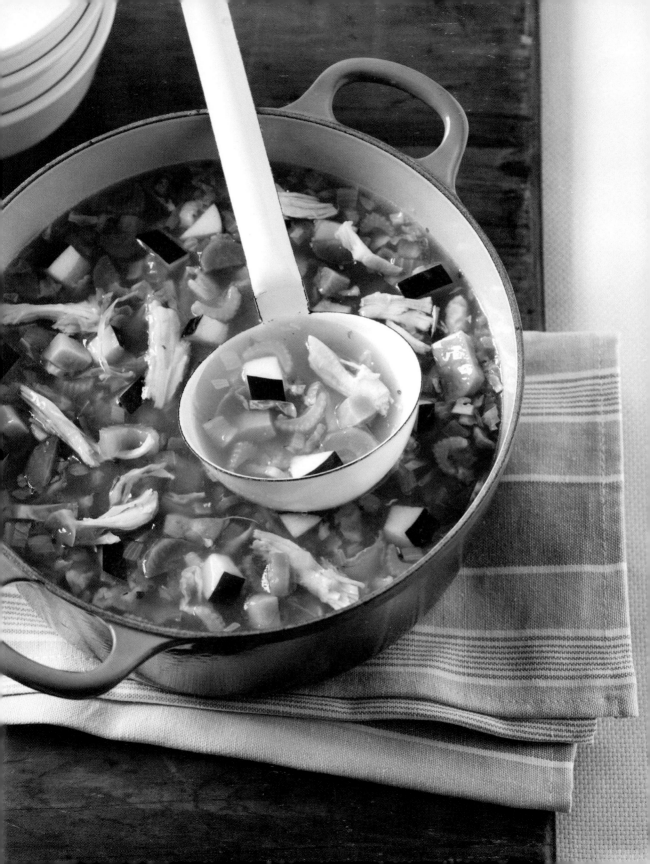

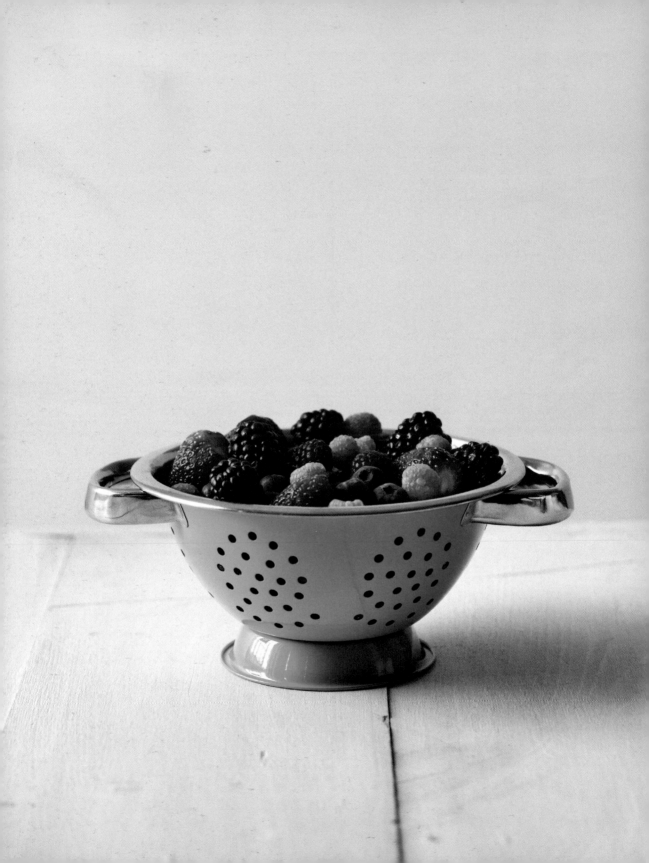

Sides

....

ITALIAN PASTA SALAD

Yield: 7 cups • Prep Time: 10 min. • Cook Time: 15 min.

Pasta salad can be a lifesaver. It packs easily for kids' lunches and can be an ideal meal. It keeps well and is not complicated to make. Teach your kids how to make this so they can feed themselves. Make it a Clean-Eating meal by adding water-packed tuna or a grilled chicken breast to the mix. Vegetarian? No problem. Add diced, cooked tofu or steamed edamame as protein alternatives.

INGREDIENTS

4 oz. / 15 g brown-rice rotini noodles

1 cup / 240 ml carrots, peeled and penny sliced or
  cubed, steamed until just tender

1 cup / 240 ml snow peas, lightly steamed

1 cup / 240 ml cauliflower florets, lightly steamed

½ cup / 120 ml chopped red pepper

1 Tbsp / 15 ml chopped fresh basil

INGREDIENTS FOR DRESSING

2 Tbsp / 30 ml rice wine vinegar

2 Tbsp/ 30 ml best-quality olive oil

1 garlic clove, passed through a garlic press

Pinch sea salt

Freshly ground black pepper

PREPARATION FOR DRESSING

1. Whisk all ingredients together in a small bowl. Pour over pasta.

PREPARATION

1. Place 4 cups of water in a pot and bring to a boil on high heat. Add pasta. While the water is coming to a boil, rinse and chop the carrots, cauliflower, snow peas, red pepper, and fresh basil.

2. Place all vegetables except the basil in a pot. Pour in just enough hot water to cover the vegetables. Cook the vegetables until tender.

3. In the meantime, mix together all ingredients for the dressing in a large bowl.

4. Drain the pasta and vegetables and place them in the bowl with the dressing.

5. Coat the salad in the dressing. Sprinkle with fresh basil.

NUTRITIONAL VALUE FOR HALF-CUP SERVING:
Calories: 56 | Calories from Fat: 20 | Fat: 2g | Saturated Fat: 0.5g | Trans Fat: 0g | Protein: 1g | Carbs: 8g | Dietary Fiber: 1g | Sodium: 70mg | Cholesterol: 0mg

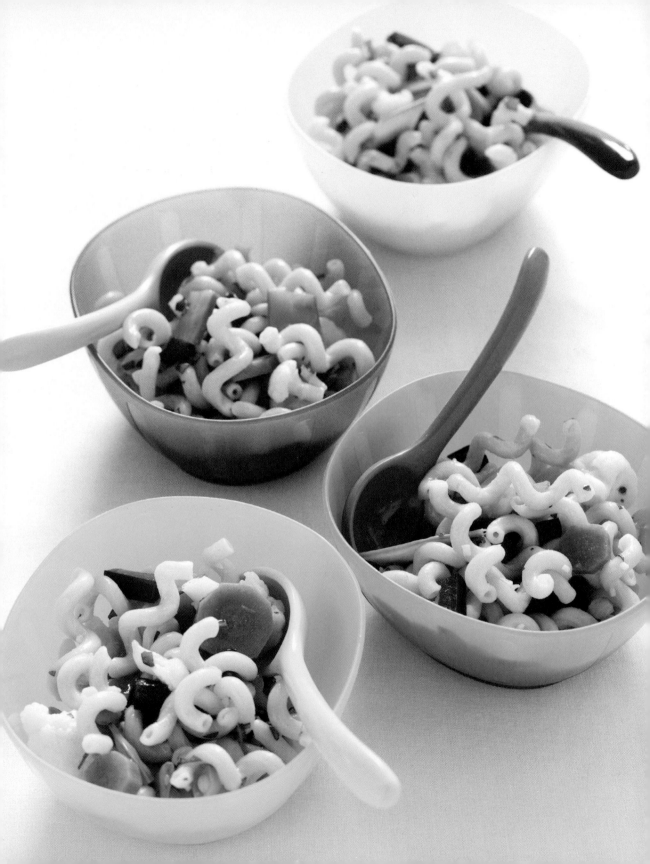

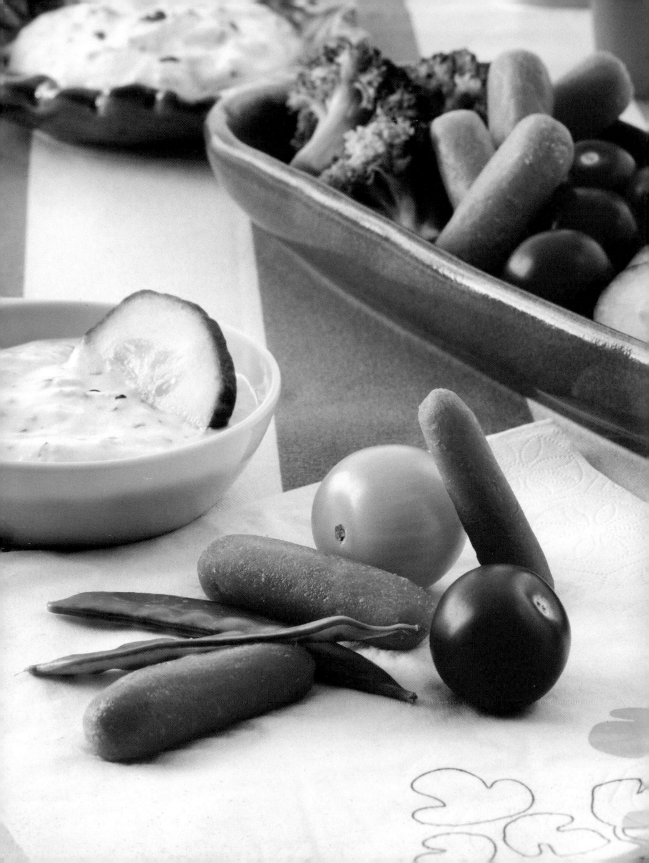

CRUDITÉS THE CLEAN EATING WAY

Yield: 1 cup • Drain Time: overnight • Prep Time: 5 min. (yogurt cheese) 30 min. (crudités)

Crisp, raw vegetables are a common side dish — usually served with a high-fat version of dip such as ranch dressing. This is akin to wearing fine white pants to a motocross event! You take gorgeous, nutritious vegetables and then you throw junk at them. I like to continue the home run with a cleaner version of dip based on nutritious low-fat yogurt ...

INGREDIENTS

Try any or all of this assortment of raw vegetables cut into bite-sized pieces:

• Peppers
• Carrots
• Broccoli
• Green beans
• Asparagus
• Turnip
• Cherry tomatoes
• Cauliflower

Arrange cut vegetables on a decorative platter. Serve with dip, recipe follows.

NOTES ABOUT YOGURT CHEESE

• Yogurt strained for 4 to 6 hours results in a sour-cream-like yogurt cheese.
• Yogurt strained for 8 to 12 hours results in a semi-solid yogurt cheese.
• Yogurt strained for 24 hours results in a firm, cream-cheese-like yogurt cheese.
• Yogurt cheese keeps for one week in the refrigerator.

In some countries you can purchase yogurt cheese already made. It goes by the name of YoCheese in Asia and Labnah in Lebanon. Apparently these folks cottoned on to the goodness of yogurt cheese a long time ago.

YOGURT CHEESE DIP

INGREDIENTS

2 cups / 480 ml **low-fat plain yogurt*** (makes one cup of yogurt cheese)
2 **cloves garlic**, passed through a garlic press
½ cup / 120 ml **fresh basil**, minced
2 Tbsp / 30 ml minced **fresh green onion**
1 tsp/ 5 ml crumbled **dried oregano**
½ tsp / 2.5 ml **sea salt**
Freshly ground black pepper
Cheesecloth for straining

* Look for a yogurt that is natural or organic and not held together with starch or gelatin. The straining process separates the whey from the liquid. If a binding agent is used, the yogurt does not separate as well.

PREPARATION OF YOGURT CHEESE

Place 2 cups / 480 ml yogurt in a colander lined with two layers of cheesecloth. Place the colander over a large bowl to catch the liquid that drips out of the yogurt. Place this set-up in the refrigerator and let stand overnight. Voilà! Discard the liquid in the bowl below, and you are left with rich, creamy yogurt cheese.

TO MAKE DIP

Place yogurt cheese in a medium-sized bowl. Add chopped green onions, garlic and spices. Mix well. Serve with crudités.

NUTRITIONAL VALUE FOR ONE TBSP:

Calories: 19 | Calories from Fat: 0.5 | Fat: 1g | Saturated Fat: 0.5g | Trans Fat: 0g | Protein: 2g | Carbs: 2.5g | Dietary Fiber: 0.1g | Sodium: 70mg | Cholesterol: 0mg

SMASHED POTATOES

Yield: 4 cups • Prep Time: 10 min. • Cook Time: 35 min.

Mashed potatoes are the stuff of dreams. The lovely texture of mashed potatoes means you can play with them on your plate, squish them between your teeth and make wells on top of your heap of mashed delight to hold the gravy. They are just plain fun!

INGREDIENTS

1 lb. / 450 g Yukon Gold potatoes, peeled and cut into chunks

1 parsnip, peeled and cut into chunks

1 cup / 240 ml cauliflower, cut into florets

3 Tbsp / 45 ml plain, low-fat yogurt

½ – ¾ cup / 120 – 180 ml low-sodium chicken or vegetable stock

Sea salt

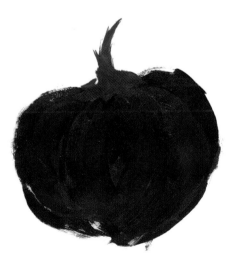

PREPARATION

1. Place potatoes and parsnips in medium-sized saucepan and cover with water. Add a dash of salt. Bring to a boil over high heat. Reduce heat to medium and continue to cook until potatoes and parsnips become soft. To test, pierce a chunk of potato and parsnip with a fork. If the fork glides in, the vegetables are ready. Otherwise continue to cook until soft. Remove from heat and drain, reserving cooking liquid for later use. Place cooked vegetables in a large mixing bowl.

2. Steam the cauliflower until tender. Cauliflower cooks faster than both potatoes and parsnips so it must be cooked separately. Once tender, add cauliflower to the potato/parsnip mix.

3. Using a potato masher, mash the vegetables well. Add the yogurt, seasonings and chicken or vegetable stock. Continue to mash until the mixture becomes smooth. My mom used to further blend with a hand-held mixer until she got it perfectly smooth. You can do the same if you like. The resultant mixture should be smooth just like you remember from your childhood.

NUTRITIONAL VALUE FOR HALF-CUP SERVING:
Calories: 62.5 | Calories from Fat: 1 | Fat: 0.1g | Saturated Fat: 0g | Trans Fat: 0g | Protein: 2g | Carbs: 14g | Dietary Fiber: 2.2g | Sodium: 49mg | Cholesterol: 0mg

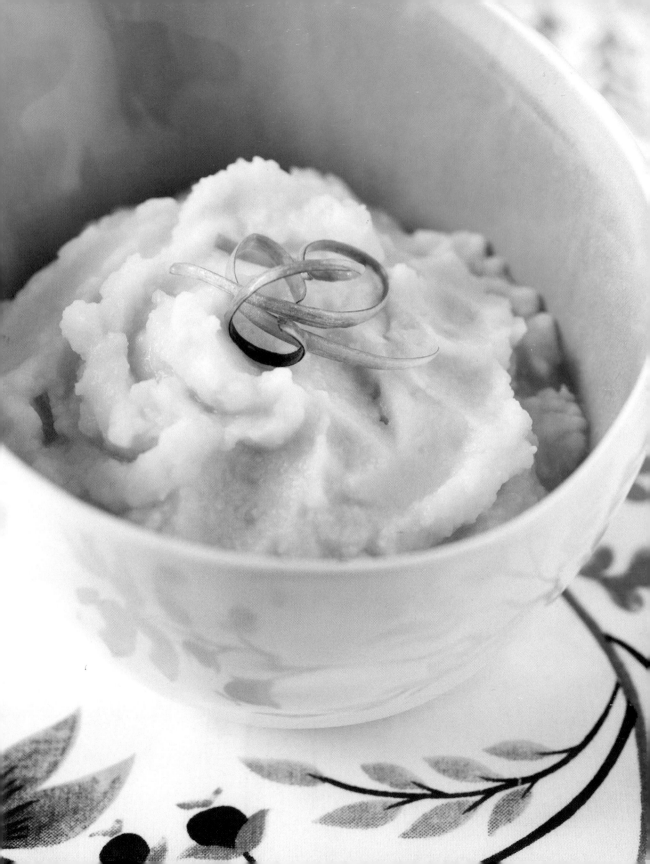

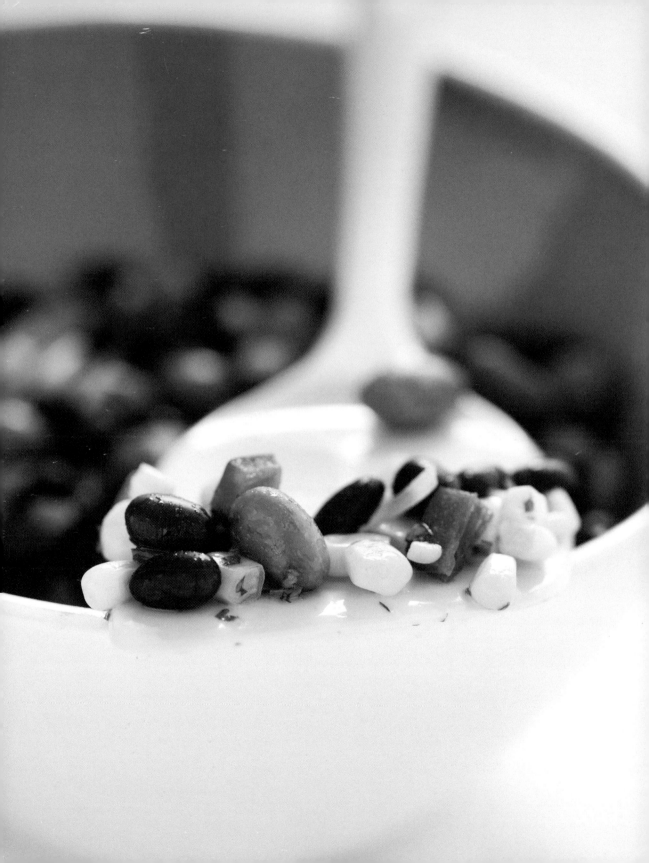

MEXICAN-STYLE BEAN SALAD

Yield: 6 cups • Prep Time: 7 min. • Cook Time: 0

With two different kinds of beans plus corn, this is a colorful salad. All it needs is crusty rolls and a plate of sliced tomatoes and cucumbers to round out the menu, but I like to use this bean salad as an accompaniment to main courses, almost like a salsa. See what you can create with your Mexican salad.

INGREDIENTS

1 can (19 oz / 540 g) black or kidney beans
1 can (19 oz / 540 g) romano beans
1 cup / 240 ml cooked corn kernels
½ cup / 120 ml thinly sliced onion
½ sweet red pepper, chopped
2 Tbsp / 30 ml chopped fresh cilantro or parsley

INGREDIENTS FOR DRESSING

⅓ cup / 80 ml lemon juice
2 Tbsp / 30 ml best-quality olive oil
Pinch sea salt
Pinch pepper

PREPARATION

1. Drain and rinse beans and place in bowl.

2. Add corn, onion and red pepper.

PREPARATION FOR DRESSING

1. In small bowl, whisk together lemon juice, olive oil, salt and pepper. Pour over bean mixture.

2. Sprinkle with cilantro; toss to coat.

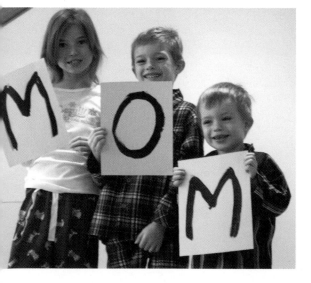

NUTRITIONAL VALUE FOR HALF-CUP SERVING:
Calories: 106 | Calories from Fat: 25 | Fat: 3g | Saturated Fat: 0.3g |
Trans Fat: 0g | Protein: 5g | Carbs: 15g | Dietary Fiber: 4g |
Sodium: 280mg | Cholesterol: 0mg

 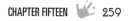

ASPARAGUS WITH A TWIST

Yield: 24-28 cooked spears • Prep Time: 5 min. Cook Time: 7 min.

Asparagus is a sure sign of spring. With its bright green tips and delicious light flavor it is one vegetable that satisfies even the pickiest eater. A light touch of honey and Asian spices kick up the "love it!" factor in this recipe.

INGREDIENTS

2 cloves garlic, passed through a garlic press

1 Tbsp / 15 ml organic honey

2 tsp / 10 ml low-sodium tamari sauce

1 Tbsp / 15 ml best-quality olive oil

1 tsp / 5 ml roasted sesame oil

2 lbs. / 900 g asparagus, trimmed and tough ends
    snapped off

1 tsp / 5 ml sesame seeds, lightly toasted

Sea salt

PREPARATION

1. In small glass bowl mix garlic, honey, tamari and oil. Heat skillet on medium and pour mixture into pan. Allow to heat until bubbling.

2. At this point add asparagus and cook until spears turn bright green and become tender crisp. Don't overcook.

3. Serve immediately, sprinkled with toasted sesame seeds and a dusting of sea salt.

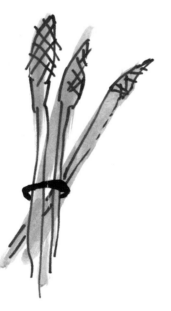

NUTRITIONAL VALUE FOR 3-4 SPEARS OF ASPARAGUS:
Calories: 55 | Calories from Fat: 23 | Fat: 2.5g | Saturated Fat: 0.5g | Trans Fat: 0g | Protein: 2.5g | Carbs: 7.5g | Dietary Fiber: 2.5g | Sodium: 180mg | Cholesterol: 0mg

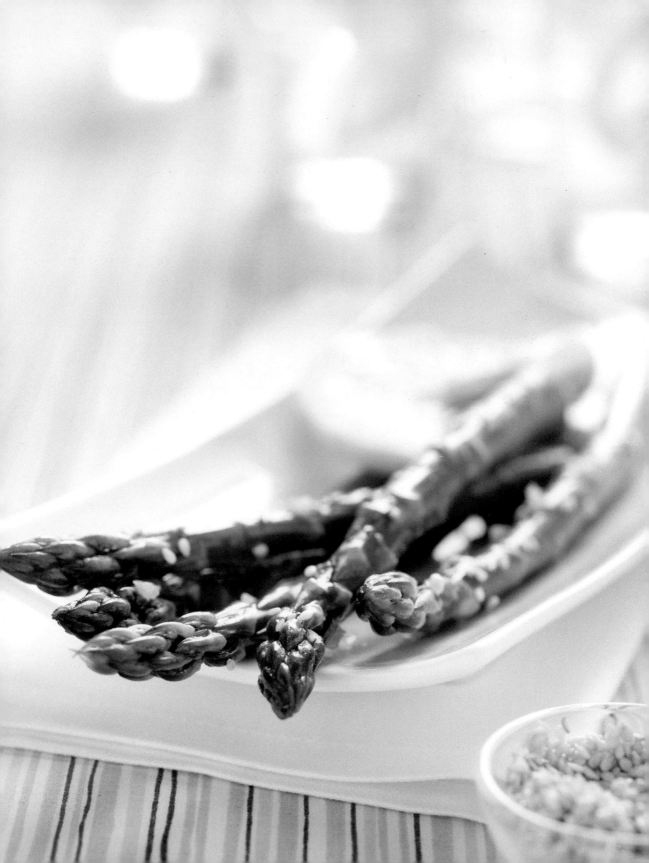

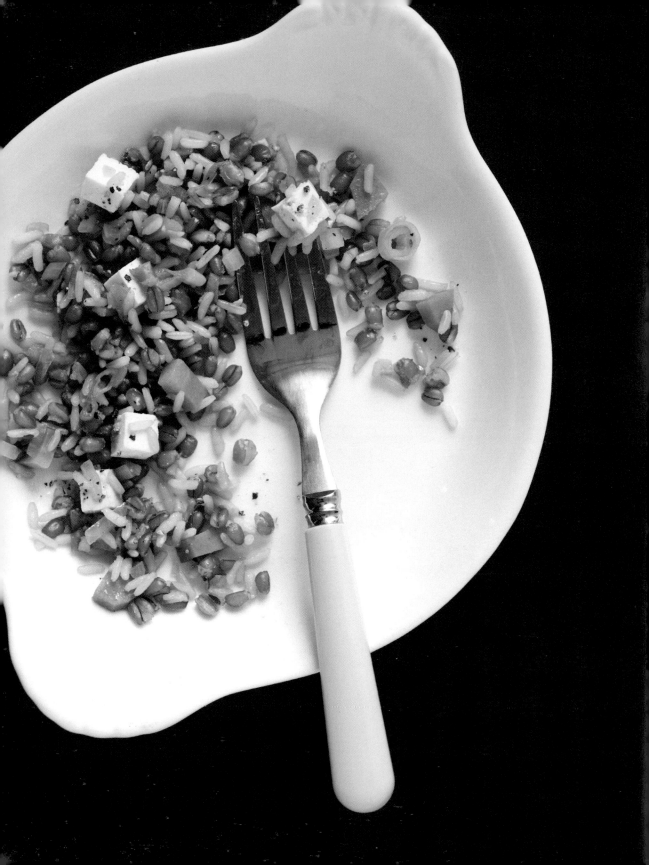

BROWN RICE AND WHEAT BERRY TOFU SALAD

Yield: 6 cups • Soak time: overnight • Prep Time: 15 min. + 20 min. • Drain time: 4 hrs. • Cook Time: 1 hr.

Don't tell your kids the ingredients… just slide a spoonful onto a plate and let them decide. I think you will be pleasantly surprised. I like to marinate the tofu overnight so the flavor really penetrates well.

INGREDIENTS

6 Tbsp / 90 ml light soy sauce or low-sodium tamari

2 tsp / 10 ml (2-inch / 5 cm piece) fresh gingerroot, peeled and finely minced

3 cloves garlic, passed through a garlic press

2 Tbsp / 30 ml best-quality olive oil

Pinch red pepper flakes

1 tsp / 5ml agave nectar

¼ tsp / 1.25 ml roasted sesame oil

½ lb. / 225 g firm tofu

4 cups / 960 ml water or low-sodium vegetable stock

½ cup / 120 ml brown rice

½ cup / 120 ml wheat berries

½ cup / 120 ml thinly sliced scallions

1 medium onion, peeled and chopped fine

1 medium carrot, peeled and chopped fine

Sea salt and fresh ground black pepper

PREPARATION

1. Place wheat berries in a glass bowl. Cover with about 4 cups / 960 ml water. Put a plate over the bowl and let stand overnight. Make tofu marinade by placing soy sauce or tamari, ginger, garlic, olive oil, red pepper flakes, agave nectar and sesame oil in small glass bowl or jar. Mix well.

2. Place tofu in a flat glass or ceramic dish. Cover with marinade and keep overnight in the refrigerator. Drain the tofu well the next day – this will take about 4 hours. Place a colander over a large bowl and put tofu in the colander. Set a heavy plate on the tofu and let the weight of it press excess liquid out. Keep the liquid.

3. Prepare rice and wheat berries for cooking at the same time. I bake them. Preheat oven to 350°F / 177°C. Place brown rice in casserole dish and add water or stock according to package instructions. Cover and bake for 35 to 40 minutes or until water is completely absorbed. Remove from oven, remove the lid and let stand until ready for use.

Prepare wheat berries. Drain in fine-mesh sieve. Place in casserole dish and add 1 ¾ cups / 420 ml water. Cover and bake for one hour or until wheat berries have absorbed all the water and look like they have split open. Remove from heat, remove the lid and let stand.

4. Meanwhile, sautée onion and carrot until soft, and set aside. Cut tofu in half-inch cubes. Put the cubes into the bowl with the marinade. Add cooked rice and wheat berries, sautéed onion and carrot and toss gently. Add chopped scallions and serve.

NUTRITIONAL VALUE FOR HALF-CUP SERVING:
Calories: 103 | Calories from Fat: 38 | Fat: 4g | Saturated Fat: 0.5g | Trans Fat: 0g | Protein: 5g | Carbs: 13g | Dietary Fiber: 2g | Sodium: 380mg | Cholesterol: 0mg

ROASTED ROOT VEGETABLES

Yield: 8 cups • Prep Time: 20 min. • Cook Time: 35 min.

Roasting is one of my favorite ways to cook vegetables. Most vegetables get a subtle and rich flavor when roasted. Roasting is also surprisingly easy to do. You can put your own combination of favorite veggies together, but remember that the cooking time of each must be similar.

INGREDIENTS

1 lb. / 455 g sweet potatoes, scrubbed and cut into two-inch chunks

1 lb. / 455 g potatoes, scrubbed and cut into two-inch chunks

2 large sweet carrots, peeled and cut into two-inch chunks

2 parsnips, peeled and cut into two-inch chunks

4 turnips, scrubbed and quartered

1 head garlic, separated into cloves, loose skin removed

Sea salt

Rosemary sprigs

2 to 3 Tbsp / 30 – 45 ml best-quality olive oil

PREPARATION

1. Preheat oven to 400°F / 205°C. Line a large cookie sheet with Silpat or parchment paper.

2. Place all scrubbed, prepared vegetables in large mixing bowl. Add sea salt and olive oil. Toss to coat.

3. Place all vegetables on baking sheet. Lay rosemary sprigs on top. Roast vegetables in hot oven for 35 minutes or until golden brown and soft.

4. Serve hot. Let your guests know they can squeeze the garlic out of the paper for an extra garlicky touch.

NUTRITIONAL VALUE FOR HALF-CUP SERVING:
Calories: 90 | Calories from Fat: 16 | Fat: 2g | Saturated Fat: 0.2g | Trans Fat: 0g | Protein: 1.5g | Carbs: 17g | Dietary Fiber: 13.5g | Sodium: 50mg | Cholesterol: 0mg

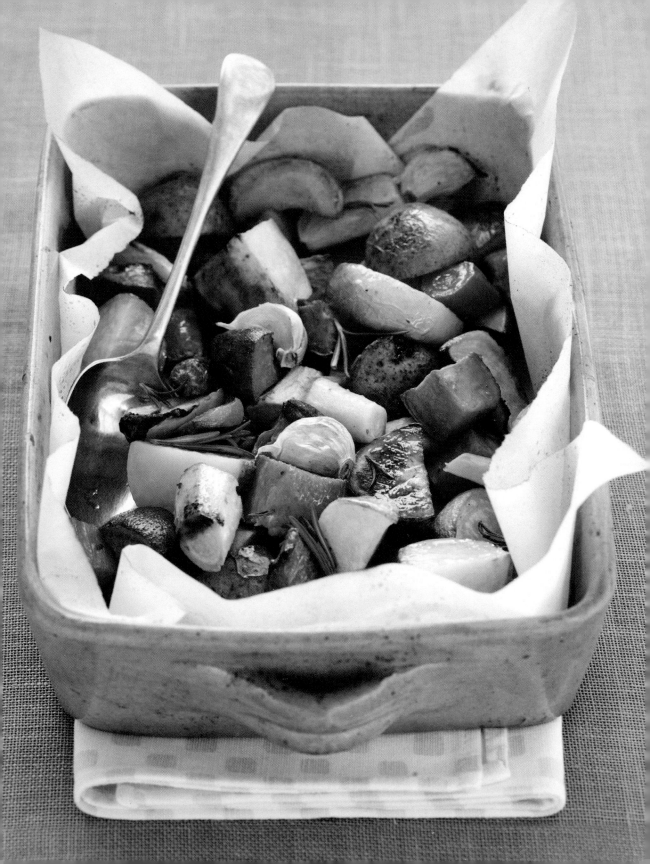

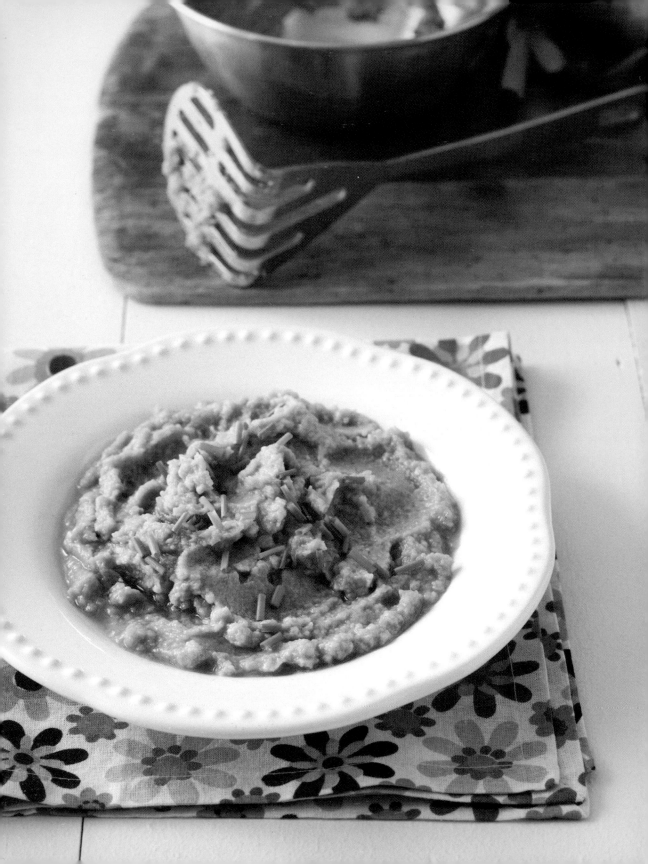

SMASHED SWEET POTATOES

Yield: 3 cups • Prep Time: 10 min. • Cook Time: 20 min.

Sweet potatoes don't have to swim in a puddle of butter and brown sugar. Their natural sweetness is enough to win over the biggest sugar fan. Make these yummy orange-colored smashed sweet potatoes to deliver nutrition and fun to your pickiest eater.

INGREDIENTS

2 medium-sized sweet potatoes, peeled and cut into chunks

1 large sweet carrot, peeled and cut into chunks

½ – 1 cup/ 120 – 240 ml low-sodium vegetable stock

1 tsp / 5 ml grated orange rind

Pinch each cinnamon and ginger

½ tsp / 2.5 ml sea salt

PREPARATION

1. Cook sweet potatoes and carrots until soft. Drain, leaving a bit of the cooking liquid.

2. Add seasonings and vegetable stock. Mash coarsely with a potato masher.

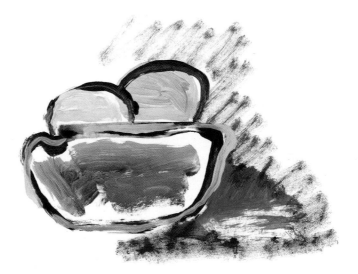

NUTRITIONAL VALUE FOR HALF-CUP SERVING:
Calories: 46 | Calories from Fat: 0.5 | Fat: 0.5g | Saturated Fat: 0g | Trans Fat: 0g | Protein: 1g | Carbs: 11g | Dietary Fiber: 1.5g | Sodium: 210mg | Cholesterol: 0mg

MOLASSES BAKED BEANS

Yield: 8 cups • Soak Time: overnight • Cook Time: 10 hrs. + 6 hrs. • Prep time: 10 min. + 25 min.

I know what song you are singing in your head: Beans, beans, the musical fruit … Come on! Give them a break! Beans are a nutritious must in everyone's diet and the sound effects can be kept at bay by soaking them overnight and by taking digestive enzymes.

INGREDIENTS

1 pound dry white beans – pea, navy or cannelini

2 medium onions, peeled and finely chopped

2 Tbsp olive oil

5.5 oz. can tomato paste

¾ cup Homemade Ketchup (see recipe page 286)

¾ cup dark, unsulfured, blackstrap molasses

4 cloves garlic, passed through a garlic press

¼ cup amber agave nectar (don't run out and buy it if you only have light at home)

2 tsp dry mustard

1 tsp sea salt

1 tsp freshly ground black pepper

PREPARATION

1. Use soaked beans only. Cover with ample water – enough to cover by at least four inches. Leave overnight. The next day, drain the beans. Place them in a large soup pot or saucepan. Again cover with clean, fresh water. Toss in a bit of sea salt or kosher salt. Bring to a boil. Reduce heat and simmer for 10 minutes. Drain and rinse.

2. Place the cooked beans in the slow cooker. Add at least 6 cups of water, again to completely cover them. Set on a long-cooking or slow setting. Cook for 10 hours. When beans are ready (when the skins split), scoop out 2 cups of cooking liquid. Set aside. Drain and discard the rest of the liquid.

3. In a medium skillet heat 2 tablespoons olive oil. Add onion and garlic. Reduce heat and sautée until soft. Add to beans in slow cooker.

4. In a small bowl combine tomato paste, ketchup, molasses, agave nectar, mustard, sea salt and black pepper. Add reserved 2 cups bean-cooking liquid. Mix well. Pour over bean/onion mixture. Cover and cook on low for 6 hours.

TIP Serve baked beans over brown rice for a complete Clean-Eating meal!

NUTRITIONAL VALUE FOR HALF-CUP SERVING:
Calories: 123 | Calories from Fat: 16.5 | Fat: 2g | Saturated Fat: 0.2g | Trans Fat: 0g | Protein: 3g | Carbs: 24g | Dietary Fiber: 3g | Sodium: 300mg | Cholesterol: 0mg

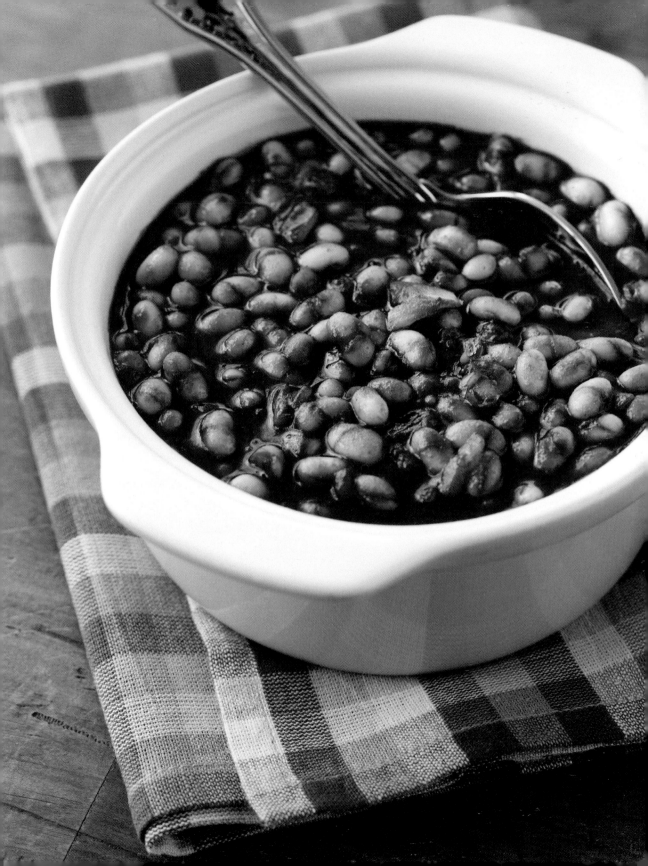

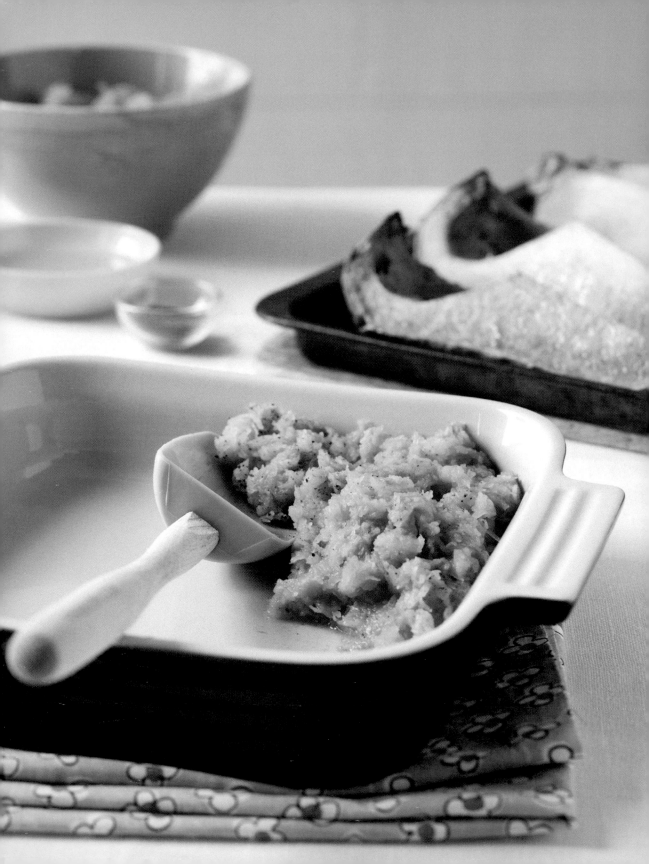

ROASTED SQUASH

Yield: 4 cups • Prep Time: 10 min. • Cook Time: 45 min.

Experiment with different varieties of squash. Butternut squash and acorn are among my favorites but hubbard squash is an interesting little number too.

INGREDIENTS

1 large butternut squash (about 3 pounds/ 1.35 kg)

2 Tbsp/ 30 ml agave nectar

Pinch cinnamon

Pinch nutmeg

Sea salt and black pepper to taste

Eat-Clean cooking spray (see page 23)

PREPARATION

1. Preheat oven to 350°F / 171°C. Line a baking sheet with parchment paper or Silpat.

2. Cut butternut squash or squash you are using in half. Using a large spoon, scoop out seeds and stringy insides. Coat squash with a light spritz of cooking spray.

3. Place the two halves of the squash cut side down on baking sheet. Place in hot oven and roast for 40 minutes. Test for doneness by piercing flesh with a fork. The flesh should be soft. Remove from oven and turn squash over.

4. Meanwhile, mix agave nectar and spices in a medium-sized bowl. Scoop cooked squash into the bowl and mash well with a potato masher.

TIP ⋯⋯ *Just thought I'd mention that you can make a mean "pumpkin" pie with the flesh of a butternut squash. Yum!*

NUTRITIONAL VALUE FOR HALF-CUP SERVING:
Calories: 89 | Calories from Fat: 1.5 | Fat: 0.2g | Saturated Fat: 0.1g |
Trans Fat: 0g | Protein: 1.6g | Carbs: 23g | Dietary Fiber: 4g |
Sodium: 105mg | Cholesterol: 0mg

 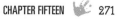

SWEET POTATO OVEN FRIES

Yield: About 25 wedges • Prep Time: 10 min. • Cook Time: 30 min.

Every kid likes fries but every doctor will tell you the trans and saturated fats are a no-no. Sweet Potato Oven Fries will keep you on friendly terms with your doctor and your kids won't even realize they are eating something totally good for them.

INGREDIENTS

2 large sweet potatoes, skin on, well scrubbed

1 ½ Tbsp / 22 ml best-quality olive oil

4 cloves garlic, passed through a garlic press

½ tsp / 2.5 ml sea salt

Freshly ground black pepper

1 Tbsp / 15 ml dried oregano, crumbled

1 Tbsp / 15 ml fresh rosemary, chopped

PREPARATION

1. Preheat oven to 450°F / 232°C. Cut the potatoes into finger-like wedges. Place them in a bowl and toss with the rest of the ingredients.

2. Line a cookie sheet with Silpat or parchment paper. Place the sweet potato wedges on the cookie sheet so the pieces remain separate from each other.

3. Bake for 30 minutes or until wedges develop a lovely golden color.

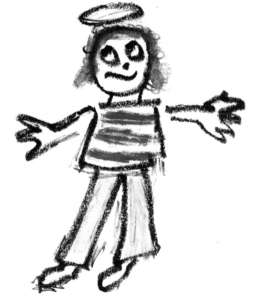

NUTRITIONAL VALUE FOR 5-6 WEDGES:
Calories: 107 | Calories from Fat: 1 | Fat: 0g | Saturated Fat: 0g |
Trans Fat: 0g | Protein: 1.5g | Carbs: 14.5g | Dietary Fiber: 2.5g |
Sodium: 232mg | Cholesterol: 0mg

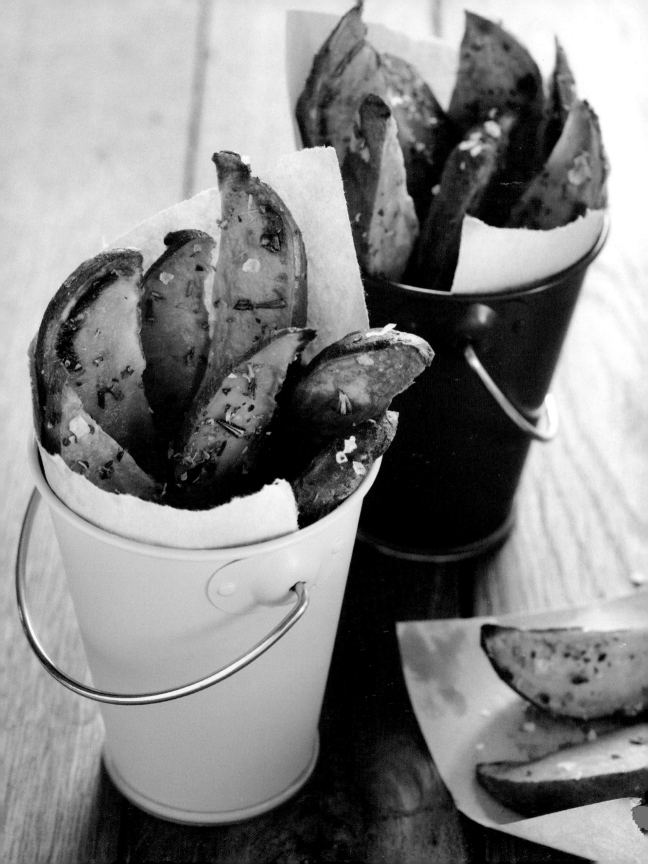

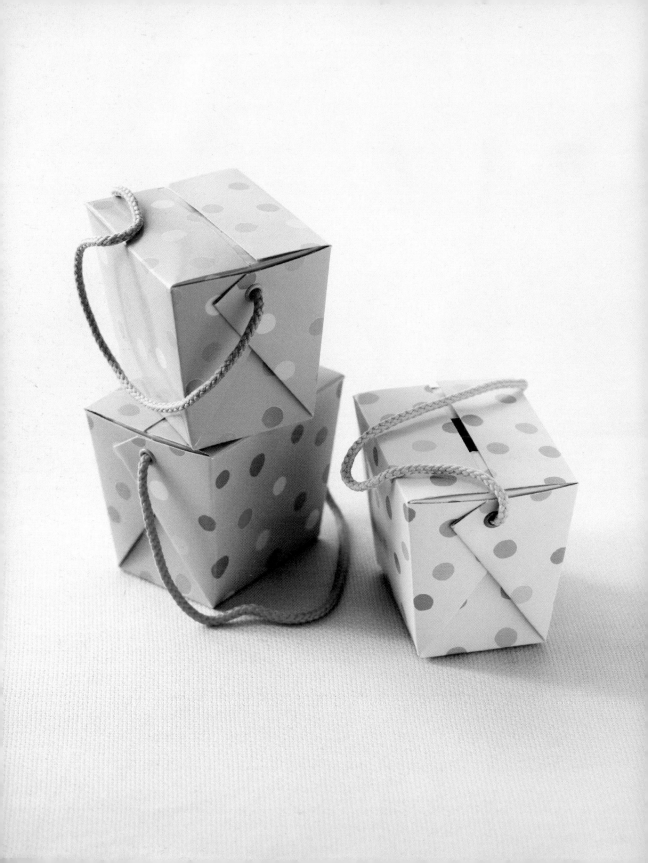

Mains

BAKED FALAFEL PATTIES

Yield: 12 patties • Prep Time: 20 min. • Cook Time: 16-20 min.

What is a falafel? It is a Middle Eastern staple made from chickpeas that tastes simply wonderful. Most recipes call for frying the patties, but I prefer to bake them. Baking keeps the fat content down and the flavor up. A falafel is an excellent source of lean protein and fiber. Your entire family will enjoy the crunchy/soft quality of this main dish and you will now have an inexpensive protein alternative.

INGREDIENTS

2 x 19 oz. / 540 g cans chickpeas

½ cup / 120 ml parsnip purée (this can be cooked and mashed beforehand)

½ tsp / 2.5 ml sea salt

2 tsp / 10 ml ground coriander

½ tsp / 2.5 ml ground cumin

Pinch nutmeg

½ tsp / 2.5 ml fresh ground black pepper

½ tsp / 2.5 ml paprika (make sure it's fresh)

¼ tsp / 1.25 ml ground cinnamon (yes you read that right)

2 cloves garlic, peeled

1 Tbsp / 15 ml fresh parsley, chopped very fine

1 Tbsp / 15 ml fresh cilantro, chopped very fine

2 Tbsp / 15 ml flax seed, ground to a very fine meal

Eat-Clean cooking spray (see page 23)

Olive oil

PREPARATION

1. Preheat oven to 375°F/ 191°C. Prepare baking sheet by lining it with parchment paper or coating with cooking spray.

2. Process the ingredients until the mixture resembles a uniformly consistent paste. Add one egg white if your mixture looks too dry.

3. Coat clean hands with a bit of olive oil and shape mixture into patties or balls. Place on baking sheet.

4. Place in oven and bake for 8 to 10 minutes on one side. Flip over and bake for another 8 to 10 minutes. The patties should be golden on both sides and the outside should be crispy while the center remains soft. Keep your eye on the oven!

TIP Add a tomato and cucumber salad on the side as a delicious Clean accompaniment.

NUTRITIONAL VALUE FOR ONE PATTY:
Calories: 118 | Calories from Fat: 13 | Fat: 1.5g | Saturated Fat: 0g | Trans Fat: 0g | Protein: 4.5g | Carbs: 22g | Dietary Fiber: 4.5g | Sodium: 4.6mg | Cholesterol: 0mg

 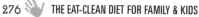

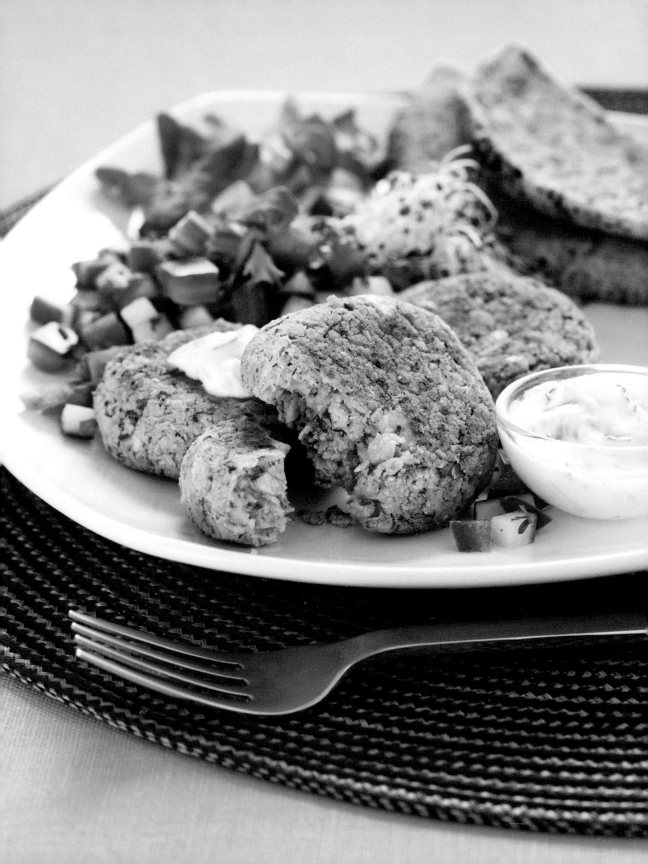

TZATZIKI BETTER THAN BEFORE

YIELD: 1 CUP • PREP TIME: 10 MIN. • COOK TIME: 0

The Greeks use this fresh-tasting sauce as an accompaniment to many dishes. Already a fairly healthy sauce built on a base of yogurt (unlike the sour cream you sometimes encounter in store-bought versions), the nutritional value – and richness of flavor – can be stepped up by using yogurt cheese. If you are planning to make this version of tzatziki, be sure to drain the yogurt overnight at least a day in advance.

INGREDIENTS

2 cups / 480 ml plain nonfat yogurt that has not been
    thickened with starch, gelatin or guar gum

1 large English cucumber, peeled and seeded, finely
    chopped

2 tsp / 10 ml sea salt

2 Tbsp / 30 ml extra virgin olive oil

Juice of one fresh lemon

5 cloves garlic, peeled and finely minced

¼ cup / 60 ml fresh cilantro, coarsely chopped*

Sea salt and black pepper to taste

*Although mint or dill is traditionally used in this recipe I prefer cilantro, but you can add whichever herbs you like.

METHOD:

6 – 24 hours in advance:

1. Set a fine-mesh sieve over a large bowl. Line it with dampened cheesecloth. Place yogurt in the sieve. Cover with a large plate and set in refrigerator. Allow to drain, preferably overnight. Discard liquid, keep thickened yogurt.

6 hours in advance:

1. Place chopped cucumber in a colander and sprinkle with sea salt. Mix the salt into the cucumber. Cover with plastic wrap or a plate and allow the liquid to drain from the cucumber for several hours.

2. Now that the main ingredients are ready you can make your tzatziki.

3. Using a paper towel, remove any excess liquid from the drained cucumber. Transfer to a mixing bowl. Add the yogurt cheese (strained yogurt). Add remaining ingredients and mix until well combined.

NUTRITIONAL VALUE PER TWO TABLESPOONS:
Calories: 56 | Calories from Fat: 31 | Fat: 3.5g | Saturated Fat: 0.5g |
Trans Fat: 0g | Protein: 2g | Carbs: 3.6g | Dietary Fiber: 0.3g |
Sodium: 0.4mg | Cholesterol: 0mg

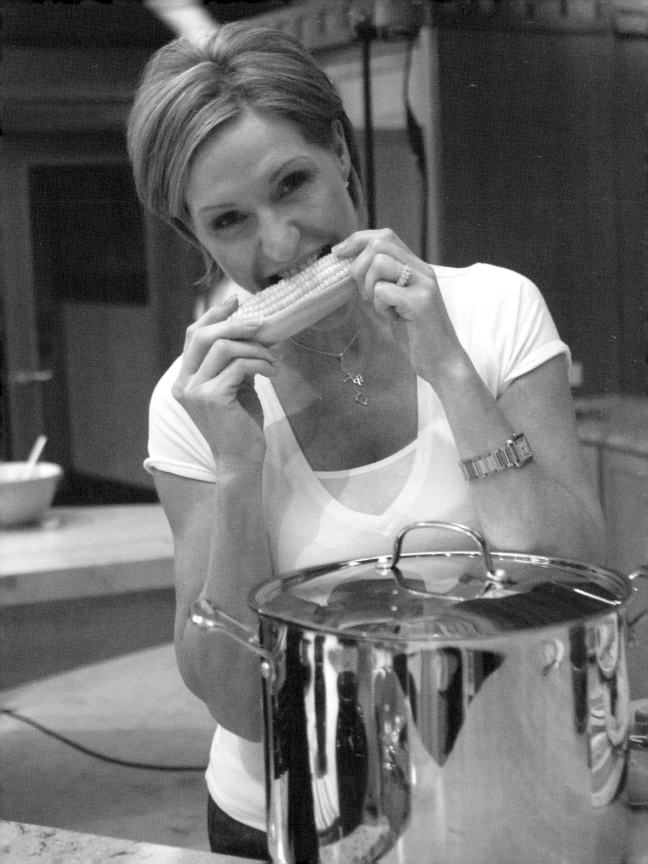

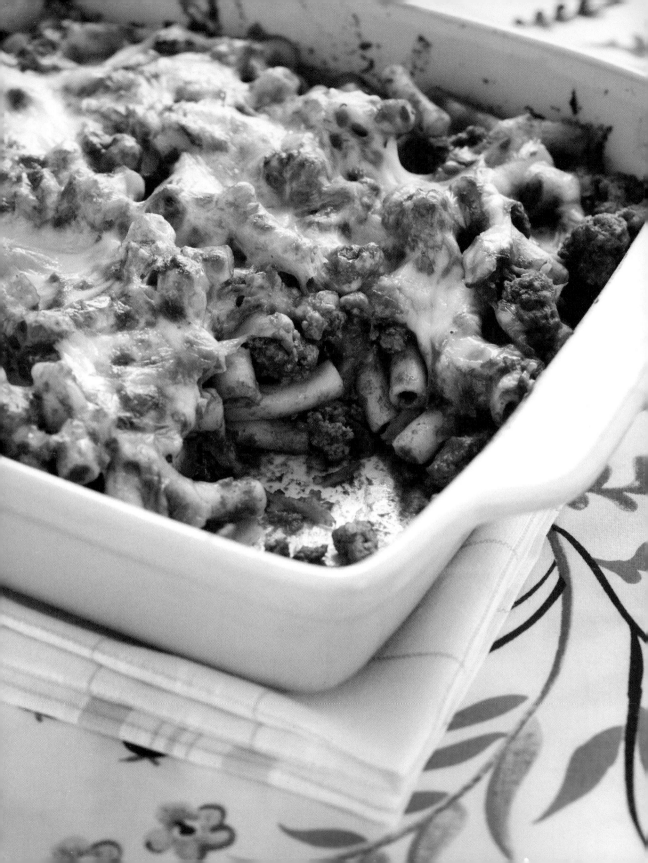

BAKED ZITI

Yield: 9 cups • Prep Time: 20 min. • Cook Time: 25 min.(Turkey) & 20 min. (Ziti)

Here is another pasta dish kids love, and there is nothing better than scooping a hot spoonful into your mouth with that crispy baked layer on top. Talk about comfort food!

INGREDIENTS

1 lb. / 455 g lean ground turkey (make sure the skin has not been ground into the meat)

2 cups / 480 ml shredded sweet carrots

1 small onion, peeled and diced fine

2 cloves garlic, passed through a garlic press

1 - 2 Tbsp / 15 -30 ml best-quality olive oil

26-oz. / 740 g can crushed tomatoes

1 cup/ 240 ml low-sodium chicken or vegetable stock

8 oz. / 225 g brown-rice penne (or other whole-grain pasta)

2 Tbsp / 30 ml fresh basil leaves, chopped fine

½ cup / 120 ml shredded low-fat mozzarella cheese *(optional)*

Eat-Clean cooking spray (see page 23)

PREPARATION

1. In a large skillet, heat olive oil over medium heat and cook ground turkey, carrots, onion and garlic until browned. Add chicken or vegetable stock, tomatoes, pasta and basil.

2. Reduce heat and simmer for 30 minutes or until pasta is al dente.

3. Preheat oven to 350°F/ 171°C. Prepare baking dish with a light coating of cooking spray. Turn pasta mixture into baking dish. Press down lightly with the back of a spoon.

4. Sprinkle with cheese, if using. Place in oven and bake for 20 minutes or until cheese is melted and golden.

NUTRITIONAL VALUE FOR ONE-CUP SERVING:
Calories: 286 | Calories from Fat: 83 | Fat: 9g | Saturated Fat: 4g | Trans Fat: 0g | Protein: 21g | Carbs: 25g | Dietary Fiber: 4.5g | Sodium: 400mg | Cholesterol: 50mg

CRISPY CHICKEN BITES

Yield: 20-24 nuggets • Prep Time: 15 min. Cook Time: 10-15 min.

Many childhood meals these days consist of countless chicken fingers consumed with French fries and gobs of ketchup. But if you watched *Super Size Me*, the breakout movie that exposes fast food for what it is, you will never touch another chicken nugget or finger. Too many unknowns in there! Try this recipe using lean chicken breast meat and yummy seasonings. Make extras for lunches. Your whole family will love them.

INGREDIENTS

3 boneless, skinless chicken breasts, weighing about
  6 oz. / 170 g each

¼ cup / 60 ml oat bran

¼ cup / 60 ml wheat germ

1 Tbsp / 15 ml coarsely ground flax seed

¼ cup / 60 ml coarsely ground almonds

½ tsp / 2.5 ml sea salt

½ tsp / 2.5 ml white pepper

Pinch garlic powder

½ cup / 120 ml water or low-sodium chicken stock

1 large egg white, lightly beaten

Eat-Clean cooking spray (see page 23)

NUTRITIONAL VALUE FOR 3-4 NUGGETS:
Calories: 100 | Calories from Fat: 32 | Fat: 3.5g | Saturated Fat: 0.5g | Trans Fat: 0g | Protein: 12g | Carbs: 7g | Dietary Fiber: 2g | Sodium: 370mg | Cholesterol: 0mg

PREPARATION

1. Preheat oven to 400°F / 205°C. Prepare baking sheet by lining with parchment paper or coating lightly with cooking spray.

2. Cut chicken breasts into nugget-sized pieces: about 1 ½ inches square. Set aside.

3. Next combine all dry ingredients in a large container with a tightly fitting lid. Shake well. This is your coating mixture. Combine water and egg in a medium bowl. Dip each chicken piece in the water/egg-white mixture and then place in the coating mixture. Make sure each piece is well coated. Place on the baking sheet. When all of your chicken has been coated and your baking sheet is full, place in oven and bake for 10 to 15 minutes or until golden.

CLEAN-EATING HONEY MUSTARD SAUCE
INGREDIENTS

1 ½ tsp / 7.5 ml honey

1 Tbsp / 15 ml Dijon mustard

PREPARATION FOR SAUCE

Mix well.

NUTRITIONAL VALUE FOR ¾ TSP:
Calories: 13 | Calories from Fat: 0 | Fat: 0g | Saturated Fat: 0g | Trans Fat: 0g | Protein: 0g | Carbs: 3g | Dietary Fiber: 0g | Sodium: 60mg | Cholesterol: 0mg

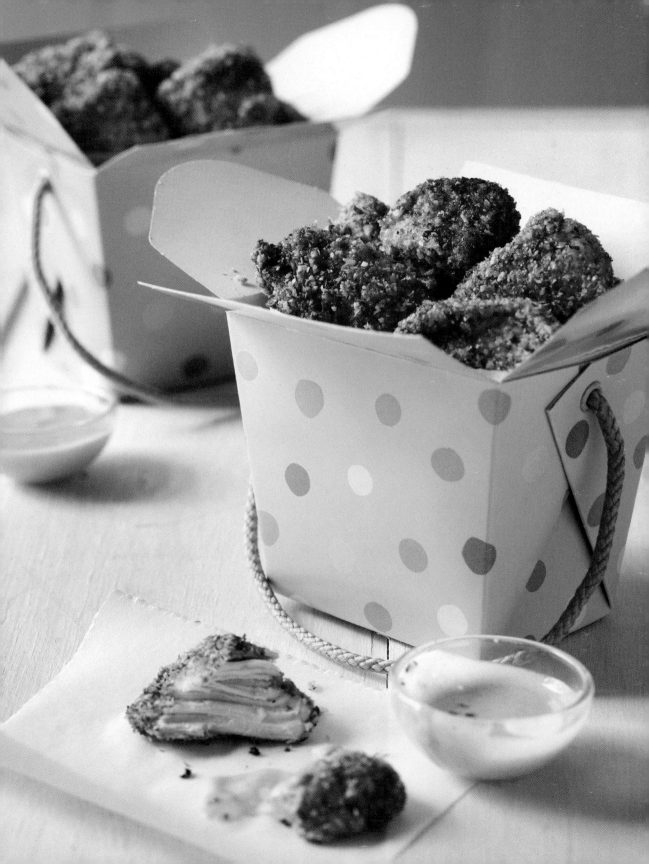

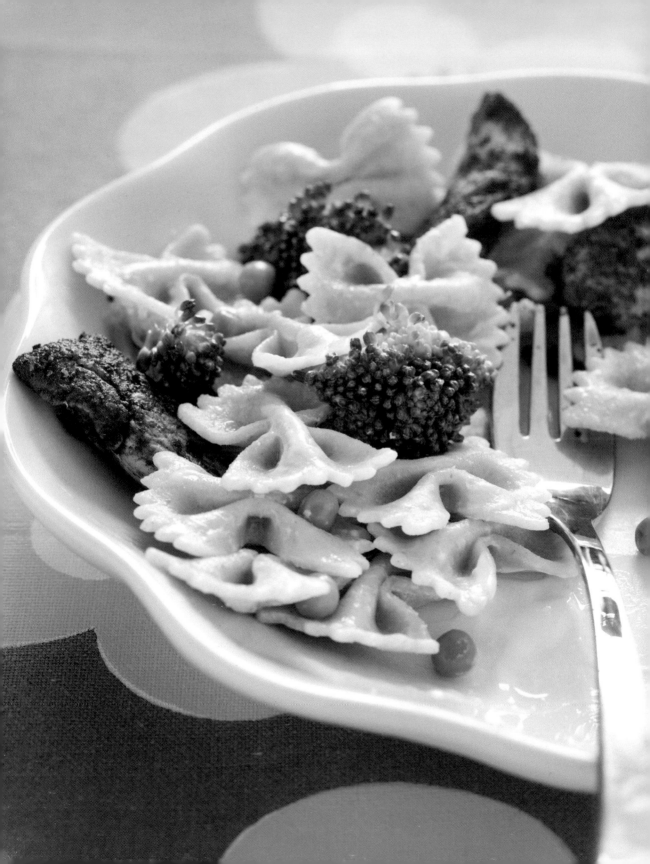

KIDS LOVE PASTA WITH CHICKEN AND BROCCOLI

Yield: 6 cups • Prep Time: 15 min. • Cook Time: 25 min.

Pasta is kid-friendly food. It is even more kid friendly when you make it using healthy grain-alternative noodles. Today you can purchase (or make if you have the time) pasta made out of everything from amaranth to zucchini. Really! So think outside of the box – your pasta box – and try a variety of these delicious pastas. You might be surprised by what your kids will eat.

INGREDIENTS

8 oz. / 225 g brown-rice pasta shapes – bow ties, penne, corkscrews or any shape you like

3 cups / 705 ml broccoli florets

1 cup / 235 ml frozen baby peas

4 lean chicken breasts, skinless and boneless, cut into ½-inch/ 1.25 cm ribbons

2 cloves garlic, passed through a garlic press

1 tsp / 5 ml chicken seasoning

¼ tsp / 1.25 ml paprika

¼ tsp / 1.25 ml chili powder (not chili pepper!)

1 tsp / 5 ml crumbled dried basil

2 Tbsp / 30 ml extra-virgin olive oil

¼ cup / 60 ml plain low-fat yogurt

Freshly ground black pepper

Sea salt

PREPARATION

1. In a large stockpot, cook pasta according to the instructions on the package. Toss the broccoli and frozen peas into the boiling pasta for the last few minutes of cooking. Drain into a large colander and return the mixture to the pot. Cover.

2. Place chopped chicken, chicken seasoning, basil, paprika and chili powder in a large Ziploc baggie. Toss until chicken is well coated. Set aside.

3. Pour olive oil into medium skillet. Heat on medium. Add chicken and cook for five minutes, stirring constantly.

4. Add cooked chicken to the pasta mixture. Add yogurt, sea salt and black pepper and toss until ingredients are evenly distributed.

IS PASTA A GOOD CARB OR A BAD CARB?

Carbohydrates are neither good nor bad. However, you do need to watch how much you eat. Complex carbohydrates are best, and these come from whole grains and vegetables. If your pasta is made from whole grains you are doing your health a favor. Keep your portion sizes in check. A reasonable serving is the size of one cupped hand.

NUTRITIONAL VALUE FOR ¾ CUP:
Calories: 200 | Calories from Fat: 12 | Fat: 5g | Saturated Fat: 0.5g | Trans Fat: 0g | Protein: 13g | Carbs: 24g | Dietary Fiber: 4.5g | Sodium: 40mg | Cholesterol: 20mg

BURGERS ARE A MUST

Yield: 3 cups/ 9 burgers • Prep Time: 20 min. • Cook Time: 10-12 min.

You would not think a burger would appear on a Clean-Eating menu, but even this all-American favorite cleans up well. Burgers are a quick meal fix too. See if your family doesn't agree.

INGREDIENTS

1 lb. / 455 g lean ground turkey or bison (Bison is a great alternative to beef.)

½ cup / 120 ml oat bran

2 Tbsp / 30 ml finely ground flax seed

2 egg whites

¼ cup / 120 ml low-fat chicken or vegetable stock

2 Tbsp / 30 ml cooked sweet potato

1 clove garlic, passed through a garlic press

Freshly ground black pepper

1 Tbsp / 15 ml low-sodium soy sauce

Dash Worcestershire sauce

NUTRITIONAL VALUE FOR ONE PATTY:
Calories: 120 | Calories from Fat: 51 | Fat: 6g | Saturated Fat: 1.3g |
Trans Fat: 0g | Protein: 12g | Carbs: 5g | Dietary Fiber: 1.5g |
Sodium: 190mg | Cholesterol: 40mg

PREPARATION

1. Combine all ingredients in a large mixing bowl. I like to use clean bare hands to mix. Just coat hands lightly with olive oil first to help prevent sticking – it's good for your skin anyway! Once everything is well mixed, form the mixture into about nine patties.

2. Meanwhile, heat a griddle over medium-high heat. Spray with Eat-Clean cooking spray. Place patties in pan. Brown on one side and then the other. It takes about 4 to 5 minutes per side.

3. Serve the burgers on toasted Ezekiel buns, rye bread or a multigrain bread of your choice. Serve with an assortment of lettuce greens, sliced tomato, sprouts, hummus and more conventional burger condiments.

MAKE YOUR OWN KETCHUP

It is not hard to do and there is a lot less salt and sugar in homemade. Yield: about 1 cup/ 240 ml

INGREDIENTS FOR KETCHUP

1 can **tomato paste**

¼ cup / 60 ml **water**

2 Tbsp / 30 ml **Sucanat sugar**

½ tsp / 2.5 ml **sea salt**

¼ tsp / 1.25 ml **cumin**

¼ tsp / 1.25 ml **dry mustard**

¼ tsp/ 1.25 ml **cinnamon**

⅛ tsp / 0.6 ml **ground cloves**

2 Tbsp / 30 ml **cider vinegar**

PREPARATION FOR KETCHUP

In a small bowl mix all ingredients together. Place in tightly sealed glass container. Delicious!

NUTRITIONAL VALUE PER ONE TBSP:
Calories: 14 | Calories from Fat: 0 | Fat: 10g | Saturated Fat: 0g |
Trans Fat: 0g | Protein: 0g | Carbs: 3.5g | Dietary Fiber: 700g |
Sodium: 80mg | Cholesterol: 0mg

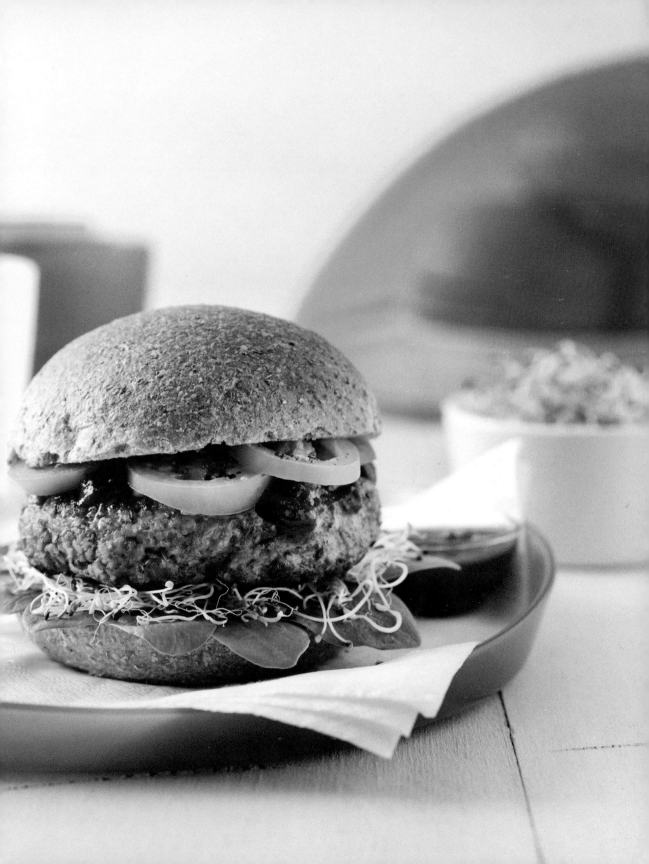

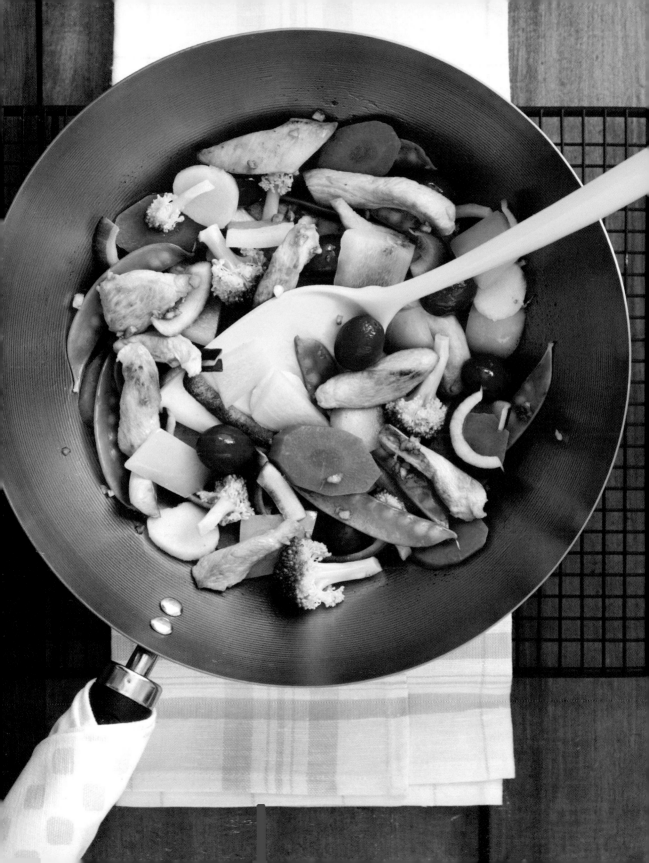

CHICKEN STIR-FRY THE WAY YOU LIKE IT

Yield: 4 cups • Prep Time: 20 min. • Cook Time: 30 min.

When I am in a panic to come up with something creative and quick for supper I almost always make a stir-fry. I start by preheating the oven and putting a batch of brown rice in there to cook while I prepare the rest of the meal.

INGREDIENTS

4 boneless, skinless chicken breasts, cut into bite-sized pieces

2 Tbsp / 30 ml tamari or low-sodium soy sauce

2 Tbsp / 30 ml best-quality olive oil, separated

1 cup / 235 ml brown rice

2 cups / 470 ml water

An assortment of fresh veggies cut into bite-sized pieces – this combination may include any of the following:

• Broccoli florets
• Cauliflower florets
• Penny or other thinly sliced carrots
• Snow peas
• Zucchini – the smaller the better, cut on the diagonal
• Celery
• Peppers of any color, seeded and de-veined
• Peas
• Bok choy
• Cabbage – especially Nappa or Chinese
• Shelled edamame
• Onions
• Mushrooms (technically it's a fungus, but you get the idea)
• Plenty of garlic, minced
• Water chestnuts, drained
• Or any vegetable your family likes

TIP Have your kids or partner chop up vegetables for you.

PREPARATION

1. Preheat oven to 350°F / 171°C. This is for the rice. Lightly coat a casserole dish with Eat-Clean cooking spray. Measure one cup brown or other whole-grain rice and enough water to cook according to package instructions. Bake in oven for 35 to 45 minutes or until all water is absorbed.

2. Meanwhile prepare all vegetables by peeling and chopping into bite-sized pieces. Place the cubed chicken in a bowl. Add soy sauce or tamari and one tablespoon of olive oil. Toss to coat. Heat remaining olive oil in large skillet over medium-high heat. Add chicken and cook until no longer pink – about 4 minutes. Place cooked chicken on plate or bowl.

3. Add a little more oil to the skillet if necessary. Cook vegetables in batches until slightly soft but still crisp. I cook my vegetables separately, since carrots have a different cooking time than zucchini, for example. Each cooked batch goes into a big oven-safe bowl in a warm oven. At the end I toss everything together.

4. Once the rice is done, scoop some into a shallow bowl and spoon hot stir-fry on top. Serve immediately with a bit of low-sodium sauce for flavor. Don't forget the chopsticks!

NUTRITIONAL VALUE FOR ONE-CUP SERVING OF CHICKEN, RICE, BROCCOLI, CARROTS, ONIONS AND MUSHROOMS:

Calories: 351 | Calories from Fat: 82 | Fat: 9g | Saturated Fat: 1.5g | Trans Fat: 0g | Protein: 21g | Carbs: 42g | Dietary Fiber: 48g | Sodium: 400mg | Cholesterol: 0mg

FRIDAY NIGHT CHILI

Yield: 12 cups • Prep Time: 10 min. • Cook Time: 40 min.

When cooler weather sets in there is something intensely warming about putting on a big pot of chili. I love to create a tummy-pleasing batch on Friday night to get me through a busy weekend. Most canned and commercial chili is heavily laced with sodium, fat and even sugar. My Friday night chili is a cleaned-up version your kids will love – not too spicy. Your family will ask for it again and again.

INGREDIENTS

1 lb. / 455 g lean ground bison or turkey

1 large onion, peeled and chopped fine

3 stalks celery, tough strings removed, chopped fine

1 thick sweet carrot, peeled and grated

3 cloves garlic, passed through a garlic press

2 Tbsp / 30 ml extra-virgin olive oil, separated

1 Tbsp / 15 ml unsulfured molasses

1 can (15 oz / 425 g) navy beans, drained and rinsed

1 can (19 oz / 540 g) diced, peeled low-sodium plum tomatoes

1 can (15 oz / 425 g) red kidney beans, drained and rinsed

¾ cup / 180 ml low-sodium chicken stock

1 medium sweet potato, peeled, cooked and mashed

1 Tbsp / 15 ml chili powder

PREPARATION

1. Put 1 tablespoon olive oil in medium skillet and heat over medium-high flame. Add ground bison or turkey and cook until browned.Transfer browned meat from skillet into a fine mesh sieve and let drain.

2. Heat remaining tablespoon olive oil over medium flame in a Dutch oven. Add garlic, onion, carrot and celery. Cook until vegetables become soft, about 5 minutes.

3. Add drained meat, chili powder, molasses, tomatoes and beans. Add chicken stock and mashed sweet potato. Bring to a boil. Reduce heat and let simmer for 20 minutes, stirring occasionally.

TIP I love to serve chili on top of a bowl of steaming brown rice to make it a perfect Clean-Eating meal.

NUTRITIONAL VALUE FOR ONE CUP:
Calories: 196 | Calories from Fat: 38 | Fat: 6.5g | Saturated Fat: 1.5g | Trans Fat: 0g | Protein: 13g | Carbs: 21g | Dietary Fiber: 5.5g | Sodium: 0.5mg | Cholesterol: 30mg

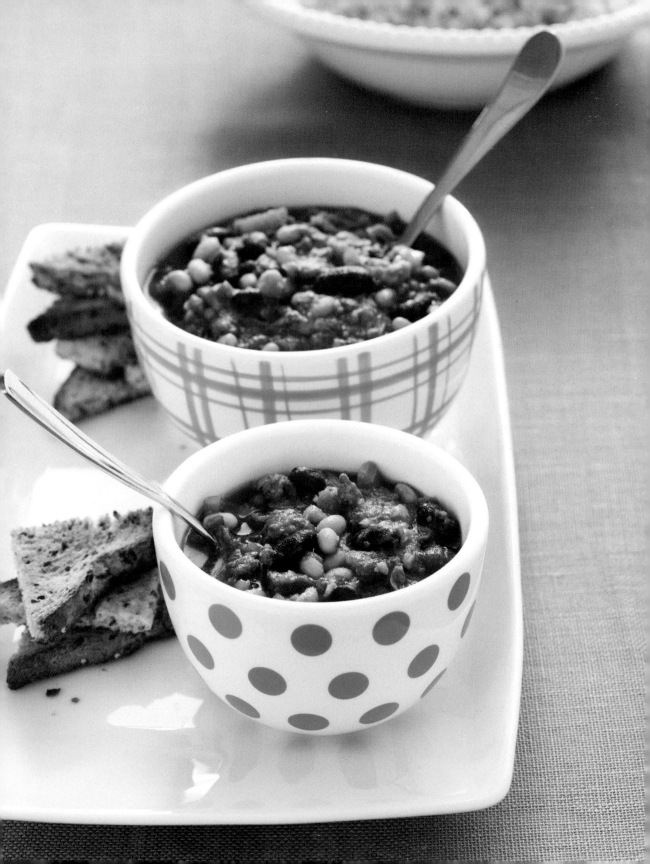

TIP In the summer serve this meal with a jug of unsweetened iced tea — green or black — alongside. Add sliced lemon for some extra zing.

WHOLE-GRAIN PASTA WITH TURKEY MEATBALLS

Yield: 8 servings • Prep Time: 20 min. (sauce) • 20 min. (meatballs) • Cook Time: 1 hr.

You'll find many new varieties of pasta on the supermarket shelves today, including buckwheat (soba noodles), spelt, kamut, amaranth and brown rice, to name just a few. What better way to enjoy the meal but with a lovely tomato sauce and turkey meatballs? Anyone hungry?

INGREDIENTS FOR SAUCE

4 Tbsp / 60ml best-quality olive oil, divided

1 large onion, peeled and chopped

Several garlic cloves, peeled and passed through a garlic press

2 stalks celery, trimmed and chopped

2 sweet carrots, peeled and grated

2 x 28-oz. / 790 g cans low-sodium diced tomatoes

¼ cup / 60 ml fresh basil, chopped fine

1 Tbsp / 15 ml dried oregano, crumbled

Sea salt and black pepper

INGREDIENTS FOR TURKEY MEATBALLS

3 Tbsp / 45 ml oat bran

1 Tbsp / 15 ml wheat germ

1 Tbsp / 15 ml very finely ground flaxseed

Sea salt and black pepper

1 large egg white

¼ to ½ cup / 60 - 120 ml chicken stock or skim milk

1 tsp / 5 ml each oregano, poultry seasoning, seasoning salt

1 ½ lbs. / 680 g lean ground turkey (make sure there is no skin in your mix)

Olive oil for hands

INGREDIENTS FOR PASTA

½ lb. / 225 g pasta noodles of your choice

PREPARATION FOR SAUCE

1. In Dutch oven or large heavy skillet, heat olive oil. Sautée onion, celery, garlic and grated carrot until soft but not browned.

2. Add tomatoes, basil, oregano, salt and pepper. Cook over low heat for one hour, stirring often. Cover and set aside.

PREPARATION FOR TURKEY MEATBALLS
(MAKE WHILE SAUCE IS COOKING):

1. Preheat oven to 350°F / 171°C. Prepare a baking sheet with parchment paper or Eat-Clean cooking spray.

2. Place oat bran, flax, wheat germ, oregano, sea salt and pepper in medium mixing bowl and mix.

3. Add egg white and milk or stock and combine thoroughly. Add ground turkey and mix well.

4. Coat clean hands lightly with olive oil. Make two-inch meatballs and place on baking sheet. Place in hot oven and bake for 25 minutes or until golden brown.

PREPARATION FOR PASTA

1. While sauce and meatballs are cooking, boil pasta according to package instructions. Serve with sauce and meatballs.

NUTRITIONAL VALUE FOR HALF-CUP PASTA, TWO MEATBALLS AND ONE CUP OF SAUCE:
Calories: 315 | Calories from Fat: 89 | Fat: 10g | Saturated Fat: 2g | Trans Fat: 0g | Protein: 9.5g | Carbs: 35g | Dietary Fiber: 8g | Sodium: 300mg | Cholesterol: 50mg

THAT'S NOT A SOY BURGER IS IT?!

Yield: 24 burgers • Soak Time: overnight • Prep Time: 30 min. • Cook Time: 2hrs. (soybeans)30-40 min. (burgers)

The health benefits of soy are substantial. My family loves this recipe so much they don't feel like they are missing out on the regular burgers at all.

INGREDIENTS

2 cups / 470 ml soybeans, soaked* (see instructions at right)

6 cups / 1.5L water

2 – 3 Tbsps / 30 – 45 ml best-quality olive oil

5 cloves garlic, passed through a garlic press

2 large sweet onions – red or Vidalia – peeled and chopped

1 thick sweet carrot, peeled and grated

2 young, firm green zucchini, washed, ends removed, grated and drained

1 small green pepper, seeded and de-veined, chopped

1 small red pepper, seeded and de-veined, chopped

1 tsp / 5 ml sea salt

1 tsp / 5 ml dried oregano, crumbled

1 tsp / 5 ml dried basil, crumbled

1 Tbsp / 15 ml fresh parsley, chopped

2 Tbsp / 30 ml tamari

2 Tbsp / 30 ml natural nut butter (you can use any kind you like, including sesame seed butter, also known as tahini)

2 cups / 480 ml cooked brown rice

NOTE: You can make these ahead of time and keep them frozen until you need them. When baking is complete, remove from heat and place the baking sheet on a wire rack to cool.

NUTRITIONAL VALUE FOR ONE PATTY:
Calories: 80 | Calories from Fat: 15 | Fat: 3g | Saturated Fat: 0.5g | Trans Fat: 0g | Protein: 4g | Carbs: 9g | Dietary Fiber: 2g | Sodium: 160mg | Cholesterol: 0mg

*PREPARATION FOR SOYBEANS

1. Soak soybeans in water overnight. Remove any floaters or stones. When ready to make the burgers, drain and rinse the soybeans well. Fill a large soup kettle with water. Add the soaked beans. Cook on low for about 2 hours or until the beans become soft. You might need to occasionally add more water.

2. Meanwhile, in Dutch oven or heavy skillet, heat olive oil over medium heat. Add garlic and onions and cook until they become translucent – about 5 minutes. Add remaining vegetables and seasonings. Cook until heated through, stirring occasionally. Remove from heat and set aside.

MAKING THE BURGERS

1. Preheat oven to 400˚F / 205˚C. Prepare a baking sheet with parchment paper or cooking spray. Remove cooked soybeans from heat and drain. Using a potato masher, mash the beans well. There should be some texture but no chunks.

2. In a large mixing bowl combine mashed soybeans and cooked vegetables. Add cooked brown rice, tamari, and nut or sesame butter.

3. Put a coating of olive oil on your clean hands and use them to mix the contents of the bowl very well.

4. Make each patty using ½ cup/ 120 ml of mixture, and place on the prepared baking sheet.

5. Place in oven. Bake for about 20 minutes on one side, then flip and cook for another 15 to 20 minutes.

TIP If your mix seems wet add 1 cup/
240 ml of oat bran.

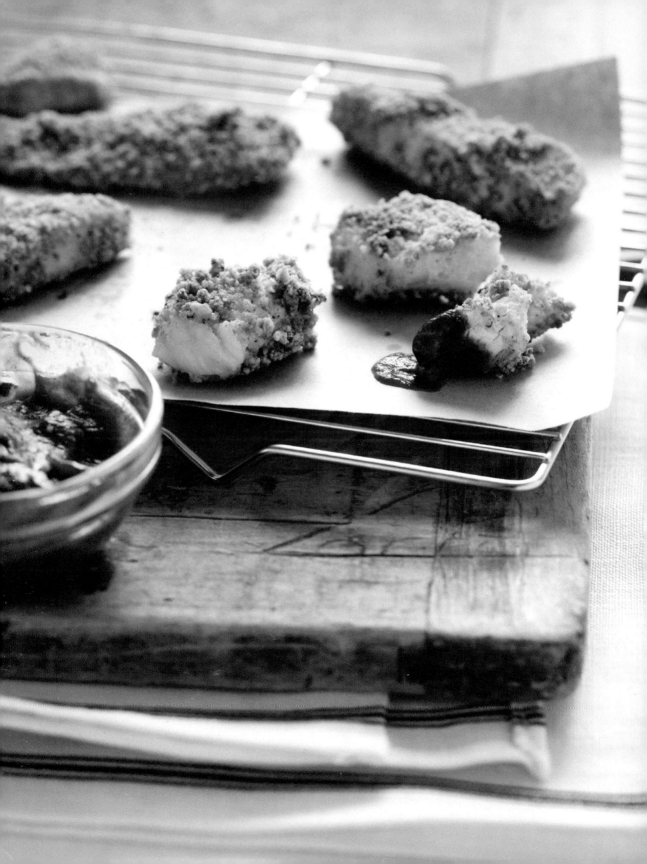

FISH STICKS

Yield: 16 Fish Sticks • Prep Time: 17 min. • Cook Time: 10 min.

It's hard to believe that fish sticks could be healthy for you. Most commercially available fish sticks with breaded coatings contain dangerous trans fats – these come from partially hydrogenated vegetable oils. Trans fats are known to cause health problems, so I encourage you to stay away from them. Most coatings are also high in unnecessary and unhealthy sugar, saturated fat and sodium. But how do you get your child to eat fish at least once a week without that yummy, crispy coating? Make your own version of breaded fish sticks. You and your family will love them.

INGREDIENTS

½ cup / 120 ml crushed Kashi High Fiber Cereal or Kashi Original 7 Grain TLC crackers (You can also use corn meal or breadcrumbs from any stale whole-grain bread.)

2 – 3 egg whites mixed with 1 Tbls water

4 x 6 oz. / 170 g white fish fillets – sole, tilapia or other mild white fish

1 clove garlic, passed through a garlic press

1 Tbsp / 15 ml herb seasoning (I like Old Bay, but prefer a lower salt content)

Eat-Clean cooking spray (see page 23)

NOTE: Serve these fish sticks with vegetable crudités and oven-baked sweet potato wedges for the ideal Clean-Eating kid meal.

PREPARATION

1. Preheat oven to 375°F/ 191°C. Prepare baking sheet by lining it with parchment paper or spray with a light coating of cooking spray. Cut fish filets into rectangles measuring about 3" x 1 ½". Try to keep a uniform size and thickness for best cooking results. Set aside.

2. In a medium-sized bowl mix crumbs with seasonings, salt and pepper. In another small bowl mix egg whites and water.

3. Dip each fish stick in egg mixture, allowing excess to drip off. Dip in crumb mixture and lay on prepared baking sheet. Discard extra breadcrumb mixture.

4. When baking sheet is full, place in oven and bake for 5 minutes or until golden on one side. Then flip and bake the other side. You may not need to bake any longer than 4 or 5 minutes, but keep an eye on the fish sticks. The ideal color is golden brown. Once baked, remove from heat and serve hot!

NUTRITIONAL VALUE FOR 2 FISH STICKS:
Calories: 195 | Calories from Fat: 29 | Fat: 3g | Saturated Fat: 1g | Trans Fat: 0g | Protein: 37g | Carbs: 5g | Dietary Fiber: 1g | Sodium: 154mg | Cholesterol: 85mg

KIDS LIKE TOFU BURRITOS

Yield: 4 wraps • Prep Time: 15 min. • Cook Time: 22 min.

Tofu is NOT YUCKY! It is a versatile, inexpensive, high-protein ingredient that can be successfully "hidden" in many dishes. The bland nature of this soybean curd means tofu works well with a variety of flavorings, including the zippy seasoning in these burritos.

INGREDIENTS

1 pkg (12 oz / 350 g) extra-firm tofu, drained

1 Tbsp / 15 ml olive oil

1 large onion, chopped

2 cloves garlic, minced

½ tsp / 2.5 ml each sea salt and pepper

½ tsp / 2.5 ml cumin

½ tsp / 2.5 ml chili powder

½ sweet green pepper, chopped

½ red bell pepper, chopped

1 jalapeno pepper, chopped

1 cup / 240 ml canned diced tomatoes, drained

4 six-inch / whole-wheat or brown rice wraps

PREPARATION

1. Preheat oven to 400°F / 205°C.

2. Pat tofu dry with paper towel. Cut into ½-inch/ 1 cm cubes. Set aside.

3. In skillet, heat oil over medium heat. Cook onion, garlic, cumin, chili powder, salt and pepper, stirring occasionally, until onion is softened, about 3 minutes. Add tofu cubes, green and jalapeno peppers and tomatoes. Cook until peppers are softened, about 4 minutes.

3. Spoon about 1 cup / 240 ml of the tofu mixture along the center of each tortilla. Fold up the bottom and top edges, then sides, until it forms a roll.

4. Bake on baking sheet lined with parchment paper in preheated oven until golden. This takes about 15 minutes. Cut diagonally into halves.

TIP Add leftover brown rice to your protein to up the complex carbs and fiber . . . and to clean out the fridge! Yum!

NUTRITIONAL VALUE FOR ONE WRAP:
Calories: 265 | Calories from Fat: 77 | Fat: 12g | Saturated Fat: 1.5g | Trans Fat: 0g | Protein: 18g | Carbs: 26g | Dietary Fiber: 6.5g | Sodium: 400mg | Cholesterol: 0mg

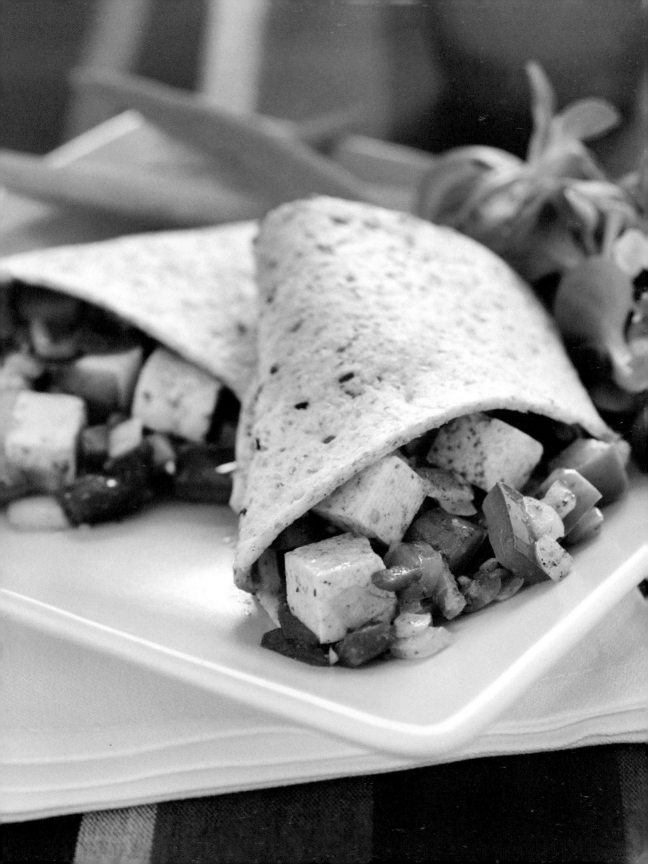

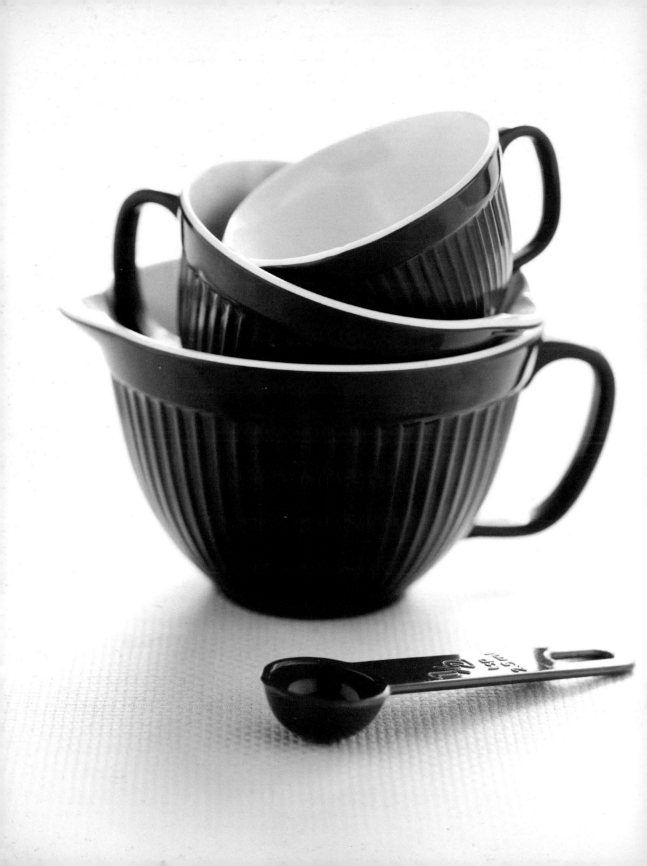

Treats

KIDS' FAVORITE APPLE BUTTER

Makes about 20 cups / 4.7 L of apple butter • Prep Time: 5 min. • Cook Time: 12 hrs + 3 hrs

Apple butter is one of my all-time favorite foods. My mother always kept apple butter in the house. The Dutch call it "appel stroop." We slathered it on everything from toast to pancakes, or just ate it off the spoon. We were kids! Give your child the chance to enjoy this down-home favorite.

KEY PIECE OF EQUIPMENT – a slow cooker or crockpot

INGREDIENTS

36 cups / 8.5 L unsweetened applesauce, divided:
  22 cups / 5.2 L for your first round of slow cooking
  and another 14 cups / 3.3 L for your second round
2 Tbsp / 30 ml ground fresh cinnamon
1 tsp / 5 ml ground cloves
½ tsp / 2.5 ml ground allspice
1 tsp / 5 ml fresh lemon juice
Pinch nutmeg
3 cups / 720 ml Sucanat or amber agave nectar,
  divided: 2 cups/ 480 ml for the first round of cooking
  and 1 cup/ 240 ml for the second round of cooking

PREPARATION

1. Place all ingredients in slow cooker. Stir until blended. Set your slow cooker on a large cookie sheet or cover the cooking area with tin foil or kitchen towels. Once the mixture heats up it will boil and splatter a bit. Set on medium-low. Set the cover so steam can escape.

2. Depending on your slow cooker, you may have to cook your apple butter for as many as 12 hours. The goal will be to have a thick, darkly colored butter of spreading consistency.

3. After this first round of cooking, add the rest of the applesauce. Add 1 more cup / 240 ml of agave nectar or Sucanat and cook for another 3 hours. Apple butter is meant to be smooth. Sometimes the butter you have stewing in your slow cooker needs to be puréed to a finer consistency. I use a hand-held blender for this.

NUTRITIONAL VALUE FOR ONE-TBSP SERVING:
Calories: 40 | Calories from Fat: 0 | Fat: 0g | Saturated Fat: 0g |
Trans Fat: 0g | Protein: 1g | Carbs: 8g | Dietary Fiber: 0.2g |
Sodium: 2mg | Cholesterol: 0mg

PLANNING ON CANNING?

You will have more apple butter than you need for immediate use, so canning the remainder is a nice idea. You will need pint-sized (470 ml) Mason jars. Put your jars in the dishwasher and give them a short wash. Leave them on a heated drying cycle – the goal here is to keep the jars as hot and sterile as possible. If you don't have a dishwasher then boil them in a large pot on the stove for at least five minutes. Reduce heat to low and let the parts sit in the hot water until you use them.

READY TO FILL

Using a large metal funnel placed atop each jar, fill to within 1/2 inch/ 1.5 cm of the top or just to the point where the neck starts. With a clean paper towel, wipe away any dribbles – any food bits left on the glass will cause the contents to spoil. Quickly place the hot lid on top, rubber side down, and then screw it in place with the ring.

HEAT IT UP!

The last step requires that you put all your jars in a very large soup kettle or canner filled with water. The water must cover the jars by at least one inch. Bring the whole thing to a boil and continue to boil the jars for 5 to 10 minutes.

ALL DONE!

Now comes the fun part. Carefully remove the jars from their water bath. Place them on a wire rack to cool. As the jars begin to cool you will hear a satisfying popping sound. Don't be alarmed. This is the sound of the jars sealing themselves. It's a good thing. I leave the jars for a long time. If any jars have not sealed properly, use them first and put the rest in a cool, dark place.

WHY BOTHER?

Homemade treats of any kind will make memories for you and your children. Make this recipe for your family, but you can also give it as a gift for friends and important people in your life.

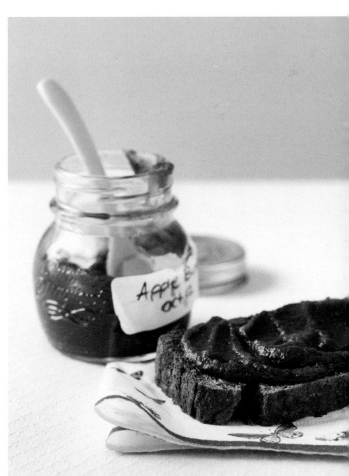

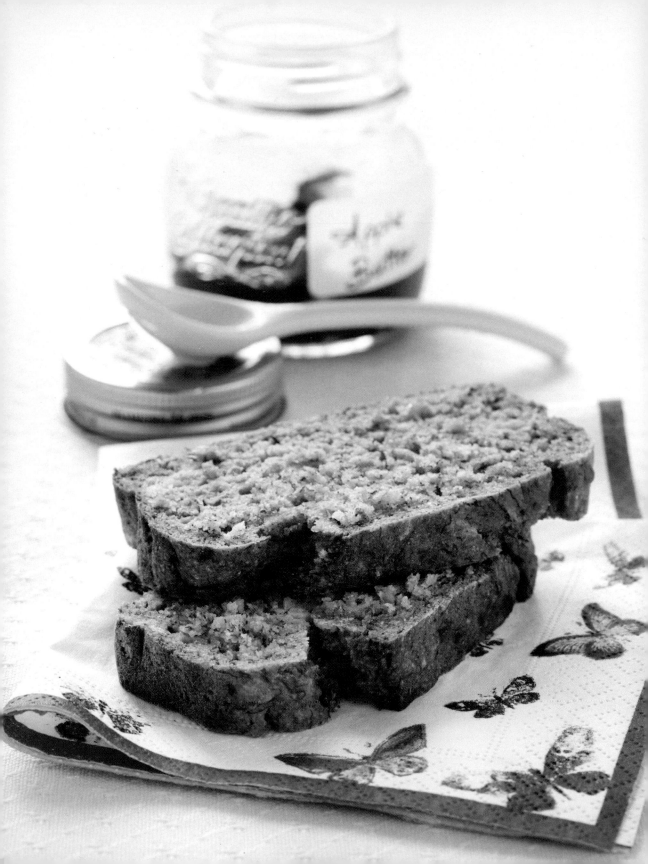

KIDS' FAVORITE BANANA BREAD

Makes 2 loaves • Prep Time: 15 min. • Cook Time: 50 min.

Virtually every kid loves banana bread. Overripe bananas can be stored in the freezer until you are ready to use them. Add sweet carrot purée to ramp up the nutritional value. Banana bread is delicious for breakfast or in your lunch pail.

INGREDIENTS

4 ripe bananas

¾ cup / 180 ml unbleached all-purpose or whole-wheat flour

½ cup / 120 ml Power Flour (see recipe page 190)

½ tsp / 2.5 ml baking soda

¼ tsp / 1.25 ml baking powder

½ tsp / 2.5 ml sea salt

1 tsp / 5 ml ground cinnamon

Pinch each cardamom and nutmeg

1 tsp / 5ml best-quality vanilla

2 large egg whites

¼ cup / 60 ml agave nectar

¼ cup / 60 ml safflower oil

½ cup / 120 ml sweet carrot purée

¼ cup / 60 ml unsweetened applesauce

Eat-Clean cooking spray (see page 23)

PREPARATION

1. Preheat oven to 350°F/ 171°C. Prepare two loaf pans with a light coating of cooking spray or line with parchment paper.

2. In medium-sized bowl combine all dry ingredients. Set aside.

3. In another bowl mash bananas until soft. Combine all wet ingredients with the bananas. Add to dry ingredients and stir until mixture is lumpy but barely blended.

4. Pour batter into loaf pans. Bake for 50 to 55 minutes or until cracked and golden brown on top. Remove from oven and set on wire rack to cool.

NUTRITIONAL VALUE FOR HALF-INCH SLICE:
Calories: 75 | Calories from Fat: 26 | Fat: 3g | Saturated Fat: 0.2g | Trans Fat: 0g | Protein: 2g | Carbs: 14g | Dietary Fiber: 2g | Sodium: 70mg | Cholesterol: 0mg

HAPPY HOT CHOCOLATE

Yield: 2 cups • Prep Time: 3 min. • Cook Time: 5 min.

This recipe for a less sugary version of hot chocolate comes from a Clean-Eating fan who shares her special brand of love on the forum at my website, www.toscareno.com. My forum gal Tasha, a fellow Kingstonian and Sister in Iron, wants you all to try this yummy version of hot chocolate. The next cold day might be a good time to try it. I'm in!

INGREDIENTS

1 cup / 240 ml skim milk or low-fat milk of your choice
  – rice, almond, soy
1 Tbsp / 15 ml raw cocoa powder – a good dark
  chocolate powder is best
4 egg whites
1 Tbsp / 15 ml agave nectar

PREPARATION

1. Place milk and cocoa powder in a saucepan and heat over a medium flame on the stove. Stir often and make sure it doesn't scald.

2. Meanwhile in a large bowl briefly whisk remaining ingredients together.

3. Remove saucepan from stove. Slowly pour the hot mixture into the egg/agave nectar mixture, whisking the whole time or blending with an electric hand blender, until slightly foamy. Pour into your favorite mug and drink steaming hot! Add a little cold milk or an ice cube to cool it down for kids.

TIP Shave some 70% or higher dark chocolate with a vegetable peeler to put on top of the hot chocolate.

NUTRITIONAL VALUE FOR ONE CUP:
Calories: 116 | Calories from Fat: 13.5 | Fat: 1g | Saturated Fat: 0.5g | Trans Fat: 0g | Protein: 12g | Carbs: 1g | Dietary Fiber: 1g | Sodium: 175mg | Cholesterol: 0mg

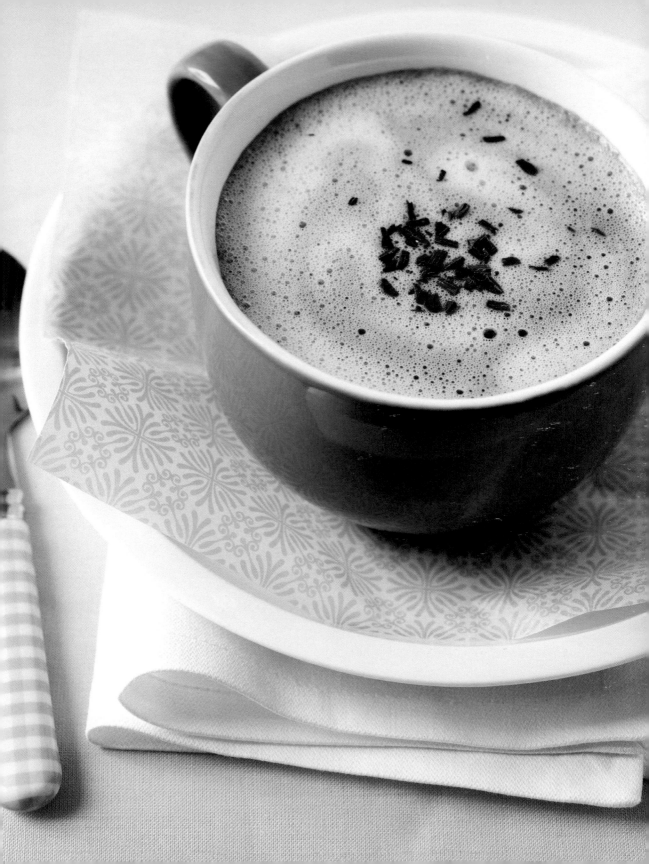

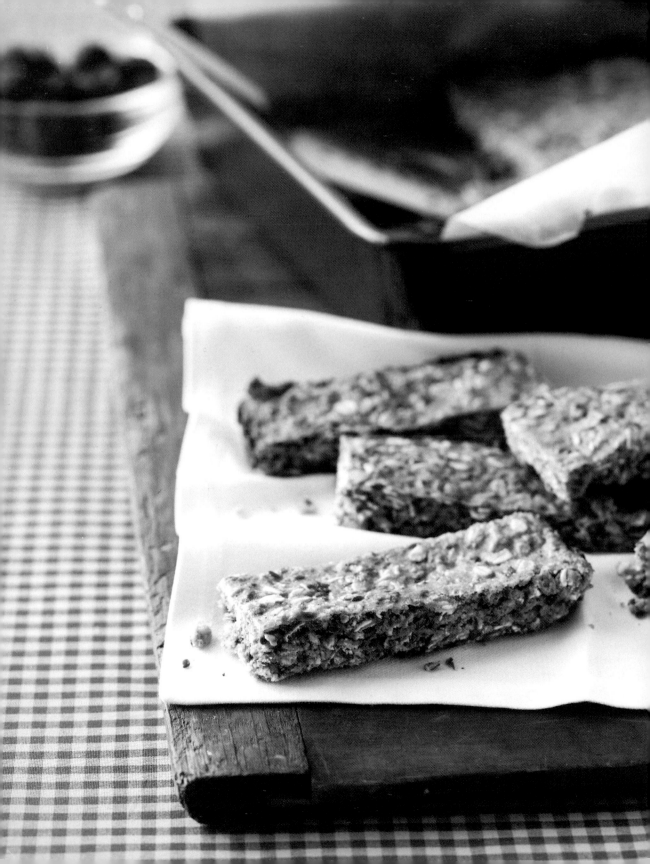

APPLESAUCE SPICE PROTEIN BARS

Makes about 18 1½" x 4" bars • Prep Time: 10 min. • Cook Time: 20-25 min.

We like to reach for a protein bar as a source of nutrition when in a hurry. Sometimes our hurried lives can leave us dependent on questionable commercial bars full of unnecessary sugars and unhealthy fats. Try these naturally sweetened bars instead. Make them up in advance, cut them into squares and freeze them individually in a sheet of wax or parchment paper. When you need one just pop it into your lunch or purse. You're all set!

INGREDIENTS

1 cup / 240 ml whey or other protein powder (remember to check for sugar on the nutrition label)

½ cup / 120 ml spelt flour

2 cups / 470 ml rolled oats – do not use instant

½ cup / 120 ml oat bran

½ cup / 120 ml coarsely ground flax seed

1 tsp / 5 ml sea salt

1 tsp / 5 ml ground cinnamon

½ tsp / 2.5 ml allspice

¼ tsp / 1.25 ml ground nutmeg

¼ tsp / 1.25 ml ground black pepper (yes, really!)

¼ cup / 60 ml apple butter (see recipe page 302)

¼ cup / 60 ml agave nectar

1 ½ cups / 360 ml unsweetened applesauce

¼ cup / 60 ml safflower oil

1 Tbsp / 15 ml vanilla

PREPARATION

1. Preheat oven to 325°F/ 163°C . Put all dry ingredients in a large mixing bowl: flours, oats, oat bran, flax seed, sea salt, cinnamon, allspice, nutmeg and ground black pepper. Mix well.

2. Beat all wet ingredients together in another medium-sized bowl until well blended.

3. Add wet to dry ingredients. Mix until all ingredients are well blended.

4. Prepare a 13 x 9 inch metal pan. Place mixture into pan and press to smooth evenly.

5. Place in oven and bake for about 20 – 25 minutes or until golden on top and firm in the middle.

NUTRITIONAL VALUE FOR ONE BAR:
Calories: 241 | Calories from Fat: 80 | Fat: 9g | Saturated Fat: 1g | Trans Fat: 0g | Protein: 16g | Carbs: 23g | Dietary Fiber: 6.5g | Sodium: 100mg | Cholesterol: 0mg

PROTEIN SMOOTHIE POPSICLES

Yield: 10 x ½ cup popsicles • Prep Time: 10 min.

Who knew popsicles could be good for you? Loading this kid favorite with protein and fruit is a little secret you can keep for yourself. The kids can just enjoy them!

INGREDIENTS

2 cups / 480ml plain low-fat yogurt

2 scoops vanilla-flavored protein powder

2 cups / 480 ml frozen berries

¼ cup / 60 ml agave nectar

PREPARATION

1. Place all ingredients in the bowl of a food processor or blender. Process until just combined.

2. Pour into popsicle molds or Dixie cups with a popsicle stick centered in the mixture. Freeze.

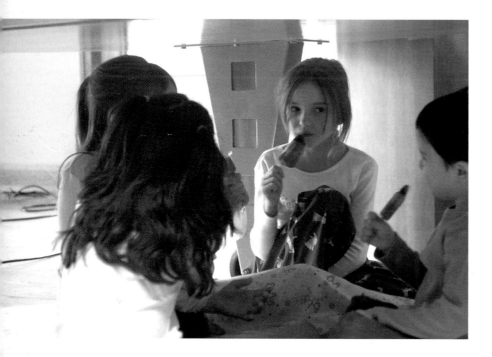

NUTRITIONAL VALUE ONE POPSICLE:
Calories: 77 | Calories from Fat: 2 | Fat: 0.2g | Saturated Fat: 0g |
Trans Fat: 0g | Protein: 5g | Carbs: 14g | Dietary Fiber: 1g |
Sodium: 40mg | Cholesterol: 0mg

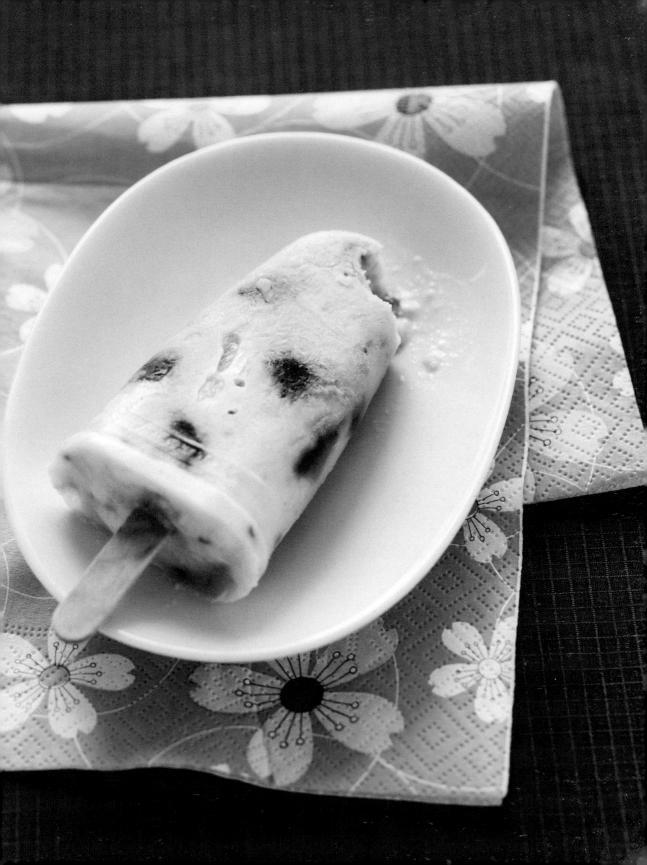

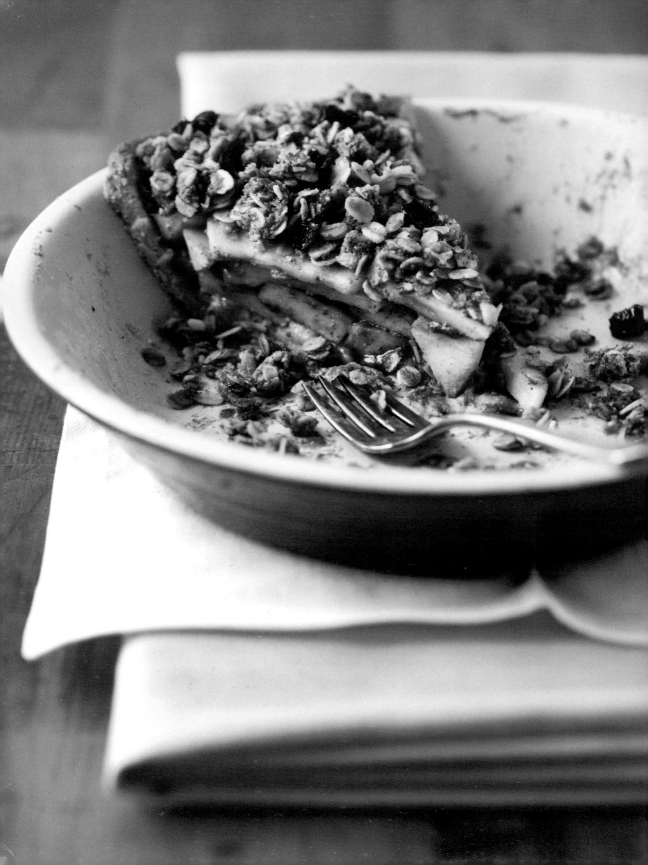

YUMMY APPLE PIE

Yield: 1 pie • Prep Time: 45 min. • Cook Time: 40 min. • Chill Time: 1 hr.

What kid – and what adult, for that matter – doesn't like apple pie? I like apple pie. But I don't like the fat value of a conventional pie. What I do like is knowing that this recipe provides a sweet treat that is not counterproductive to Clean Eating. Try this recipe the next time you are putting on a festive meal.

INGREDIENTS FOR PASTRY CRUST

1 ½ cups / 360 ml unbleached all-purpose or spelt flour

1 tsp / 5 ml sea salt, not too coarse

¾ cup / 180 ml agave nectar

2 oz. / 57 g skim milk or milk of your choice

INGREDIENTS FOR APPLE FILLING

4 large crisp tart baking-type apples – Spy, Granny
    Smith, Macintosh, Mutsu, Empire or other

Juice of one lemon

Water

2 Tbsp / 30 ml Sucanat

1 Tbsp / 15 ml agave nectar

1 tsp / 5 ml ground cinnamon

½ tsp / 2.5 ml ground cloves

⅛ tsp/ 0.6 ml ground nutmeg

1 oz. / 28.5 g unbleached all-purpose or spelt flour

1 tsp / 5 ml best-quality vanilla

INGREDIENTS FOR STREUSEL TOPPING

½ – ¾ cup / 120 ml – 180 ml rolled oats – large flake is
    best

½ cup/ 120 ml Sucanat

½ – ¾ cup / 120 ml – 180 ml unbleached all-purpose
    or spelt flour

1 Tbsp / 15 ml agave nectar

⅓ cup / 80 ml dried cranberries

1 tsp / 5 ml ground cinnamon

½ tsp / 2.5 ml ground cloves

⅛ tsp / 0.6 ml ground nutmeg

2 Tbsp / 30 ml of olive-oil based margarine

PREPARATION FOR PASTRY CRUST

1. Combine all ingredients in a medium-sized mixing bowl. Mix until ingredients are just combined. The resulting mixture should look crumbly and lumpy. Cover dough with plastic wrap and refrigerate. It will need about one hour of chilling time.

2. Remove dough from refrigerator. Roll out with a rolling pin, cut and place in a 9-inch pie dish. Cover with plastic wrap and chill.

PREPARATION FOR APPLE FILLING

1. Peel and core apples. Slice and place in a medium bowl containing the lemon juice and enough water to cover.

2. Place the rest of the filling ingredients in another bowl. Mix well. Toss the apples in the mixture until well coated. Remove crust from refrigerator and pour filling into crust.

Preheat oven to 375°F/ 191°C.

PREPARATION FOR STREUSEL TOPPING

1. Toss all ingredients together in a small bowl. The resulting mix should be crumbly. Sprinkle the streusel mixture over the apple pie.

2. Bake at 375°F / 191°C for 40 minutes or until the apple mixture begins to bubble on top and the streusel turns golden. Remove from oven and let cool on a wire rack. Don't cut into the pie until it has set a bit.

NUTRITIONAL VALUE FOR ONE-EIGHTH OF PIE:
Calories: 372 | Calories from Fat: 11 | Fat: 1g | Saturated Fat: 0.3g |
Trans Fat: 0g | Protein: 6g | Carbs: 60g | Dietary Fiber: 8g |
Sodium: 240mg | Cholesterol: 0mg

FUN PUMPKIN HERMITS

Yield: 24 cookies • Prep Time: 25 min. • Cook Time: 15 min.

What child does not love hermits? They are loads of fun to make … and eat! The added antioxidant power of pumpkin along with raw pumpkin seeds and dates makes these New England favorites better than ever.

INGREDIENTS

⅔ cup / 160 ml whole-wheat flour

⅔ cup / 160 ml unbleached all-purpose flour

⅓ tsp / 1.5 ml baking soda

⅓ tsp/ 1.5 ml sea salt

2 tsp / 10 ml ground cinnamon

1 tsp / 5 ml ground allspice

¼ tsp / 1.25 ml fresh ground nutmeg

¼ tsp / 1.25 ml ground cloves

¼ cup / 1.25 ml Sucanat or agave nectar

1 cup / 240 ml pumpkin purée

½ cup / 120 ml apple butter (see recipe on page 302)

½ cup / 120 ml safflower oil

3 – 4 egg whites, whipped till stiff peaks form

1 ½ cups / 360 ml chopped dates

1 cup / 240 ml raw pumpkin seeds

PREPARATION

1. Preheat oven to 375˚F / 191˚C.

2. In large mixing bowl, combine agave nectar or Sucanat, pumpkin purée, whipped egg whites, apple butter and safflower oil. Beat until all ingredients are well blended.

3. In another medium-sized bowl, mix all dry ingredients: whole-wheat flour, unbleached all-purpose flour, baking soda, sea salt, cinnamon, allspice, nutmeg and cloves. Stir until all ingredients are well blended.

4. Combine wet and dry ingredients. Add chopped dates and pumpkin seeds. Mix until all ingredients are evenly distributed.

5. Line a cookie sheet with parchment paper. Drop cookie dough onto baking sheet with a tablespoon.

6. Bake for 10 to 15 minutes or until golden brown and firm.

NUTRITIONAL VALUE FOR ONE COOKIE:
Calories: 163 | Calories from Fat: 66 | Fat: 7.5g | Saturated Fat: 1g | Trans Fat: 0g | Protein: 3g | Carbs: 22g | Dietary Fiber: 2.5g | Sodium: 50mg | Cholesterol: 0mg

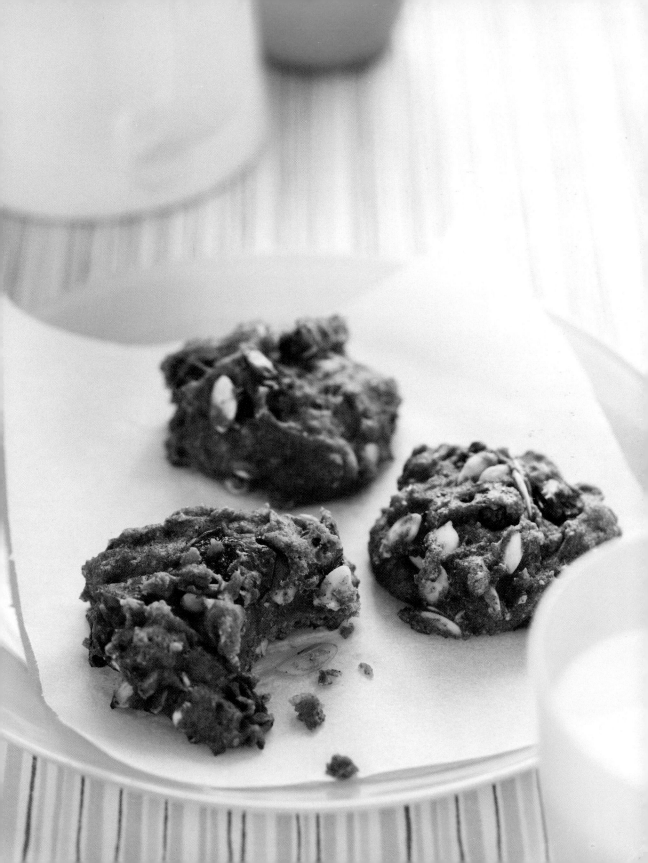

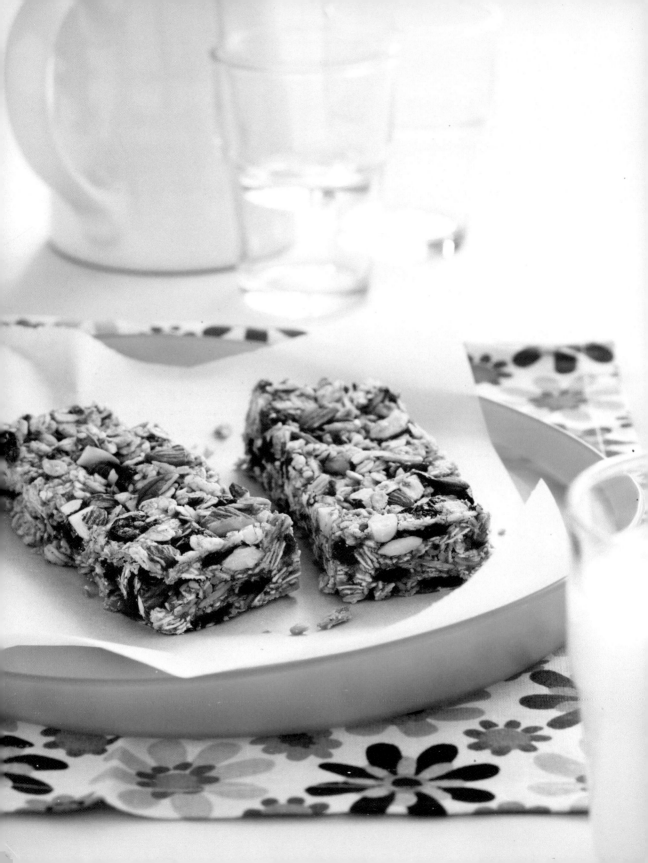

BEST GRANOLA BARS

Yield 16 bars • Prep Time: 15 min. • Cook Time: 25 min.

These bars are perfect for packing into your child's lunch pail for a treat. Make a batch and cut it into squares. Wrap each square individually and store in the freezer. When you need one it's ready to go. You will never eat another commercial granola bar again!

INGREDIENTS

1 cup / 240 ml rolled oats

1 cup / 240 ml dry muesli

½ cup / 120 ml whole-wheat flour

2 scoops* protein powder

½ cup / 120 ml raw, unsalted sunflower seeds

¼ cup / 60 ml raw, unsalted sesame seeds

¼ cup / 60 ml raw, unsalted almonds, chopped

⅓ cup / 80 ml sultana raisins

⅓ cup / 80 ml dried cranberries

2 egg whites, lightly beaten

3 Tbsp / 45 ml dark agave nectar

3 Tbsp / 45 ml organic honey

3 Tbsp / 45 ml safflower oil

Pinch ground nutmeg

½ tsp / 2.5 ml ground cinnamon

* Serving size will depend on what kind of protein
   you use.

PREPARATION

1. Preheat oven to 325°F / 163°C. Line an 8-inch square baking pan with parchment paper. Set aside.

2. Combine all dry ingredients in a large mixing bowl. In a smaller bowl, mix cinnamon, nutmeg, honey, agave nectar, oil and egg.

3. Add wet to dry ingredients and mix until just blended. Mixture should be lumpy.

4. Press mixture into prepared pan. Bake for 25 minutes. The edges will be lightly brown.

5. Remove from oven and set on wire cooling rack to cool. When cool, cut into 1"x 4" bars.

NUTRITIONAL VALUE FOR ONE BAR:
Calories: 171 | Calories from Fat: 70 | Fat: 8g | Saturated Fat: 1g |
Trans Fat: 0g | Protein: 6g | Carbs: 23g | Dietary Fiber: 1.5g |
Sodium: 20mg | Cholesterol: 0mg

LUCKY GINGER SPICE COOKIES

Yield: 30 cookies • Prep Time: 12 min. • Cook Time: 12-15 min.

Many spices help the body burn fat faster. These include cinnamon, nutmeg and cloves. What better way to add these to your diet than with these little gems? Ginger spice cookies are peppered with these delicious ingredients. Try them for your next treat.

INGREDIENTS

¼ cup / 60 ml olive-oil-based margarine
½ cup / 120 ml Sucanat
¼ cup / 60 ml molasses, unsulfured is best
3 large egg whites
1 ¼ cup / 300 ml unbleached all-purpose flour
⅓ cup / 80 ml whole-wheat pastry flour
1 tsp / 5 ml baking soda
1 tsp / 5 ml ground cinnamon
Pinch ground cloves
⅛ tsp / 0.6 ml ground ginger
Pinch ground nutmeg

PREPARATION

1. Preheat oven to 350°F / 171°C. Prepare cookie sheets with Silpat or parchment paper.
2. In a medium-sized mixing bowl beat margarine until soft. Add sugar and molasses and continue to mix well. Add egg whites and continue to mix until batter is creamy in texture.
3. Combine all dry ingredients in a separate bowl.
4. Add dry ingredients to wet and stir until well blended. Drop large spoonfuls of dough onto prepared cookie sheets. Bake for 12 to 15 minutes.

NUTRITIONAL INFORMATION FOR ONE COOKIE:
Calories: 71 | Calories from Fat: 7 | Fat: 1g | Saturated Fat: 1g |
Trans Fat: 0g | Protein: 1g | Carbs: 10g | Dietary Fiber: 1g |
Sodium: 50mg | Cholesterol: 0mg

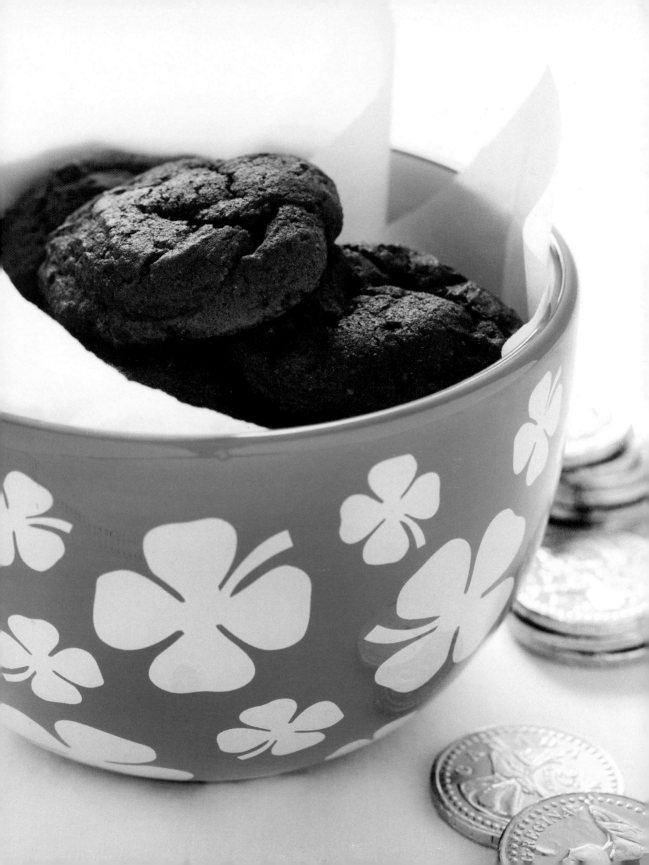

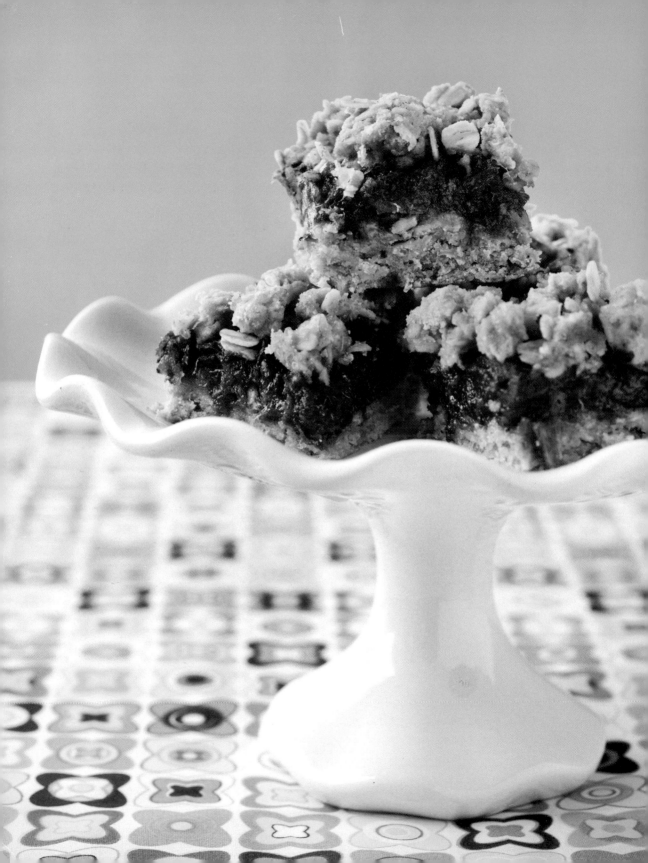

IT'S A DATE! DATE SQUARES

Makes about 24 small squares • Prep Time: 10 min. (Filling) & 10 min. (Base) •
Cook Time: 20 min. (Filling) & 25 min. (Squares)

When Grandma put dates and oats together she knew what she was up to. It turns out dates are full of antioxidant goodness, fiber and complex carbohydrates and naturally low in fat – in fact, a Superfood. Dates also happen to be delicious. Hook them up with oatmeal, another Superfood plump with protein, fiber and goodness and you have an unbeatable combination. I find this gooey square irresistible. I love it with my morning coffee, I have to admit. Your family will enjoy it in lunches and after school. Make up a batch at the beginning of your week so you'll have plenty on hand. Make an extra batch for your freezer – they keep well.

INGREDIENTS FOR FILLING

1 lb. / 455 g pitted dates (much less work for you if they are pitted)

2 Tbsp / 30 ml agave nectar, maple syrup or honey

1 ½ cups / 360 ml water

1 Tbsp/ 15 ml fresh lemon juice

1 tsp/ 5 ml grated lemon rind

INGREDIENTS FOR BASE AND TOPPING

½ cup / 120 ml olive-oil-based margarine, Do It Yourself Olive Butter Spread* or olive oil

¾ cup / 180 ml unsweetened applesauce

3 Tbsp / 45 ml agave nectar

1 cup / 240 ml Power Flour (see recipe page 190) or other unrefined flour

1 cup / 240 ml large-flake rolled oats

¼ tsp / 1.25 ml baking soda

PREPARATION FOR FILLING

1. Preheat oven to 350˚F/ 171˚C . Prepare 9-inch square baking dish with a light coating of cooking spray or line it with parchment paper.

2. Using kitchen scissors, cut your dates into smaller pieces. You will have about 3 cups / 720 ml when you have finished. Set aside.

3. In a small saucepan, place water, lemon juice

* See page 117 in The Eat-Clean Diet Cookbook.

and rind, agave nectar and dates. Bring to a boil. Reduce heat and let simmer for about 10 minutes. You will notice the mixture becoming thick, which is exactly what you want. Stir as it cooks so it doesn't stick to the pan. Remove from heat and let cool.

4. In a large bowl combine olive-oil ingredient with applesauce and agave nectar and mix well. Set aside.

5. In a medium-sized bowl combine oatmeal, flour and baking soda. Add to applesauce mixture and combine until the mixture looks crumbly. Don't over blend.

6. Using about ⅔ of the crumbly mixture, make a layer on the bottom of your baking dish. Pat it down firmly so the base is fairly dense. Spread the cooked date mixture over the base. Now sprinkle the remaining crumb mixture over the date layer. Bake in your preheated oven for 25 minutes. The top should be nicely browned but not too dark. If it looks too light after 25 minutes, bake a little longer. Remove from heat and let cool on a wire cooling rack. Cut into 1"x1"squares. Makes about 24 small squares.

NUTRITIONAL VALUE FOR ONE SQUARE:
Calories: 92 | Calories from Fat: 9 | Fat: 1g | Saturated Fat: 0g | Trans Fat: 0g | Protein: 2g | Carbs: 25g | Dietary Fiber: 1.2g | Sodium: 30mg | Cholesterol: 0mg

LUNCH PAIL MUFFINS

Yield: 12 muffins • Prep Time: 10 min. • Cook Time: 20 min.

I remember packing endless lunches for my children. I would line lunch bags up on the counter and start filling. The trouble was none of my girls ate the same way and they all had a sweet tooth. What could I possibly pack into their lunch pail that would satisfy their sweet tooth that they all would eat? This recipe was my solution.

INGREDIENTS

1 ½ cups / 360ml Power Flour (see page190) or unbleached all-purpose flour
1 cup / 240 ml old-fashioned rolled oats
1 tsp / 15 ml baking powder
½ tsp / 2.5 ml baking soda
½ tsp / 2.5 ml cinnamon
Pinch nutmeg
½ tsp / 2.5 ml sea salt
1 cup / 240 ml unsweetened applesauce
2 egg whites + one yolk
½ cup / 120 ml skim milk soured with 1 tsp lemon juice
½ cup / 120 ml puréed sweet carrots
½ cup / 120 ml agave nectar
¼ cup / 60 ml safflower oil
1 Tbsp / 15 ml best-quality vanilla
½ cup / 120 ml raisins, *optional*

PREPARATION

1. Preheat oven to 400°F / 205°C. Prepare muffin tin by lining with Silpat reusable liners or parchment liners.

2. In one large bowl combine Power Flour with oats, baking powder, baking soda, sea salt and spices. Use a wire whisk to mix ingredients well. In another bowl combine wet ingredients: applesauce, egg yolks and whites, soured milk, carrot purée, agave nectar, vanilla and oil. Mix well.

3. Add wet to dry ingredients. Mix until just blended. Your batter will look lumpy if you have done it correctly.

4. Fill muffin cups with batter. Bake for 20 minutes or until golden brown. Remove from oven and place on wire rack to cool. Serve with apple butter or unsweetened applesauce.

NUTRITIONAL VALUE FOR ONE MUFFIN:
Calories: 93 | Calories from Fat: 10 | Fat: 1g | Saturated Fat: 0g | Trans Fat: 0g | Protein: 4g | Carbs: 18g | Dietary Fiber: 3g | Sodium: 180mg | Cholesterol: 20mg

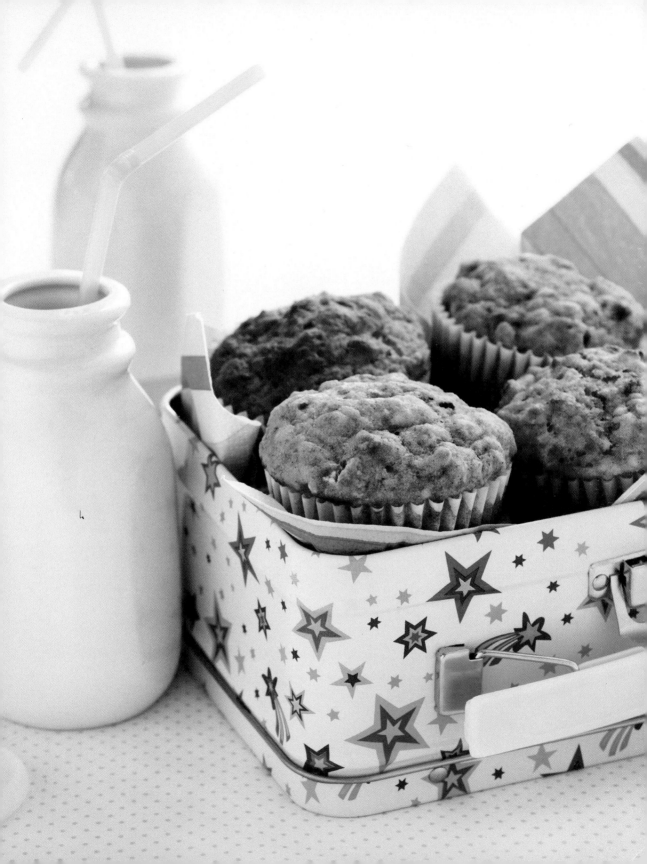

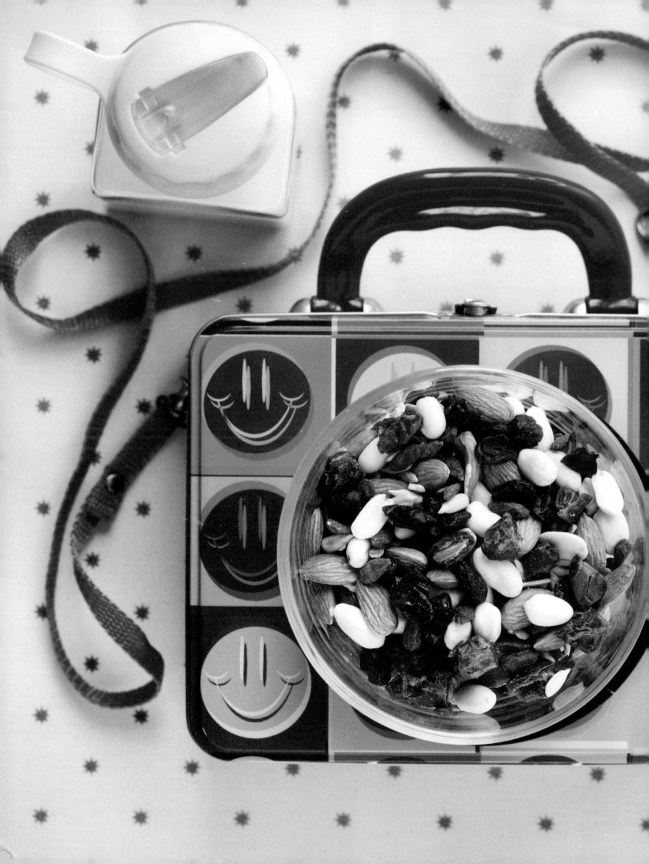

TRAIL MIX FOR ALL TRAILS

Makes 6 x 1/4 cup servings • Prep Time: 5 min.

Trail mix has evolved to be more than just trail-friendly food. A long-time standard of hikers and skiers, this energy-dense food is now also the favorite of urban commuters, school children, travelers and anyone looking for a highly portable nutritious food. Most mixes contain loads of nut and seed proteins as well as dried fruit complex carbohydrates. Keep an airtight container filled with trail mix on hand for emergency snack food.

INGREDIENTS

¼ cup / 60 ml raw, unsalted almonds (look for almonds with the brown peel attached to the nut)

¼ cup / 60 ml unsalted Jungle peanuts* or regular, unsalted raw peanuts

¼ cup / 60 ml unsalted, raw sunflower seeds

¼ cup / 60 ml dried, unsulfured cranberries

¼ cup / 60 ml pitted dates, cut into pieces

¼ cup / 60 ml Goji berries**

PREPARATION

1. Making trail mix is a cinch! Just combine all ingredients in an airtight container, preferably a glass Mason jar or other glass container with a tight-fitting lid.

*WHAT ARE JUNGLE PEANUTS?

In contrast to ordinary peanuts, jungle peanuts contain none of the pesky mold called aflatoxin. Jungle peanuts do contain a hefty dose of complete protein — 26 percent! That's significantly more than hemp seed, or even my favorite flax seed. This peanut varies from the common peanut in appearance and color. Jungle peanuts are a chestnut brown color with reddish stripes. They taste amazing and contain loads of skin-beautifying oleic acid.

**WHAT ARE GOJI BERRIES?

Berries high in antioxidants help the body fight cancer and other diseases. Goji berries, from high in the Himalayas, contain concentrated levels of antioxidants as well as significant protein. Tossing these into your trail mix will increase the protein and complex carbohydrate value of this snack, making it a perfect Clean-Eating meal.

NUTRITIONAL INFORMATION FOR A QUARTER-CUP:
Calories: 165 | Calories from Fat: 83 | Fat: 9g | Saturated Fat: 1g | Trans Fat: 0g | Protein: 5g | Carbs: 19g | Dietary Fiber: 3g | Sodium: 30mg | Cholesterol: 0mg

PUMPKIN BREAD

Makes 2 loaves • Prep Time: 15 min. • Cook Time: 50 min.

The pumpkin holds a place of esteem in the North American diet. Rich in antioxidants, the brilliant orange flesh offers a super array of nutrients. Besides, pumpkin is a fun food to eat!

INGREDIENTS

¾ cup / 60 ml unbleached all purpose flour

¾ cup / 180 ml Power Flour (page 190) , spelt, kamut, amaranth or other whole-grain flour of your choosing

½ tsp / 2.5 ml sea salt

1 tsp / 5 ml baking powder

¼ tsp / 1.25 ml baking soda

½ tsp / 2.5 ml ground cinnamon

⅛ tsp / 0.6 ml ground cardamom

¼ tsp / 1.25 ml ground nutmeg

⅛ tsp / 0.6 ml fresh ground black pepper

⅛ tsp / 0.6 ml ground cloves

½ cup / 120 ml dark organic sultana raisins reconstituted (let raisins sit in hot water for 10 minutes and drain)

OR ½ cup / 120 ml chopped pitted dates

1 cup / 240 ml plain puréed pumpkin flesh

4 egg whites and one yolk

¼ cup / 60 ml agave nectar

½ cup / 120 ml safflower oil

PREPARATION

1. Preheat oven to 375°F / 191°C. Prepare two 8 ½" x 4 ½" loaf pans – coat it lightly with cooking spray and then dust lightly with flour.

2. Sift dry ingredients together in a medium-sized mixing bowl. Whip egg whites stiffly in a separate bowl.

3. In another bowl combine raisins, pumpkin purée, egg yolks, egg whites and oil. Combine wet and dry ingredients until just blended. Do not over-mix. Place batter in the loaf pan, place in the hot oven to bake for about 50 minutes or until loaves are golden and just beginning to crack on top.

4. Remove from oven and let cool on wire racks. Slide loaves out of pans and let cool further before slicing.

NUTRITIONAL VALUE FOR HALF-INCH SLICE:
Calories: 64 | Calories from Fat: 32 | Fat: 3.6g | Saturated Fat: 0.3g | Trans Fat: 0g | Protein: 1g | Carbs: 7g | Dietary Fiber: 0.6g | Sodium: 17mg | Cholesterol: 10mg

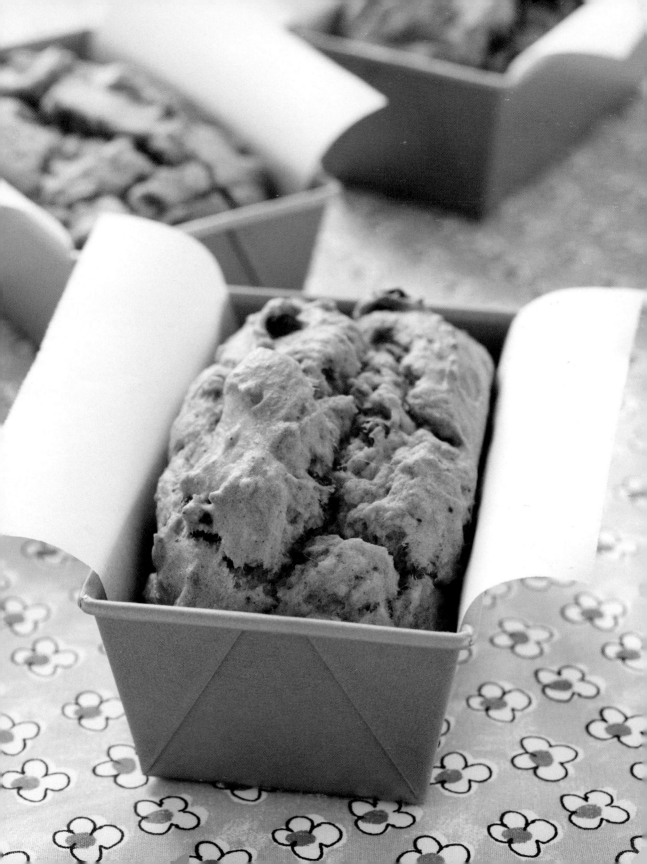

Acknowledgments

✳ ✳

MY FAMILY MEMBERS WHO MODELLED FOR THE BOOK ON A SNOWY WINTER WEEKEND:

Martina and Warren Edwards with children Alissa and Tayler

Rene and Jody Van Diepen with children Anika, William and Ethan

Ron and Tammy Van Diepen with children Ryan and Reid

MY OWN BEAUTIFUL DAUGHTERS for MODELLING AND SUPPORT

Rachel, Kiersten, Kelsey-Lynn and Chelsea

OUR BABY MODEL:

Emma Simpson with Mom, Tracy Collins

A few years ago I wrote a book, *The Eat-Clean Diet*. No one could have predicted its success. Our team, a bare bones but enthusiastic and talented bunch, has consistently surprised me with their Woman Power. I can only be as good as my team. The fact that the first book and the second *(The Eat-Clean Diet Cookbook)* are bestsellers is due in large part to my team:

Gabriella Caruso Marques, who adds life to my words, Rachel Corradetti, who creates concise, thorough reading out of chaos, Vinita Persaud, who carries the load when the rest of us cannot, and Wendy Morley, who tames the motley crew. I am indebted to you.

The idea of Eating Clean came from my ingenious husband, Robert Kennedy, who planted that seed in my brain and helped me grow this garden of books. I thank you for your persistent support when I needed it.

Eating Clean happens every day at our house. Our family is a happy mix of brothers, sisters, stepchildren, moms, dads, and cousins, oh, and dogs! Each of you has carried me. I thank you. My inspiration comes from you Rachel, Kiersten, Kelsey-Lynn, Chelsea, and Braden, the very people who drive me to be the best person I can be.

I thank my own brothers and sisters and their children for devoting an entire winter weekend to shooting for the book. We worked hard, ate a lot, laughed like crazy, and then got snowed in. So we did more of the same for the next two days. What fun!

A big thank you to all of you who read my books and columns. Your emails, letters, and words teach me to continually Raise my own Bar. When I feel I have written enough, you ask for more. I dig deep and give because it is You who show me I can. I am always listening!

And finally, a special thank you to my mother. This woman has borne much in life and still manages to smile. She can't walk anywhere without giving a little skip hop every so often. At 73 years of age she looks fabulous and is in perfect health. That's what Clean Eating can do for you too. Thanks Mom. You are my friend.

Credits

* * * * * * * * * *

FRONT COVER PHOTO CREDIT
Donna Griffith (Make-up & hair by Franca Tarullo)

BACK COVER PHOTO CREDIT
Donna Griffith
(Food styling - Marianne Wren)

INTERIOR PHOTO CREDITS

All black and white photos by **Robert Kennedy**
(Make-up & hair by Franca Tarullo)

All photos in the recipe section by **Donna Griffith.**
(Food styling - Marianne Wren)

Donna Griffith: Page 10, 114-115, 143, 146, 191, 194
(Make-up & hair by Franca Tarullo)

PaulBuceta.com: Page 56, 88, 106, 126
(Make-up & hair by Franca Tarullo)

Cathy Chatterton: Page 20, 67, 81
(Make-up & hair by Franca Tarullo)

All other photos from istockphoto.com

PROP-STYLING CREDITS
Rachel Corradetti & Gabriella Caruso Marques

CHILDREN'S DRAWINGS:
Kelsey-Lynn Corradetti (age 17)
Kira Daniels (age 6)
Blake Daniels (age 4)
Luke Nocera (age 5)
Samantha Nocera (age 7)
Alissa Edwards (age 9)

RESEARCH CREDIT
Robyn Simpson, BA Honours Kinesiology

TIPS:
Kiersten Corradetti, Queen's University

ASSISTANT WRITING:
Rachel Corradetti, B.Sc. Honours Kinesiology

* Images of Tosca shopping were photographed in Zehrs, Orangeville, ON.